Professional
Nursing Practice

Professional Nursing Practice

Marilyn H. Oermann, PhD, RN, FAAN
Professor
College of Nursing
Wayne State University
Detroit, Michigan

With Contributors

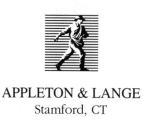

APPLETON & LANGE
Stamford, CT

Copyright © 1997 by Appleton & Lange
A Simon & Schuster Company

97 98 99 00 01 / 10 9 8 7 6 5 4 3 2 1

Prentice Hall International (UK) Limited, *London*
Prentice Hall of Australia Pty. Limited, *Sydney*
Prentice Hall Canada, Inc., *Toronto*
Prentice Hall Hispanoamericana, S.A., *Mexico*
Prentice Hall of India Private Limited, *New Delhi*
Prentice Hall of Japan, Inc., *Tokyo*
Simon & Schuster Asia Pte. Ltd., *Singapore*
Editora Prentice Hall do Brasil Ltda., *Rio de Janeiro*
Prentice Hall, *Upper Saddle River, New Jersey*

ISBN 0-8385-8114-5
90000
9 780838 581148

Acquisitions Editor: David P. Carroll
Production Editor: Eileen L. Pendagast
Designer: Mary Skudlarek
Cover Designer: Mike Kelly

PRINTED IN THE UNITED STATES OF AMERICA

Dedicated to
My parents, Laurence and Dorothy Haag,
and
In memory of Dr. Dorothy E. Reilly,
mentor, former colleague, and dear friend

Contents

Contributors

Nancy T. Artinian, PhD, RN
Associate Professor
College of Nursing
Wayne State University
Detroit, Michigan

Marlyn D. Boyd, PhD, RN, CHES
Research Professor
College of Nursing
University of South Carolina
Columbia, South Carolina

Patricia A. Brown, PhD, RNC
Author and Editor
Professional Development Software, Inc.
Chapel Hill, North Carolina

Marjorie A. Isenberg, DNSc, RN, FAAN
Professor and Associate Dean for Academic Affairs
College of Nursing
Wayne State University
Detroit, Michigan

Sally S. Kellum, MSN, CCRN
Clinical Coordinator, Hospital Informatics
Veterans Affairs Medical Center
Durham, North Carolina

Shaké Ketefian, EdD, RN, FAAN
Professor and Director of Doctoral and Postdoctoral Studies
School of Nursing
University of Michigan
Ann Arbor, Michigan

Kate Moore, PhD, RN
Assistant Professor
College of Nursing
Wayne State University
Detroit, Michigan

Laurel L. Northouse, PhD, RN, FAAN
Associate Professor
College of Nursing
Wayne State University
Detroit, Michigan

Fredericka P. Shea, PhD, RN, FAAN
Associate Professor
College of Nursing
Wayne State University
Detroit, Michigan

Linda Kay Tanner Strodtman, PhD, RN
Assistant Professor
School of Nursing
Clinical Nurse Specialist
University of Michigan
Ann Arbor, Michigan

Preface

Professionals serve an essential role in society. Through their specialized knowledge and skills and acceptance of a set of values and ethics related to their practice, professionals serve on behalf of clients and ultimately meet the needs of society. Professional nursing practice addresses a wide range of health problems that require of its practitioners specialized knowledge and skills to reflect the complexity of care needed by clients. The goal of *Professional Nursing Practice* is to enable students to develop an understanding of their role as professionals in providing this care to clients.

The purpose of this book is to present concepts and theories underlying professional nursing practice. The book was written particularly for registered nurses entering baccalaureate or master's programs to introduce them to concepts and theories underlying professional nursing practice and assist them in developing their own roles as professional practitioners. The book is intended for beginning nursing courses for registered nurses, for example, in a transition or introductory course for RNs entering a baccalaureate or master's nursing program, as well as in later courses in the program in which students again examine these theories and other aspects of professional nursing practice. The book also may be used by generic students in baccalaureate and higher degree programs as an introduction to concepts underlying professional nursing practice. For these students the book is valuable in an introductory concepts course in a baccalaureate or master's nursing program or to complement a foundations of nursing course. Students in other types of nursing programs may find the textbook useful as a resource or reference book.

Professional Nursing Practice builds on the nurse's previous education. Theory and research are emphasized throughout to promote the development of a beginning theoretical framework for practice and a "different" way of thinking about nursing. The book examines professional nursing practice and the role of the nurse in the context of nursing's history; nursing models and theories and their relationship to practice; the individual, family, and community as client; nursing process within the context of clinical judgment and critical thinking; the communication process, with an emphasis on collaboration and communicating with other providers within the health care system; health education and the role of the nurse in teaching clients; computers in nursing practice; moral and ethical dimensions of nursing; nursing research and its impact on practice; leadership; and future perspectives on professional nursing. Some chapters, such as nursing research and leadership, introduce content important as students progress through their programs but with the assumption that further courses will be completed in these areas to extend the students' knowledge base.

The book provides a scholarly perspective intent on enabling the student to move from a technical view of nursing and its practice to a professional view. In addition, the text provides a transition for the student to professional literature in nursing.

Chapter 1 explores nursing as a profession. It examines characteristics of nursing as a profession, dimensions of professional nursing practice, and present and future roles of the professional nurse. Socialization for professional practice is discussed in terms of theory and research. The nursing education system is considered as it relates to the roles and competencies of different levels of practitioners; a historical perspective is provided of the development of the nursing education system. Research on the registered nurse returning for a baccalaureate or other advanced nursing degree is integrated within the discussion of issues associated with returning to school.

Chapter 2, written by a nurse-historian, describes the development of nursing as a profession from the pre-Nightingale era, through the Nightingale era and development of modern American nursing, to the present time. This chapter is an important addition to the text as students frequently lack an understanding of the social, economic, and other factors that influenced the development of the profession and role of the nurse.

Chapter 3 describes theory development in nursing and its relationship to practice and research. It discusses the development of nursing as a science and the nursing models and theories of Martha Rogers, Imogene King, Dorothea Orem, Sister Callista Roy, and Betty Neuman, particularly as they relate to nursing practice. The nursing theories of human care of Madeleine Leininger and Jean Watson also are examined. How the nursing process is conceptualized within selected models is discussed in the chapter on nursing process, and examples of assessment forms based on the models are included to demonstrate their use in practice.

Professional nursing practice involves care of the individual, family, and community. Chapter 4 examines these client populations and emphasizes family theories and their use in nursing practice as a way of preparing the registered nurse to care for the family as a client. Related nursing research is integrated in the discussion. The chapter also explores concepts associated with the community and the role of the nurse in community health.

Chapter 5, which presents the nursing process, builds on the nurse's knowledge base of and experience with the nursing process. The phases of the nursing process are discussed, and related research is integrated throughout. The development of nursing diagnoses and related issues and the evolving nature of nursing diagnoses and classification systems are discussed. This chapter also explores the cognitive processes used by the nurse in carrying out the nursing process, differing theoretical perspectives of clinical judgment, and the relationship of critical thinking to the nursing process.

Chapter 6 examines the communication process and provides information to help nurses communicate with clients and other health professionals. The chapter discusses the importance of communication in health care, and a theoretical basis for communication is provided. The developmental phases of the nurse–client relationship are discussed, as are specific factors that promote effective communication with clients and other health professionals. In keeping with trends in health care and skills nurses need to develop to practice within multidisciplinary models of care delivery, this chapter emphasizes the importance of collaboration and communicating with other health providers.

Chapter 7 focuses on health education and the role of the nurse in teaching clients. It presents the knowledge and skills needed to teach clients particularly in the context of promoting health and teaching them in multiple settings. The chapter emphasizes the mandate for health teaching by nurses, concepts of learning and motivation, assessment of learning abilities of clients, plans for teaching, teaching and behavioral strategies, and evaluation and documentation of health teaching.

The nurse of today and tomorrow must have a sound knowledge base in computer technology and its nursing practice applications. Chapter 8 provides a discussion of computers and their use in the health care system and a beginning point for the development of computer literacy. Computer technology is described and illustrated. The clinical practice applications of this technology are examined in terms of medical diagnosis and treatment and health care information systems, including hospital information systems, nursing information systems, and patient data management systems. Computer use in other areas of nursing is described.

Chapter 9 deals with ethical concerns in the profession. Ethical practice is considered as integral to professional nursing practice; it is the essence of professional nursing practice. Examined in this chapter are moral reasoning, ethical theories and principles, professional codes and guidelines, ethical decision making, and other ethical aspects of nursing practice.

The purpose of nursing research and its importance in terms of nursing practice are presented in Chapter 10. The chapter provides an understanding of the research process and the role of the nurse in different phases of research. The relationship of nursing research to practice is emphasized. This chapter is not intended to replace a course in nursing research but instead to introduce the reader to the research process and use of research findings in practice. It provides a basis for subsequent courses in which research findings are integrated and the student is asked to read research literature.

Chapter 11 examines concepts of leadership and the leadership role of the nurse in a changing health care system. It presents different perspectives of leadership, enables the students to gain an understanding of how to develop his or her own role as leader, and discusses models of nursing care delivery and the nurse's role within them. As with the chapter on research, this chapter is intended as an introduction to these concepts, with the assumption that students will complete an additional course on nursing leadership and management.

The final chapter provides a future perspective of professional nursing practice. Current major changes occurring in the health care system are discussed, including technology, costs of health care, acuity of client care in hospitals, and need for professional nursing care in the home and community settings. Other major forces, such as the increasing age of the population, are explored in terms of health care resources and nursing practice.

Many individuals have made contributions during the writing and preparation of this book. Special acknowledgment is extended to David Nelson of Nelson's Graphics (Riverview, Michigan) for his expert typing, ability to develop graphics to complement the text, commitment, and willingness to devote extensive time to typing and formatting the manuscript. David, Ross, and Eric Oermann were supportive during the preparation of this book and other manuscripts.

MARILYN H. OERMANN, PhD, RN, FAAN

Foreword

In *Professional Nursing Practice*, Marilyn Oermann and her panel of authors provide an appropriate text for nurses whose career goals change from technical to professional practice. Professionals change career directions, and each change requires new knowledge and skills. The challenge to faculty is to identify the new knowledge and skills to be included in the educational experiences of nurses returning to school and of nursing students beginning their education and to select the professional literature that will lead them into new domains of learning. Through deliberately designed programs of study in nursing education, nurses have an opportunity to change career goals and acquire knowledge and skills for their new practice.

The content of this book is primarily theoretical. It includes concepts and theories that are fundamental to the practice of professional nursing while introducing bodies of knowledge that reflect the changing role of nursing and the evolving milieus where nursing is practiced.

Many chapters reflect the changing role of the nurse. The early chapters highlight the meaning of this change, and one chapter provides an historical context within which to view present directions for nursing practice. Nursing models and their use in practice are described. The family and community as client is emphasized as an important direction for nursing practice and health care. Communication among professionals is developed within the broader scope of collaboration, a process most appropriate to the multidisciplinary models of health care delivery. A chapter on health education addresses the critical role of professional nursing in teaching clients about health and illness. The emphasis of research in nursing focuses on its relevance to nursing practice and its impact on practice itself. This approach provides the basis for further study of the research process in nursing. Other chapters on nursing process, computers in nursing, and moral and ethical dimensions of nursing practice build on the learner's previous education and experience and provide a transition to professional nursing education.

Developing models of health care delivery give new meaning to the concepts of leadership and management. The final chapter examines the movement of health care toward the community, the assets and liabilities of this movement, and the economic and social forces that are directing much of health care. The nurse thus can develop a framework for examining his or her own role as a professional within the health care system.

The material is well presented, substantive, and reflective of the learner's already acquired knowledge base. The text incorporates extensive references and bibliographies for greater in-depth study by the student.

This text is timely and enters the nursing literature at a crucial period when nursing programs are addressing the changing role of the nurse. It is an outstanding reference not only for those nurses who are undertaking a career change, but also for those students who are not yet in practice and those in practice who wish to update their nursing knowledge. Many areas of content in this text lend themselves remarkably well to in service programs meant to enhance professional practice in health care agencies.

Dr. Oermann and her panel of authors are presenting a timely text. It recognizes both present needs and the knowledge base essential for nursing practice into the next century. I highly recommend the book.

†Dorothy E. Reilly, EdD, RN, FAAN
Professor Emeritus
College of Nursing
Wayne State University
Detroit, Michigan

† deceased
The book is dedicated to Dorothy Reilly, who wrote the foreword shortly before her death.

Professional Nursing Practice

Marilyn H. Oermann

Professionals play an essential role in society. Through their specialized knowledge and skills and adherence to a set of values and ethics, professionals serve on behalf of particular clients and ultimately meet the needs of society as a whole. Professional nursing practice involves deliberately planned actions in response to the needs of clients for whose care nurses are responsible. The professional makes a commitment of service to the client; this commitment represents a lifetime career. As society and the needs of clients change, the professional's knowledge and skills also must expand and become more differentiated in terms of the services required (Reilly & Oermann, 1992).

Professionals practice in society and in many ways can be said to be owned by society (American Nurses Association, 1995, p. 2). Professionals perform their services for the benefit of society, and society, in turn, expects them to possess the knowledge and skills needed for carrying out these services. Professionals practice because of a need they meet in society that grants the authority and autonomy essential for that practice.

Nursing is a profession that serves the needs of society in the area of health. The practice of nursing addresses a wide range of health problems, both actual and potential, requiring of its practitioners a specialized body of knowledge and skills to meet client needs and a value system that recognizes the client as an autonomous human being with rights. As a profession, nursing has played a vital role in the health care system throughout history, and it continues to do so today.

This chapter explores the concept of nursing as a profession. Socialization into the profession is examined from the perspectives of theory and research, and the development of a professional self-concept and need for career growth in nursing are discussed. The chapter also considers the role of the nursing education system in developing nursing as a profession and teaching the knowlege and competencies required of practitioners at different educational levels. Educational programs for the registered nurse (RN) returning for a baccalaureate or other advanced nursing degree and related research also are discussed.

NURSING AS A PROFESSION

Definitions of nursing throughout its history have been influenced by the social context in which nursing was practiced and the status of the delivery of health care services at the time. More than 100 years ago, Nightingale (1859) wrote that nursing involved having "charge of the personal health of somebody" with the goal "to put the patient in the best condition for nature to act upon him" (cited in ANA, 1995, p. 5). Abdellah, Beland, Martin, and Matheney (1964) described nursing as a service to individuals and families that helps them, when ill or well, to cope with their health needs (p. 24). Henderson and Nite (1978) believed that the function of the nurse was to assist sick or well clients in performing activities that would contribute to the clients' health, recovery, or peaceful death—activities that they could perform unaided if they had the necessary strength, will, or knowledge (p. 34). Schlotfeldt (1981) defined nursing as "assessing and enhancing the general health status, health assets, and health potentials of human beings" (p. 298). Throughout time, nursing has been viewed as providing care to others—individuals, groups, and communities—with a focus on promoting health.

In the American Nurses Association's (ANA) social policy statement (1980), nursing is defined as "the diagnosis and treatment of human responses to actual or potential health problems" (p. 9). Nursing is concerned with the experiences and responses of individuals, families, groups, and communities to birth, health, illness, and death (ANA, 1995). These experiences and responses are considered the phenomena of concern to nurses, such as self-care limitations, impaired physiological and pathophysiological processes, pain, and emotional problems, to name a few. Nurses use theory to understand these phenomena and determine interventions or actions to take. Nursing interventions should benefit the individual, family, group, or community, and evaluation of the effectiveness of these interventions in terms of outcomes of care is an important nursing responsibility (ANA, 1995).

Nursing is rapidly becoming a scientific discipline through the work of nurse theorists and other researchers in nursing who have defined more clearly its practice and theory base. Commitment to the development of a theoretical base for nursing is essential to the continued evolution of nursing as a discipline and profession. The discipline dimension of nursing is concerned with the development of nursing as a science; the professional dimension is concerned with the practice of nursing, delivering care to meet societal health needs.

Recently, definitions of nursing have reflected the views of nurse theorists. Table 1–1 compares definitions of nursing according to five leading nurse theorists.

Dimensions of Nursing Practice

Professional nursing practice today requires specialized knowledge and skills to reflect the complexity of care required by clients in most health care settings. Depth of knowledge, skill in carrying out the technical aspects of care, expertise in clinical judgment, skill in prioritizing and organizing care for groups of clients, and concern with providing humanistic care are only a few of the competencies essential for professional nursing practice. Nursing has emerged as a specialized clinical field with much of its practice independent of physicians. Some care functions, such as those associated with prescribed medical treatments, medication administration, and other medical interventions, are determined by others, but the majority of nursing care is in the control of nurses. Nurses decide which data to collect from a client, analyze the data to derive nursing diagnoses, plan and modify interventions appropriate for the client's health problems, and evaluate outcomes and the effectiveness of care. Nursing interventions continue to be developed and tested through nursing research.

In professional practice, the nurse carries out multiple roles, depending on the client, state of the client's health, setting, and nurse's expertise. These roles include provider of care, counselor, manager, leader, educator (of clients, staff, and others), consultant, and advocate. The effective implementation of these roles requires skill in developing relationships with patients, families, and others inside and outside of the clinical setting and in maintaining effective communication with them.

Clearly, the most fundamental role of the nurse is that of provider of care. Through the provider role, the nurse assesses, plans, delivers, and evaluates the effectiveness of care for clients. Changes in health care have expanded this role of the nurse. In some settings nurses are the sole providers of client care such as in the role of nurse practitioner; in other settings the nurse assumes responsibility for managing care of individuals and groups of patients and delivering care to communities. The caregiving role of the nurse includes the provision of care to individual patients, families, groups, and communities; delegation of activities to other care providers, including professional nursing staff and nonprofessional personnel; supervision of others in the delivery of care; and managing the client's care.

In the role of counselor the nurse assists the client to cope with health problems and acquire knowledge and behaviors to promote health. The

TABLE 1-1. DEFINITION OF NURSING ACCORDING TO FIVE NURSING THEORISTS

Imogene King	Betty Neuman	Dorothea Orem	Martha Rogers	Sister Callista Roy
Nursing is a helping profession involving a process of action, reaction, interaction, and transaction whereby nurse and client share their perceptions in the nursing situation through purposeful communication; identify specific goals, problems, or concerns; explore means to achieve the goal; agree to these means; and both move toward goal attainment.	Nursing is a unique, wholistic profession concerned with all variables affecting a client's response to environmental stressors. Nursing actions are appropriate to the total needs of the client on his/her own wellness/illness continuum toward providing optimum client/client system stability or wellness.	Nursing is a human service whose concern is the individual's need for self-care and the provision and management of it on a continuous basis in order to sustain life and health, recover from disease or injury, and cope with their effects. Conditions that validate the requirement for nursing as an adult are the absence of ability to maintain continuously that amount and quality of self-care which is therapeutic in sustaining life and health, in recovery from disease or injury, or in coping with their effects. In children, the condition is the inability of parent (or guardian) to maintain continuously for the child the amount and quality of care that is therapeutic.	Nursing (nursing science) is the science of irreducible human and environmental energy fields arrived at by a synthesis of facts and ideas commensurate with a new worldview; [it is] an organized system of abstract knowledge. The practice of nursing is the imaginative and creative use of nursing knowledge for human betterment. The science of irreducible human beings basic to nursing requires a new worldview and an abstract system specific to nursing's phenomenon of concern. People and their environments are perceived as irreducible, pandimensional energy fields integral with one another and continuously creative in their evolution. It is postulated that people have the capacity to participate knowingly in the process of change.	Nursing is a scientific way of providing care for the ill or potentially ill person that acts through the nursing process to promote adaptation in each of the four modes of adaptation in situations of health and illness.

Adapted from Reilly, D. E., & Oermann, M. H. (1992). Clinical teaching in nursing education. New York: National League for Nursing, pp. 80–81, with permission.

counseling role is important in helping patients to weigh different treatments and options available and making informed decisions about their care. The nurse's interpersonal skills are critical in counseling patients and families.

The manager role of the nurse varies greatly with the nurse's position in the organization. In delivering care to individuals and groups of clients and delegating and supervising care, the nurse is functioning in the manager role. As a case manager the nurse assesses patients and families, develops care plans, delegates interventions and activities to others as needed, coordinates care through the course of a client's illness, collaborates with other health providers, and evaluates outcomes of care. Other management positions include clinical nurse manager, nursing supervisor, and vice president for nursing. The role of the nurse as manager and leader are described more fully in Chapter 11.

Regardless of the position the nurse assumes and agency in which he or she is employed, the nurse serves as a leader for patients and staff. In this leadership role the nurse assists the client to make decisions and influences other nurses and health providers toward achieving their goals and those of the organization. Leaders in nursing communicate effectively, develop trusting relationships with others, balance the needs of the individual with organizational goals, and encourage people to work toward their goals.

In the educator role, the nurse teaches individuals, families, groups, and staff. Teaching is an interactional process that facilitates the development of knowledge, skills, and values. In teaching clients, the nurse improves understanding of underlying health problems, related interventions, how to integrate them in their own lifestyle, and strategies for promoting health. The ultimate goal of health education is to foster the knowledge and skills necessary for self-care. The health educator role is critical as patients and families assume greater responsibility for care in homes and community agencies. In terms of staff education, the nurse helps the staff develop further knowledge and skills in caring for patients and reinforcing their learning. In some settings the nurse has an important role in multidisciplinary education.

As nurses acquire advanced knowledge and skills and gain expertise in their own areas of practice, they are frequently called upon to consult with other nurses and health providers. In the consultant role the nurse provides information, guidance, and advice to others. Nurses serve as consultants because of their expertise and specialized knowledge and skills in a particular area.

In the advocacy role, the nurse helps patients to become autonomous in their decision making and to make informed decisions about treatments and other aspects of care. To achieve this goal, the nurse provides sufficient information for the client to make an informed decision. At times the nurse may be called upon the protect the client's rights in the health care system. Boughn (1995) emphasizes that nurses are positioned to be the "primary and most effective advocates for patients within the health care system" (p. 112).

Another perspective of advocacy relates to the nurse's role in promoting and maintaining a professional practice environment. Young, Hayes, and Morin (1995) describe workplace advocacy, challenging nurses to address issues associated with their professional practice to create and maintain a professional work environment.

The nurse cares for clients with varying degrees of illness and types of health problems and for people who are healthy. In periods of illness, the nurse serves the individual and family in the hospital, the clinic, the home, and other community and health care settings by providing nursing management for the health problem and assistance in coping with it. Professional nursing practice also involves providing information to clients about their health practices and counseling to promote health. Health promotion focuses on increasing and maintaining the level of well-being of individuals, families, other groups, and the community. Health-related interventions include activities such as stress management; breast self-examination, hypertension, and other educational programs; exercise and physical fitness programs; and health screening. As health care becomes increasingly focused on health promotion and primary health care, the nurse's role will continue to shift in this direction. Hills and Lindsey (1994) emphasize the importance of nurses incorporating the principles of health promotion into their care of clients for nursing to be a leader in health care in the future.

Along with this emphasis on health promotion, the nurse's practice is shifting toward the community, in the workplace, clinics, homes, schools, and other community-based settings (de Tornyay, 1993; Oermann, 1994a, b). These settings are oriented toward maintaining the client's health and preventing illness. Peters and Hays (1995) suggest that this shift affords nurses an opportunity to "grasp newly defined and expanded roles for themselves" (p. 359).

Characteristics of a Profession

Over time, many definitions of professions have been offered. In the 1930s, Carr-Saunders and Wilson (1933) described professions in terms of the extent of knowledge associated with preparing for an occupation requiring rigorous, lengthy study. Other definitions of a profession also emphasized knowledge as a requirement. The knowledge base of a profession is specialized and well defined, setting the professional off from other individuals. Professionals apply this knowledge to solving instrumental problems of their practice (Schön, 1990, pp. 32–33). Knowledge, therefore, is considered one requirement of a profession. The development of nursing knowledge and its application in practice are essential in moving nursing forward in its professionalization.

The knowledge base for nursing is derived from nursing science and concepts and theories from other fields such as the physical, biomedical, behavioral, and social sciences; philosophy; and ethics (ANA, 1995, p. 7). Nurses develop this knowledge base by generating and testing new nursing theories, conducting research in nursing, and applying research findings in practice.

The chief difference between a professional and a nonprofessional is in the body of theory possessed by the professional. This theory, or knowledge base, describes the phenomena of concern to the professional. Greenwood (1984) writes that preparation for a profession requires prior or simultaneous mastery of theory, which is limited in the training of the nonprofessional, as well as practice experience (p. 15). The development of nursing theory, a unique body of knowledge for nursing, has promoted the movement of nursing toward full professional status. Nursing is committed to building a body of knowledge through research (Mohr, 1995).

In addition to knowledge, other views of professions have emphasized the autonomy of the professional group in terms of controlling its practice. This autonomy, control over one's own practice, is essential for nurses to make decisions and judgments about nursing interventions and practice. Nursing as a profession regulates its own practice by defining its practice base, developing its own system for nursing education, establishing the structure within which nursing care is delivered, and assuring the public that quality care is provided (ANA, 1995, p. 17). Because of their knowledge and skills gained through education, professionals expect to make independent judgments about proper courses of actions for clients (Brint, 1994, p. 83).

Nurses exercise autonomy and freedom to make decisions and clinical judgments within their scope of practice. Nurses have autonomy in delivering nursing care to their clients, and they also are held accountable for that care. Moloney (1992) suggests, however, that in some settings, such as hospitals, nurses lack autonomy and authority over practice, leading her to conclude that autonomy is one attribute of a profession not fully developed in nursing. Wiens (1990) identified strategies for increasing nurses' autonomy in rural hospitals such as expanded clinical ladders, which specify increasingly complex practice levels and independence in decision making, and shared governance, which provides staff nurses with significant input into decisions about nursing practice.

Although control over professional practice is essential, in health care collaboration among professionals also is needed to provide effective care. One of the competencies needed for health professionals identified by the Pew Health Professions Commission (1991) is the ability to work with other health providers and participate in coordinated care of clients. Skill in collaboration, combined with ability to exercise control over nursing decisions in the interdisciplinary team, are important to maintain the autonomy and authority of nurses for decisions involving nursing care of clients (Oermann, 1994a).

The professional has a certain degree of authority, derived from his or her extensive body of knowledge, which is acknowledged by the clients served. In addition, communities sanction the authority of the profession by approving its powers and privileges. Greenwood (1984) cites the following examples of such sanctions: professional regulation of its schools through accreditation, such as accreditation of nursing programs by the National League for Nursing (NLN); control of entry into the profession by requiring graduation from one of its professional schools and through licensing, as with the state boards for nursing; and professional privileges, such as confidentiality of information between the professional and client, the setting of standards of practice by the profession, and immunity from community judgment on technical matters (pp. 18–19). These requirements contribute to establishing the status of a profession, as do professional organizations that influence the educational system and credentialing for practice as a professional (Brint, 1994).

Professionals also have a code of ethics that helps to regulate their relationships with clients and each other. The code of ethics can be formal, that is, written, such as the ANA (1985) Code for Nurses, or informal, that is, unwritten. The code of ethics is highly developed in nursing. As a profession, nursing throughout its history has developed and adhered to a strong code of ethics to guide practice. Moloney (1992) in comparing nursing with other professions suggests that nursing has a highly developed code of ethics (p. 20).

A related attribute of a profession is the existence of a professional culture, the values and norms accepted by the profession. As part of this culture, professionals are inclined to value education and demonstrate a strong commitment to education for practice as a professional, emphasize autonomy and self-direction, attempt to balance competing values, and expect certain behavior of individuals within their professional group (Brint, 1994, pp. 82–83).

One final characteristic applied to professions is the standardization of educational preparation for entry into the profession. The education of professionals in other fields occurs typically within institutions of higher education, colleges, and universities, and in some professions such as medicine, dentistry, and law, to name a few, at the postbaccalaureate level. Higher education provides the credentials, skills, and training necessary to practice as a professional and authority within an organization (Brint, 1994). Because professional practice greatly depends on education, professionals as a group value education as the means of entering the profession and keeping current in their practice.

Nursing continues to educate for entry into practice at varied levels, leading Moloney (1992) to express concern over nursing's lack of standardization of education. Although there is a lack of standardization for entry into practice, the growth of nurses prepared at the master's and doctoral levels and the independence of advanced practice nurses have contributed to the development of nursing as a profession.

Deciding whether or not nursing is a profession by applying a list of characteristics has been of minimal value. Perhaps more important than these external criteria is the internal set of beliefs and values held by the nurse about the nature, purpose, and outcomes of nursing. As nursing develops its theory base and gains greater autonomy over practice, nursing will continue to move further toward a profession regardless of which set of criteria is applied. This effort to develop nursing knowledge is essential, given the extensive knowledge and skills needed for providing care in health care settings today. In turn, developing the knowledge base of nursing will promote greater control over practice. A distinct body of knowledge that differentiates nursing practice from the practice of other health professionals will enable nursing to control its own practice more effectively.

PROFESSIONAL SOCIALIZATION

Socialization is the process through which a person acquires the knowledge, skills, and values necessary to become a functioning member of society. Although there are various theoretical perspectives on this process, consistent among them is the notion that, through socialization, the individual learns socially relevant behaviors. The process of socialization involves learning motor and language skills, social roles, moral norms and values, and other ways of functioning within society (Hurley-Wilson, 1988, p. 75). Family, friends, and other people, as well as institutions, through their interactions with an individual, promote the social learning needed to perform specific roles as an adult. Socialization is an interactional process that ultimately prepares the individual to function in particular roles within society.

In general, the two phases of socialization are: (1) childhood socialization and (2) adult socialization. *Childhood socialization* focuses on developing language and motor skills and learning about the values and standards of society and the child's own social group. The family serves as the primary agent in this early socialization. *Adult socialization* provides the means through which a person develops new role behaviors and values associated with roles assumed as an adult. In adult socialization, in contrast to childhood socialization, the individual brings to the new situation a set of values and beliefs as well as preconceived notions about the role. Adults are concerned with learning new role behaviors and role-specific expectations, whereas in childhood, the focus is on acquiring societal values and general role demands of society.

Socialization frequently has been viewed within the perspective of role theory. *Role theory* is a "collection of concepts . . . that predict how actors will perform in a given role, or under what circumstances certain types of behaviors can be expected" (Conway, 1988b, p. 63). Through socialization, then, an individual develops the knowledge, skills, and values he or she needs to perform as an adult in certain roles. These roles may be those associated with an occupation as well as marital and parental roles. Whenever an adult assumes a new role, such as that of student, nurse, or parent, or one associated with a change in job, the individual becomes socialized for that role. In the process of socialization, other people in the role assist the individual in learning necessary behaviors, values, and norms for assuming the new role.

An individual learns role behaviors through two processes that occur simultaneously: (1) interaction and (2) learning. The interaction process, which involves interaction with others, enables a person to master specific role behaviors and prerequisites for learning about the role. These prerequisites include the acquisition of language skills, which are a prerequisite for learning most roles; the learning of role-taking skills, which enable the person to take on the role of another person; development of the self, the process in which the person becomes an object to himself or herself by first responding to attitudes of others and then developing an organized set of attitudes; and development of interpersonal skills, which enable an individual to present himself or herself through social interaction (Hurley-Wilson, 1988). The learning process through which socialization occurs includes reinforcement of behavior, direct instruction, observing the behavior of others, imitative learning, modeling, and role playing. Many of these learning processes are apparent in preceptorships in nursing in which a student, new graduate, or other nurse works closely with a clinical preceptor, a staff nurse, or other practitioner who serves as a role model. Preceptorships are based on the concept of modeling. Learners acquire or modify role behaviors by observing a model who has the behaviors needed by the person and by then practicing those behaviors (Oermann, 1996; Reilly & Oermann, 1992). By working on a one-to-one basis with a practitioner functioning in the role, the learner is able to model behaviors of the nurse and become socialized into the role.

Professional socialization, an important type of adult socialization, is the process of learning the roles and values of a professional. From the perspective of nursing, professional socialization represents the process through which the student or nurse acquires the knowledge and skills needed for practice and internalizes the norms and values of the nursing profession into his or her own behavior. Through professional socialization the student develops a view of self as a member of the nursing profession. The process of socialization occurs when students learn about the practice of nursing in their initial educational programs, new graduates enter the work setting in which different norms and values exist from those in the educational setting, nurses return for advanced nursing degrees, and individuals change roles within nursing and need to learn new role behaviors and expectations.

Conway (1988a) defined professional socialization as a process of becoming, which begins with the individual's recognition of what attributes identify the ideal professional and is followed by an attempt to model himself or herself after the professional. Through this socialization, the student develops a self-concept associated with the role and acquires the role behaviors and expectations needed for carrying out the role in practice. These role behaviors enable the student to develop a professional identity. In many ways professional socialization is a process of role transition that occurs when a person moves from one major position to another, such as when a college student enters the nursing program or when the student graduates and enters the workplace (Hardy & Hardy, 1988; Strader & Decker, 1995). Professional education is designed to shape the values, attitudes, self-concept, and role behaviors of the student, thereby enabling the learner to assume the new role of a professional practitioner.

Models of Socialization

A number of models have been developed to describe the process of professional socialization. Early on, Simpson (1967) proposed that professional socialization in nursing occurred in three phases: (1) a shift in attention from broad, societal goals, which might have led the individual to choose nursing as a profession, to becoming proficient in certain tasks associated with practice of nursing; (2) a selection of others in the work setting as the main referent group; and (3) an internalization of the values of the professional group and adoption of the behaviors of the professional (p. 47). Hinshaw (1986) described the socialization process in nursing as the transition of anticipatory role expectations to the actual role expectations of the people now setting the standards for the individual entering the profession; attachment to significant others who are practicing in the professional role; the labeling of inconsistencies between anticipated roles and those of significant others, including faculty in the initial professional socialization and then colleagues in the work setting; and internalization of role behaviors and values associated with the new role (pp. 21–22).

Tracy, Samarel, and DeYoung (1995) suggest that the socialization process in nursing involves socialization into the practice and professional roles. Socialization into the practice role involves acquiring the knowledge and skills needed for practice. Socialization into the professional role includes developing an understanding of the need for continual learning as essential to personal and professional development and becoming actively involved in professional organizations and activities.

A model developed by Cohen (1981) and associates describes professional socialization in nursing in terms of the cognitive development of the student, thus representing a different view of professional socialization. Drawing on theories of child development and cognitive development, Cohen proposes that a similar progression occurs in the learning of professional skills and in becoming socialized into the role. There are four stages in this model:

- **Stage 1.** *Unilateral dependence.* The learner relies entirely on external controls and searches for the one right answer.

- **Stage 2.** *Negative/independence.* Learners begin to question the instructor and ideas presented to them; as part of this process, they develop an ability to question the ideas of others.
- **Stage 3.** *Dependence/mutuality.* Students begin to think more abstractly, are able to evaluate the ideas of others rather than to merely accept them, and begin to demonstrate empathy and commitment to others.
- **Stage 4.** *Interdependence.* In the final stage, students are able to exercise independent judgment and weigh alternatives. Cohen described this stage as the one in which the student has become a professional. (pp. 16–18)

Cohen's developmental model of professional socialization was examined in a study by McCain (1985). In McCain's research, beginning nursing students were more dependent than graduate students; older students were less dependent and more interdependent than younger students; students with concurrent work experience in nursing tended to be highly interdependent; and all students in the sample had an interdependence stage. McCain concluded from her findings that students did not progress through these four developmental stages as clearly as described in the model.

Others (Frisch, 1990; Reilly & Oermann, 1992; Valiga, 1983; Zorn, Ponick, & Peck, 1995) have described the cognitive development of nursing students in terms of Perry's theory. Perry (1970) proposes that the ability to think and reason develops over time through a series of stages. The developmental stage influences the student's ability to make independent judgments, deal with ambiguity in the clinical setting, and accept differing points of view. Cognitive development, according to Perry, progresses along a continuum of nine positions grouped into four stages:

- **Stage 1.** *Dualism.* In the beginning, students think in terms of absolutes and are unable to deal with multiple points of view.
- **Stage 2.** *Multiplicity.* In this stage, students are able to examine different perspectives, although they are not yet at the point at which they can evaluate them.
- **Stage 3.** *Relativism.* Students who have progressed to this stage are able to evaluate their own ideas and those of others. There is an improved understanding of different alternatives and their consequences of them.
- **Stage 4.** *Commitment in relativism.* The most advanced stage is one in which the student has developed a personal and professional value system and his or her own identity. Learners are able to act according to their own values and beliefs about nursing.

According to Perry (1970), students move from dualistic thinking, that is, simplistic and categorical, to a way of thinking that enables them to evaluate and accept diverse perspectives and deal with ambiguities. Not all learners, however, progress through these four stages in their cognitive development. Some remain at a particular stage or retreat to dualism or absolute thinking rather than develop a commitment to their own values and beliefs. A higher level of cognitive development is essential, considering the complexity of nursing practice in a society characterized by ambiguities rather than absolutes.

Socialization to Work Setting

When a new graduate enters the work setting, the socialization process begins again, this time enabling the nurse to modify the professional nursing role learned in an educational setting to fit the workplace. Although most nursing students select an instructor as their role model, with continued employment, they gradually begin to identify with a work-related nurse. Kramer (1974) described the transition from school to work and the need for new graduates to resolve role conflict as they adapt the values and skills learned in school to the work setting. In this process, nurses need to integrate the professional values acquired as part of their educational preparation into those associated with the bureaucratic health care system. Ideally, the new graduate is able to use the role behaviors and values of the professional in the workplace, but often conflict arises because of incongruities among these values.

Strader and Decker (1995) view this period as one of role transition during which the new graduate learns behaviors appropriate to the position and group with whom she or he is working. In effective role transition, the new graduate accepts the role and develops behaviors associated with it (Strader & Decker, 1995, p. 62). Role models in the work setting facilitate this transition to the professional nurse role.

Green (1988) surveyed 25 senior baccalaureate nursing students to examine the relationships between their role models and role perceptions. Findings indicated that the faculty role models of new graduates were replaced by work-related models within the first 3 months of employment. The most important characteristic of the role model chosen by subjects was clinical experience and performance. Findings also revealed a decrease in *professional role orientation* (an emphasis on professional standards rather than institutional policies) and an increase in both *bureaucratic orientation* (an emphasis on rules and regulations of the institution) and *service orientation* (an emphasis on the dignity and humanity of the client) after graduation (pp. 246–247). These findings are consistent with other studies in this area. Role transition for the new graduate seems to be promoted by adapting the professional role and values to the work setting and by demonstrating an increase in bureaucratic and service orientations.

Extensive research has been conducted on the socialization of nurses. Researchers have examined the process through which students are socialized into the profession as well as the socialization of nurses in practice. Some nurses experience difficulty in developing their professional role because of the demands of the bureaucratic work setting and of other health professionals.

Socialization Through Education

Returning to school for advanced nursing education represents another period of socialization for the student. Associate degree and diploma nursing graduates returning for a baccalaureate or other advanced degree, baccalaureate-prepared nurses returning for a master's degree, and nurses engaged in doctoral study go through a period of socialization as they acquire new knowledge and skills and the behaviors of the new practice role for which they are preparing. When RNs enter baccalaureate programs, for instance, they initially may reject aspects of the program, particularly those that differ significantly from their previous educational experiences. In time, however, they are able to resolve most, if not all, of these conflicts and integrate values and norms of the workplace with their developing view of self as a professional practitioner.

Research has been conducted on the role socialization of RNs returning for baccalaureate and higher degrees. Lawler and Rose (1987) examined the concept of professionalism among seniors in a generic baccalaureate nursing (BSN) program, senior RN students, and senior associate degree nursing (ADN) students. The RN students demonstrated more professional orientation than the other groups. Lynn, McCain, and Boss (1989) studied the effect of a BSN program on professional socialization. Although RN students did not demonstrate significant differences in their professional orientation, generic students had higher socialization scores on graduation than when they entered the nursing program.

The nurse's re-entry into the academic setting may be considered a period of role transition. This transition entails both learning new role behaviors and expectations associated with the professional nursing role and combining school with existing roles and obligations. When an individual is confronted with multiple roles and competing demands, particularly in terms of time, role conflict can occur. Multiple roles can exhaust time and energy and eventually result in role strain (Campaniello, 1988, p. 136). A study of 155 RNs enrolled in a baccalaureate completion program, however, indicated that, for these nurses, having multiple roles did not increase role conflict. Being a parent, though, was a major source of conflict (p. 138). Apparently, the number of roles may be less significant than the particular role and its obligations. Findings from the study also indicate that multiple roles may enhance the well-being of the student; school provides more benefits for the student than the stresses created.

Lengacher (1993b) tested a model for predicting role strain in RN students ($N = 86$) returning to school. Findings indicated that the student's personality, stage of career development, and marital status were related to the role strain experienced by RNs. Support systems need to be developed for students as they reenter the educational system to assist them in adjusting to the educational environment and coping with stresses and role strain they might experience as they return to school (Dick & Anderson, 1993; Lengacher, 1993a, 1996).

PATTERNS OF NURSING EDUCATION

Historical Perspectives

Some type of nursing care has always existed. Early on, care of the sick was provided typically by women in the family. No particular education or experience was needed to provide this care. Over time, however, nurses became recognized as care givers for the ill, and training programs for nurses were then developed. The first such program was initiated in 1860 by Florence Nightingale at St. Thomas's Hospital in London. This training program for nurses was designed to prepare nurses for practice and as such met educational goals rather than the needs of the hospital. An apprenticeship model of nursing education was used in which students worked under the tutelage of ward sisters.

Nightingale's emphasis on autonomy for the school enabled it to pursue its educational mission and develop a systematic approach to teaching the theory and practice dimensions of nursing. Nightingale, through her writings and practice, offered recommendations on the role and responsibilities of the nurse in an attempt to improve patient care.

In the United States, nurses were first prepared for their professional role in the 1870s. At that time, patients were cared for primarily in the home, either by women within the family or by hired nurses. Throughout the history of nursing, an assumption has been that nurses would substitute for family members in the provision of care, thereby transferring "the job of 'caring for another' from the family to nursing" (Lynaugh & Fagin, 1988, p. 184). Initially, nurses cared for patients who did not have family members, who were poor, or who were considered threats by their families because of illness or insanity. By the end of the 19th century, however, it was more common for families to delegate care to nurses because "it was safer or more convenient and because they could afford it" (p. 184).

In 1873, three schools of nursing were established: (1) the Connecticut Training School, (2) the Boston Training School, and (3) the Bellevue Training School; these schools adopted the Nightingale system of nursing education (Chapter 2, page 42). Other training schools followed suit. The educational value of these training schools, however, soon was diminished when hospitals realized that students could be used to care for the ill. The Goldmark Report (Goldmark, 1923) and Committee on the Grading of Nursing Schools Report (1934) described the problems in nursing education, particularly the combined service and educational purposes of the schools at that time.

Before the Depression, most trained nurses worked in private duty, but by the end of the 1920s, many private duty nurses were finding it difficult to maintain their employment. After the Depression, potential employers no longer had the financial resources for private duty nursing care. Hospital care of patients became increasingly more common, with nursing students rather than graduate nurses providing the care. Students subsidized hospitals that had minimal financial resources. Lynaugh and Fagin (1988) reported that "pupil nurses" were willing to trade their time and labor for the title "graduate nurse" (p. 185). Hospitals tended to operate under rather simple budgets, and, by using students as providers of service, they were able to reduce the real costs of nursing care. With the closing of diploma schools and the shift of nursing education to colleges and universities, beginning in the 1960s and continuing over the years, the costs of nursing care became a reality and remain so today.

World War II greatly increased the demand for nurses to care for military personnel and mothers and children in the community and schools. The introduction of federal funding into nursing education, through programs such as the Cadet Nurse Corps, was seen as one solution to the nursing shortage and was an impetus in upgrading many schools of nursing.

Accompanying the growth of colleges and universities following World War II was an increase in collegiate programs in nursing. In 1951, Mildred Montag proposed an additional level of nursing education—that of preparing RNs in community colleges. She conceptualized associate degree programs as technical programs that would prepare the nurse for immediate employment. The growth of associate degree programs compounded concerns regarding the educational preparation needed for nursing practice and for developing nursing as a profession and the issues associated with differentiating practice among graduates of these varied programs. Specific differences in nurses' roles and responsibilities based on their educational background were yet to be identified, and the addition of ADN programs to the nursing education system resulted in one more level of practitioner with similar, and in many cases the same, functions.

In 1965, the ANA published its position paper on education for nursing, recommending the baccalaureate degree as the minimum preparation for professional nursing, associate degree for technical nursing, and short preservice programs in vocational education for health service occupations. Even today, the level of educational preparation needed for entry into professional nursing practices remains an issue. The desire to promote the development of nursing as a profession is basic to the recommendation of the baccalaureate degree as the entry-level degree for professional nursing. With this degree, professionals are prepared in university settings for entry into practice. Other reasons for supporting the baccalaureate degree for entry into professional nursing include the need for a greater theoretical base, drawing on nursing science and a range of theories from other fields, to reflect the rapidly changing and complex health care system of today; the need to differentiate more clearly levels of nursing practice and related roles and responsibilities of the nurse; and the need to enhance the status of nursing as a profession. On the other hand, opponents argue that opportunities for career mobility for RNs prepared in associate and diploma programs are lacking in some geographical areas and, when available, sometimes require nurses to repeat content and experiences from their previous educational programs.

Types of Educational Programs

Nursing, unlike most professions, has a variety of educational programs that prepare students for entry into practice. These often are referred to as basic or generic programs. The three major types of educational programs that lead to RN licensure are: (1) diploma, (2) associate degree, and (3) baccalaureate degree programs. Other types of basic professional programs, although less common, include the generic master's degree and nurse doctorate.

Technical education is provided in a variety of programs that are hospital based or in community colleges. Most diploma programs are 2 years in length, and most of the education is provided in the hospital; associate degree programs, offered by community colleges, also typically last 2 academic years. There is a limited number of diploma programs in the United States, 124 programs, or 8.3% of basic RN programs. The most common type of nursing program is associate degree, 868 programs, which represent 57.8% of basic nursing programs. There are 509 baccalaureate programs in the United States, 33.9% (NLN, 1995, p. 21).

Professional nursing education is provided in baccalaureate programs in colleges and universities and in generic master's and nurse doctorate programs. Graduates of baccalaureate programs are prepared as generalists in the care of individuals, families, groups, and communities. Traditional generic baccalaureate programs prepare students for entry into practice after approximately 4 years of study, including both nursing and liberal arts components. There also is a growing number of programs designed specifically for college graduates with non-nursing degrees. These programs are of two types: (1) accelerated programs that offer a second bachelor's degree, in nursing, in fewer than 18 months on the average, and (2) generic master's programs that award the master's degree in nursing following approximately 3 years of study. McDonald (1995) reported on the successful performance of graduates of an accelerated nursing program for students with non-nursing college degrees. The nurse doctorate programs at Case Western Reserve University and the University of Colorado award a professional nursing doctorate (ND) to college graduates as the entry degree for nursing practice. These innovative programs are viewed by many as a step in developing nursing as a profession that offers a status equal to those of other health professionals.

Graduate nursing education occurs at two levels: (1) master's and (2) doctoral. Master's programs vary in length, generally between 1 and 2 years, and the type of degree awarded. They prepare students for advanced clinical practice in an area of nursing specialization. Advanced practice nurses prepared at the master's level have consistently demonstrated their ability to provide cost-effective and high-quality care (Watson, 1995). For many decades master's programs prepared clinical nurse specialists (CNS), focusing on a specialized area of nursing practice, and nurse practitioners (NP), prepared to provide a full range of primary care services. These health services include: (1) health promotion and disease prevention and (2) assessment, diagnosis, and management of acute and chronic illness, including prescription of medications and other treatments (Thraikill & Domine, 1993, p. 11). Watson (1995) has noted the growing trend toward graduate programs that blend clinical nurse specialist and nurse practitioner preparation for advanced practice. Along with advanced nursing practice, master's programs prepare graduates to provide leadership in the delivery of care, identify researchable problems and participate in the research process, and contribute to the improvement of nursing and health care and advancement of nursing as a profession (NLN, 1987).

Doctoral nursing programs generally consist of 3 years of study beyond the master's degree, although some programs admit baccalaureate graduates and include master's study within the doctoral requirements. At the doctoral level, nurses are prepared as researchers and advanced practitioners who are able to contribute to the development of nursing theory and the testing of that theory in clinical practice. A variety of doctoral degrees, both academic and professional, are offered in nursing (Marriner-Tomey, 1990). The doctor of philosophy (PhD) is an academic degree that prepares nurses to become researchers who are able to contribute to the development of nursing as a science. A professional degree, doctorate of nursing science (DNS), emphasizes the application of nursing research and testing of nursing theories in the clinical setting.

Differences in Practice

One of the major issues that continues to face nursing education is entry into professional practice. Since the ANA's (1965) first position paper on nursing education that called for the baccalaureate degree as a minimum requirement, there has been controversy over the outcomes of associate and baccalaureate degree nursing programs in terms of professional nursing practice. Over the years, many different routes have been available in nursing to become licensed as an RN. Currently, graduates from diploma, associate degree, and baccalaureate degree programs, as well as from nontraditional nursing education programs (such as the New York Regents External Degree, which grants a baccalaureate degree after students complete a series of tests), generic master's programs, and others all take the RN licensing examination for entry into practice.

In 1985, the ANA recommended that the state associations establish the baccalaureate degree in nursing as the minimum education for professional practice and licensure as an RN and associate degree in nursing for licensure at the technical level (Lewis, 1985). The NLN and other nursing groups also have supported the baccalaureate degree for entry into professional practice. North Dakota was the first state to establish these two entry levels of practice (Wakefield-Fisher, Wright, & Kraft, 1986). Further development of nursing as a profession requires that its professionals be educated at least at the baccalaureate level, as with other professions.

A major difficulty in implementing two levels of practice has been in differentiating the role and competencies of graduates from diploma, associate degree, and baccalaureate degree programs. Both the ANA and NLN have published documents describing the competencies of these different levels. Other nurse educators and leaders in nursing over the years also have described the levels of practice and how they should differ in terms of role and abilities in the health care setting. Overall, the baccalaureate graduate is viewed as possessing a liberal education as well as knowledge and skills in nursing. This background enables the graduate to deliver care to individuals, families, groups, and communities with multiple and complex needs in a range of settings. Practice at the technical level focuses more on the individual client with common, well-defined health problems.

Differentiated practice focuses on structuring the roles and responsibilities of nurses according to educational preparation and clinical competence. Differentiated nursing roles along the continuum of care match the knowledge and skills of nurses to the needs of patients (American Association of Colleges of Nursing, 1995, p. 26).

Identifying the roles and competencies of nurses prepared at the ADN and BSN levels serves as one means of differentiating nursing practice. The role of the ADN is to care for individuals and members of a family consistent with the identified goals of care. The ADN functions within structured health care settings, where policies, procedures, and protocols are established. Care of patients by the ADN graduate focuses on common, well-defined nursing diagnoses giving consideration to the client's relationship within the family. The ADN uses basic communication skills, coordinates care with other health care members, modifies standard teaching plans, recognizes the relationship of research to practice, and plans and implements care consistent with the overall admission to discharge plans (AACN, 1995, pp. 28–29).

The BSN cares for individuals, families, groups, and communities in structured and unstructured health care settings. Unstructured health care settings may not have established policies, procedures, and protocols. The BSN uses complex communication skills, collaborates with other providers, plans and delivers comprehensive teaching to clients, incorporates research into practice, and manages care from admission to postdischarge (AACN,

TABLE 1–2. COMPETENCIES OF ASSOCIATE DEGREE NURSE VERSUS BACCALAUREATE DEGREE NURSE

Associate Degree Nurse	Baccalaureate Degree Nurse
Differentiated Competency Statements	
The ADN cares for focal clients who are identified as individuals and members of a family. The level of responsibility of the ADN is for a specified work period and is consistent with the identified goals of care. The ADN is prepared to function in structured health care settings. The structured settings are geographical or situational environments in which the policies, procedures, and protocols for provision of health care are established and there is recourse to assistance and support from the full scope of nursing expertise.	Ths BSN cares for focal clients who are identified as individuals, families, aggregates, and community groups. The level of responsibility of the BSN is from admission to postdischarge. The BSN is prepared to function in structured and unstructured health care settings. The unstructured setting is a geographical or situational environment that may not have established policies, procedures, and protocols and has the potential for variations requiring independent nursing decisions.
Provision of Direct Care Competencies	
The ADN provides direct care for the focal client with common, well-defined nursing diagnoses by	The BSN provides direct care for the focal client with complex interactions of nursing diagnoses by
A. Collecting health pattern data from available resources using established assessment format to identify basic health care needs	A. Expanding the collection of data to identify complex health care needs
B. Organizing and analyzing health pattern data to select nursing diagnoses from an established list	B. Organizing and analyzing complex health pattern data to develop nursing diagnoses
C. Establishing goals with the focal client for a specified work period that are consistent with the overall comprehensive nursing plan of care	C. Establishing goals with the focal client to develop a comprehensive nursing plan of care from admission to postdischarge
D. Developing and implementing an individualized nursing plan of care using established nursing diagnoses and protocols to promote, maintain, and restore health	D. Developing and implementing a comprehensive nursing plan of care based on nursing diagnoses for health promotion
E. Participating in the medical plan of care to promote an integrated health care plan	E. Interpreting the medical plan of care into nursing activities to formulate approaches to nursing care
F. Evaluating focal client responses to nursing interventions and altering the plan of care as necessary to meet client needs	F. Evaluating the nursing care delivery system and promoting goal-directed change to meet individualized client needs
Communication Competencies	
The ADN uses basic communication skills with the focal client by	The BSN uses complex communication skills with the focal client by
A. Developing and maintaining goal-directed interactions to encourage expression of needs and support coping behaviors	A. Developing and maintaining goal-directed interactions to promote effective coping behaviors and facilitate change in behavior
B. Modifying and implementing a standard teaching plan to restore, maintain, and promote health	B. Designing and implementing a comprehensive teaching plan for health promotion

TABLE 1–2. COMPETENCIES OF ASSOCIATE DEGREE NURSE VERSUS BACCALAUREATE DEGREE NURSE (continued)

Associate Degree Nurse	Baccalaureate Degree Nurse
The ADN coordinates focal client care with other health team members by	The BSN collaborates with other health team members by
A. Documenting and communicating data for clients with common, well-defined nursing diagnoses to provide continuity of care	A. Documenting and communicating comprehensive data for clients with complex interactions of nursing diagnoses to provide continuity of care
B. Using established channels of communication to implement an effective health care plan	B. Using established channels of communication to modify health care delivery
C. Using interpreted nursing research findings for developing nursing care	C. Incorporating research findings into practice and by consulting with nurse researchers regarding identified nursing problems to enhance nursing practice
Management Competencies	
The ADN organizes those aspects of care for focal clients for whom the ADN is accountable by	The BSN manages nursing care of focal clients by
A. Prioritizing, planning, and organizing the delivery of standard nursing care to use time and resources effectively and efficiently	A. Prioritizing, planning, and organizing the delivery of comprehensive nursing care to use time and resources effectively and efficiently
B. Delegating aspects of care to peers, licensed practical nurses, and ancillary nursing personnel, consistent with their level of education and expertise, to meet client needs	B. Delegating aspects of care to other nursing personnel, consistent with their levels of education and expertise, to meet client needs and to maximize staff performance
C. Maintaining accountability for own care and care delegated to others to ensure adherence to ethical and legal standards	C. Maintaining accountability for own care and care delegated to others to ensure adherence to ethical and legal standards
D. Recognizing the need for referral and conferring with appropriate nursing personnel for assistance to promote continuity of care	D. Initiating referral to appropriate departments and agencies to provide services that promote continuity of care
E. Working with other care personnel within the organizational structure to manage client care	E. Assuming a leadership role in health care management to improve client care

Reprinted from Midwest Alliance in Nursing. (1984). Facilitating competency development. Indianapolis, IN: Author, with permission; competencies part of AACN. (1995). A model for differentiated nursing practice. Washington, DC: AACN.

1995, pp. 28–29). Competencies of ADN and BSN graduates are listed in Table 1–2.

Another approach to differentiating practice is based on the clinical competence of the nurse. Clinical ladders, for instance, are designed to differentiate varying levels of clinical practice (McClure, 1990).

Considering the explosion of knowledge, changes within the health care system, and community orientation, the need exists for more nurses prepared at the baccalaureate level. Fagin and Lynaugh (1992) recommend the BSN, among other qualifications, for entry into nursing practice, with expanded access to generic baccalaureate programs and partnerships between community colleges and baccalaureate programs. "Asserting the baccalaureate as the norm for nursing practice recognizes the reality of nursing as an occupation (i.e., a vital work serving the public), as well as a profession (i.e., a living body of knowledge and skills)" (p. 217).

Educational programs in nursing need to address present and future health needs: preparing graduates for an important role in health promotion, delivering community-based primary care, exercising leadership in the health care system, practicing in new systems of care, and being able to use and manage technology. Graduates need at least a baccalaureate degree to develop this knowledge and these skills and be prepared for the changes they will encounter in the health care system (Oermann, 1994a, b).

Returning to School

There has been an influx of RNs returning for baccalaureate and other advanced nursing degrees. Many of these nurses are looking ahead to the time when the baccalaureate degree in nursing may be required for entry into professional practice. Others return to school to improve their chances of advancement in nursing, to develop their knowledge base and skills further, to change positions within nursing, and for a variety of other reasons.

Nurse executives report their desire for a majority of staff nurses prepared at the baccalaureate level to meet the complex needs of patients and families. In 1980, 55% of RNs held a diploma as their highest degree; 22% of nurses were prepared at the baccalaureate level, and 18% at the associate degree level. By 1992, the percentage of RNs with diplomas decreased to 34. At the same time, the percentage of nurses with bachelor's degrees increased to 30 and those with associate degrees to 28 (AACN, 1994). Recent studies suggest that by the year 2000, there will be half as many nurses prepared at the baccalaureate and higher degree level as needed and an excess of nurses prepared at the associate degree level (Oermann, 1994a; U.S. Public Health Service, 1990). In addition, there is increasing demand for nurses with master's and doctoral degrees for advanced practice.

RNs represent a heterogeneous student population with needs and backgrounds different from generic, or basic, students (Baj, 1985; Mattson, 1990; McClelland, & Daly, 1991). These differences need to be considered in the design of the educational program. King (1988), in a comparison of RN and generic students, found that RNs had advanced further along in their stage of life and development and were more concerned about their careers than generic students. RNs favored programs that provided flexibility and autonomy. As adult learners, RNs bring to the educational setting a wealth of nursing and life experiences; the knowledge and skills they want to develop often are quite specific to their career goals. Learning experiences, therefore, need to be individualized, with the teacher serving as the resource person. Self-direction and independence in learning are important.

When RNs return for a baccalaureate degree, they can choose from a variety of types of educational programs. Many baccalaureate programs have tracks for RNs. Other programs are designed for RNs only, often providing greater flexibility for meeting their needs as adult learners. These RN-only programs have become more common over the years. In Beeman's (1988) study, RNs in RN-only programs reported that their programs encouraged independence in learning and self-direction more than traditional baccalaureate nursing programs. In addition, RNs in traditional programs suggested that certain aspects of the program, such as the need to repeat previously learned material and the costs of education, interfered with their learning (p. 369).

Cragg (1991) interviewed RN students who had taken distance education in nursing courses. Findings indicated that the students were cognizant of professional nursing issues and had professional values and attitudes about nursing even though they had limited contact with faculty from the main campus. Recent reviews of research on educational reentry for RNs document outcomes and benefits of programs for registered nurses (Lengacher & VanCott, 1992; VanCott & Lengacher, 1993).

One newer model of RN education involves RN-MSN programs that enable the RN to combine the baccalaureate and master's programs in nursing. RN-MSN programs provide one option for qualified RNs seeking an advanced degree in nursing, enabling them to receive a master's degree in less time than completing the baccalaureate followed by the master's program. Creasia (1994) described the development and benefits of an RN-MSN track.

Even with the emergence of programs geared specifically for the RN and alternate types of curricula, problems remain in returning for a baccalaureate and master's degree. Some of these include the cost of education; the need to combine school with ongoing responsibilities including work, family, and others; the lack of accessibility to programs in certain areas of the country; and problems in scheduling work and classes. The nursing literature also suggests that the stress that some RNs experience as students may be a contributing factor in their decision not to continue in the program and even perhaps not to enroll. Assuming a dependent role as a student may be stressful in itself, particularly when work and family life demand independent thinking and decision making. Derstine (1988) concluded from her study of 203 RNs enrolled in baccalaureate degree programs that most cope effectively with the demands of returning to school. Even with problems associated with returning to school, the benefits outweigh the difficulties.

CAREER DEVELOPMENT

The decision to return to school often marks the beginning of another phase in the career development of the nurse. There are both personal and professional rewards for advanced education, and many nurses view education as one means of promoting their careers. Nurses need to identify their personal and professional goals and seek opportunities that improve their chances of advancement. Setting goals is essential for the nurse to plan future activities more carefully and take advantage of opportunities for advancement in the workplace and in other settings.

A job is different from a career. In a job the nurse carries out a role and responsibilities associated with a particular position. A career, however, is a chosen path to fulfill personal and professional goals (Henderson & McGettigan, 1994, p. 2). When they view nursing as a career, nurses identify what they want to accomplish, develop personal and professional goals to be achieved, and plan activities to meet these goals. Nurses need to capitalize on career opportunities. Career advancement reflects personal and professional goals, as each nurse's career path may differ, as may their satisfaction with their chosen path and related accomplishments. Henderson and McGettigan (1994) view a nursing career as "a *developmental process*, a *personal experience*, and a *self-directed pursuit* within a *social context*" (p. 3). Career development in nursing is important not only to the individual nurse but also to the profession as a whole.

SUMMARY

Whether nursing can be characterized as a profession has been debated for years. Nursing has made substantial progress in developing itself as a profession. Research continues on the generation and testing of nursing theory, and nurses, both individually and as a profession, are exerting greater control over practice. The ANA Social Policy Statement (ANA, 1995) describes nursing as a profession and scientific discipline. The need for education at the baccalaureate level for entry into professional practice has been accepted by many individual nurses and nursing groups and is recognized as important to achieving full professional status in the health care system.

In professional socialization (the process through which one acquires the knowledge, skills, and values of the profession) the values and norms of the profession become internalized into the nurses' own behavior. The nursing professional possesses a set of attitudes and values that distinguishes her or him as a professional. The true test of whether the student has developed a concept of self as a professional occurs in the workplace. Socialization occurs not only during the initial preparation for nursing practice but also when the new graduate enters the work setting and the nurse returns to school and acquires behaviors associated with other roles in nursing.

Controversy over the minimum educational requirements for entry into different levels of nursing practice and the roles and competencies of practice at these levels has persisted. Differences in the roles and competencies of graduates of diploma, associate degree, and baccalaureate degree programs have been described in the literature, although in practice in some health care settings these differences may not be readily apparent. Research in nursing has attempted to explicate these differences. Registered nurses are returning for baccalaureate and advanced degrees in nursing in record numbers, thus creating the need in nursing for programs that are flexible and designed for the adult learner. Even when problems associated with returning to school are taken into consideration, the benefits outweigh the stresses involved, and, for many nurses, education is one of the means of promoting their careers in nursing. Advanced education also benefits nursing in its goal of professionalism.

REFERENCES

Abdellah, F. G., Beland, I., Martin, A., & Matheney, R. (1964). *Patient-centered approaches to nursing*. New York: Macmillan.

American Association of Colleges of Nursing. (1994, May). Nursing fact sheet. Washington, DC: Author.

American Association of Colleges of Nursing. (1995). *A model for differentiated nursing practice*. Washington, DC: Author.

American Nurses Association. (1965). American Nurses Association's first position on education for nursing. *American Journal of Nursing, 65*(12), 106–111.

American Nurses Association. (1980). *Nursing: A social policy statement*. Kansas City, MO: Author.

American Nurses Association. (1985). *Code for nurses with interpretive statements*. Kansas City, MO: Author.

American Nurses Association. (1995). *Nursing's social policy statement*. Washington, DC: Author.

Baj, P. A. (1985). Demographic characteristics of RN and generic students: Implications for curriculum. *Journal of Nursing Education, 24*, 230–236.

Beeman, P. (1988). RNs' perceptions of their baccalaureate programs: Meeting their adult learning needs. *Journal of Nursing Education, 27*, 364–370.

Boughn, S. (1995). An instrument for measuring autonomy-related attitudes and behaviors in women nursing students. *Journal of Nursing Education, 34*, 106–113.

Brint, S. (1994). *In an age of experts: The changing role of professionals in politics and public life*. Princeton: Princeton University Press.

Campaniello, J. A. (1988). When professional nurses return to school: A study of role conflict and well-being in multiple-role women. *Journal of Professional Nursing, 4*, 136–140.

Carr-Saunders, A. M., & Wilson, P. A. (1933). *The professions*. Oxford: Clarendon Press. Cited in M. M. Moloney, *Professionalization of nursing* (2nd ed.). Philadelphia: J. B. Lippincott.

Cohen, H. A. (1981). *The nurse's quest for a professional identity*. Menlo Park, CA: Addison-Wesley.

Committee on the Grading of Nursing Schools. (1934). *Nursing schools today and tomorrow*. New York: Author.

Conway, M. E. (1988a). Curriculum, the professional person, and accountability. *Journal of Professional Nursing, 4*, 74.

Conway, M. E. (1988b). Theoretical approaches to the study of roles. In M. E. Hardy

& M. E. Conway (Eds.), *Role theory: Perspectives for health professions* (2nd ed., pp. 63–72). Norwalk, CT: Appleton & Lange.

Cragg, C. (1991). Professional resocialization of post-RN baccalaureate students by distance education. *Journal of Nursing Education, 30,* 256–260.

Creasia, J. L. (1994). Issues in designing an RN-MS track. *Nurse Educator, 19*(1), 27–32.

de Tornyay, R. (1993). Nursing education: Staying on track. *Nursing & Health Care, 14,* 302–306.

Derstine, J. B. (1988). Anxiety in the adult learner in an RN to BSN program: Real or imagined. *Health Education, 19* (4), 13–15.

Dick, M., & Anderson, S. (1993). Job burnout in RN-to-BSN students: Relationships to life stress, time commitments, and support for returning to school. *The Journal of Continuing Education in Nursing, 24,* 105–109.

Fagin, C. M., & Lynaugh, J. E. (1992). Reaping the rewards of radical change: A new agenda for nursing education. *Nursing Outlook, 40,* 213–220.

Frisch, N. C. (1990). An international nursing student exchange program: An educational experience that enhanced student cognitive development. *Journal of Nursing Education, 29,* 10–12.

Goldmark, J. (1923). *Nursing and nursing education in the United States.* New York: Macmillan.

Green, G. J. (1988). Relationships between role models and role perceptions of new graduate nurses. *Nursing Research, 37,* 245–248.

Greenwood, E. (1984). Attributes of a profession. In B. Fuszard (Ed.), *Self-actualization for nurses* (pp. 13–26). Rockville, MD: Aspen.

Hardy, M. E., & Hardy, W. L. (1988). Role stress and role strain. In M. E. Hardy & M. E. Conway (Eds.), *Role theory: Perspectives for health professions* (2nd ed., pp. 159–239). Norwalk, CT: Appleton & Lange.

Henderson, F. C., & McGettigan, B. O. (1994). *Managing your career in nursing.* New York: National League for Nursing.

Henderson, V., & Nite, G. (1978). *Principles and practice of nursing* (6th ed.). New York: Macmillan.

Hills, M. D., & Lindsey, E. (1994). Health promotion: A viable curriculum framework for nursing education. *Nursing Outlook, 42,* 158–162.

Hinshaw, A. S. (1986). Socialization and resocialization of nurses for professional nursing practice. In E. C. Hein & M. J. Nicholson (Eds.), *Contemporary leadership behavior: Selected readings* (2nd ed., pp. 19–34). Boston: Little, Brown.

Hurley-Wilson, B. A. (1988). Socialization for roles. In M. E. Hardy & M. E. Conway (Eds.), *Role theory: Perspectives for health professions* (2nd ed., pp. 73–110). Norwalk, CT: Appleton & Lange.

King, J. E. (1988). Differences between RN and generic students and the impact on the educational process. *Journal of Nursing Education, 27,* 131–135.

Kramer, M. (1974). *Reality shock: Why nurses leave nursing.* St. Louis, MO: Mosby.

Lawler, T., & Rose, M. (1987). Professionalization: A comparison among generic baccalaureate, ADN, and RN/BSN nurses. *Nurse Educator, 12*(3), 19–22.

Lengacher, C. A. (1993a). Comparative analysis of role strain and self-esteem across academic programs. *Nursing Connections, 6*(3), 33–46.

Lengacher, C. A. (1993b). Development of a predictive model for role strain in registered nurses returning to school. *Journal of Nursing Education, 32,* 301–308.

Lengacher, C. A. (1996). Role strain, role stress, and anxiety in nursing faculty and students: Theory and research analysis. In K. R. Stevens (Ed.), *Review of Research in Nursing Education* (Vol. VII, pp. 40–66). New York: National League for Nursing.

Lengacher, C., & VanCott, M. L. (1992). Nursing research related to educational reentry for the registered nurse. In L. R. Allen (Ed.), *Review of research in nursing education* (Vol. V, pp. 75–106). New York: National League for Nursing.

Lewis, E. P. (1985). Taking care of business: The ANA house of delegates, 1985. *Nursing Outlook, 33,* 239–243.

Lynaugh, J. E., & Fagin, C. M. (1988). Nursing comes of age. *Image: Journal of Nursing Scholarship, 20,* 184–190.

Lynn, M., McCain, N., & Boss, B. (1989). Socialization of RN to BSN. *Image, 21,* 232–237.

Marriner-Tomey, A. (1990). Historical development of doctoral programs from the Middle Ages to nursing education today. *Nursing & Health Care, 11,* 133–137.

Mattson, S. (1990). Coping and developmental maturity of RN baccalaureate students. *Western Journal of Nursing Research, 12,* 514–524.

McCain, N. L. (1985). A test of Cohen's developmental model for professional socialization with baccalaureate nursing students. *Journal of Nursing Education, 24,* 180–186.

McClelland, E., & Daly, J. (1991). A comparison of selected demographic characteristics and academic performance of on-campus and satellite-center RNs: Implications for the curriculum. *Journal of Nursing Education, 30,* 261–266.

McClure, M. L. (1990). Introduction. In E. Goertzen (Ed.), *Differentiating nursing practice into the twenty-first century* (pp. 1–11). Washington, DC: American Academy of Nursing.

McDonald, W. K. (1995). Comparison of performance of students in an accelerated baccalaureate nursing program for college graduates and a traditional nursing program. *Journal of Nursing Education, 34,* 123–127.

Mohr, W. K. (1995). Multiple ideologies and their proposed roles in the outcomes of nurse practice settings: The for-profit psychiatric hospital scandal as a paradigm case. *Nursing Outlook, 43,* 215–223.

Moloney, M. M. (1992). *Professionalization of nursing* (2nd ed.). Philadelphia: Lippincott.

National League for Nursing. (1987). *Characteristics of master's education in nursing.* New York: Author.

National League for Nursing. (1995). *Nursing Datasource 1995.* New York: Author.

Nightingale, F. (1859). *Notes on nursing: What it is and what it is not.* London: Harrison and Sons. (Facsimile edition, Lippincott, 1946.)

Oermann, M. H. (1994a). Professional nursing education in the future: Changes and challenges. *Journal of Obstetric, Gynecologic, and Neonatal Nursing, 23,* 153–159.

Oermann, M. H. (1994b). Reforming nursing education for future practice. *Journal of Nursing Education, 33,* 215–219.

Oermann, M. H. (1996). Research on teaching in the clinical setting. In K. R. Stevens (Ed.), *Review of research in nursing education* (Vol. VII, pp. 91–126). New York: National League for Nursing.

Perry, W. G., Jr. (1970). *Forms of intellectual and ethical development in the college years.* New York: Holt, Rinehart, & Winston.

Peters, D. A., & Hays, B. J. (1995). Measuring the essence of nursing: A guide for future practice. *Journal of Professional Nursing, 11,* 358–363.

Pew Health Professions Commission. (1991). *Healthy America: Practitioners for 2005.* Durham, NC: Author.

Reilly, D. E., & Oermann, M. H. (1992). *Clinical teaching in nursing education* (2nd ed.). New York: National League for Nursing.

Schlotfeldt, R. M. (1981). Nursing in the future. *Nursing Outlook, 29,* 295–301.

Schön, D. A. (1990). *Educating the reflective practitioner.* San Francisco: Jossey-Bass.

Simpson, I. H. (1967). Patterns of socialization into professions: The case of student nurses. *Sociological Inquiry, 37*(1), 47–54.

Strader, M. K., & Decker, P. J. (1995). *Role transition to patient care management.* Norwalk, CT: Appleton & Lange.

Thraikill, A., & Domine, L. (1993). Council of Nurses in Advanced Practice Alliance Meets. *ANA Council Perspectives, 2*(2), 10–11.

Tracy, J., Samarel, N., & DeYoung, S. (1995). Professional role development in baccalaureate nursing education. *Journal of Nursing Education, 34,* 180–182.

U.S. Public Health Service. (1990). *Nursing: Seventh report to the President and Congress on the status of health personnel.* Washington, DC: U.S. Department of Health and Human Services, Public Health Service.

Valiga, T. M. (1983). Cognitive development: A critical component of baccalaureate nursing education. *Image, 15,* 115–119.

VanCott, M. L., & Lengacher, C. (1993). Review of research related to educational reentry for the registered nurse: 1985–1991. In N. L. Diekelmann & M. L. Rather (Eds.), *Transforming RN education* (pp. 79–96). New York: National League for Nursing.

Wakefield-Fisher, M., Wright, M. M., & Kraft, L. (1986). A first for the nation: North Dakota and entry into nursing practice. *Nursing & Health Care, 7,* 135–141.

Watson, J. (1995). Advanced nursing practice . . . and what might be. *Nursing & Health Care, 16,* 78–83.

Wiens, A. G. (1990). Expanded nurse autonomy: Models for small rural hospitals. *Journal of Nursing Administration, 20*(12), 15–22.

Young, S. W., Hayes, E., & Morin, K. (1995). Developing workplace advocacy behaviors. *Journal of Nursing Staff Development, 11,* 265–269.

Zorn, C. R., Ponick, D. A., & Peck, S. D. (1995). An analysis of the impact of participation in an international study program on the cognitive development of senior baccalaureate nursing students. *Journal of Nursing Education, 34,* 67–70.

BIBLIOGRAPHY

Alspach, J. G. (1990). Critical care nursing in the 21st century. *Critical Care Nurse, 10,* 8–16.

American Association of Colleges of Nursing (AACN). (1993, March). *Addressing nursing education's agenda for the 21st century [Position statement].* Washington, DC: Author.

Angelini, D. (1995). Mentoring in the career development of hospital staff nurses: Models and strategies. *Journal of Professional Nursing, 11,* 89–97.

Barger, S. E. (1988). Child development center—Nursing center partnership: A win-win arrangement. *Nursing & Health Care, 9,* 147–149.

Barger, S. E., & Crumpton, R. B. (1991). Public health nursing partnership: Agencies and academe. *Nurse Educator, 16*(4), 16–19.

Billingsley, M. (1995). From the editor. The differentiated nurse. *NursingConnections, 8*(2), 12–13.

Brodie, B. (1994). Nursing's quest for professionalism. In J. C. McCloskey & H. K. Grace (Eds.), *Current issues in nursing* (4th ed., pp. 559–565). St. Louis: Mosby.

Brooten, D., Brown, L. P., Munro, B. H., York, R., Cohen, S. M., Roncoli, M., & Hollingsworth, A. (1988). Early discharge and specialist transitional care. *Image: Journal of Nursing Scholarship, 20*, 64–68.

Bunkers, S., & Geyer, C. (1988). The nursing portfolio of prior learning: Access and credibility for the RN. *Journal of Nursing Education, 27*(6), 280–282.

Clinton, H. R. (1993). Nurses in the front lines. *Nursing & Health Care, 14*, 286–288.

Cohen, B. J., & Jordet, C. P. (1988). Nursing schools: Students' beacon to professionalism? *Nursing & Health Care, 9*, 39–41.

Corcoran, S. (1988). Toward operationalizing an advocacy role. *Journal of Professional Nursing, 4*, 242–248.

Coudret, N. A., Fuchs, P. L., Roberts, C. S., Suhrheinrich, J. A., & White, A. H. (1994). Role socialization of graduating student nurses: Impact of a nursing practicum on professional role conception. *Journal of Professional Nursing, 10*, 342–349.

de Tornyay, R. (1992). Reconsidering nursing education: The report of the Pew Health Professions Commission. *Journal of Nursing Education, 31*, 296–301.

Diekelmann, N. L., & Rather, M. L. (Eds.). (1993). *Transforming RN education.* New York: National League for Nursing.

Diers, D. (1987). When college grads choose nursing. *American Journal of Nursing, 87*, 1631–1635.

Donley, R., Sr., & Flaherty, M. J., Sr. (1989). Analysis of the market driven nursing shortage. *Nursing & Health Care, 10*, 183–187.

Ellis, J. R., & Hartley, C. L. (1995). *Nursing in today's world.* Philadelphia: Lippincott.

Fagin, C. M., & Diers, D. (1983). Nursing as metaphor. *New England Journal of Medicine, 309*(2), 116–117.

Fagin, C. M., & Maraldo, P. J. (1988). Feminism & the nursing shortage: Do women have a choice? *Nursing & Health Care, 9*, 365–367.

Fields, W. L. (1988). The PhD: The ultimate nursing doctorate. *Nursing Outlook, 36*, 188–189.

Goldenberg, D., & Iwasiw, C. (1993). Professional socialization of nursing students as an outcome of a senior clinical preceptorship experience. *Nurse Education Today, 13*(1), 3–15.

Harrington, C. (1991). Why we need a teaching home care program. *Nursing Outlook, 39*, 10–29.

Hegyvary, S. T. (1992). Nursing education for health care reform. *Journal of Professional Nursing, 8*, 3.

Higgs, Z. R. (1988). The academic nurse-managed center movement: A survey report. *Journal of Professional Nursing, 4*, 422–429.

Green, C. P. (1987). Multiple role women: The real world of the mature RN learner. *Journal of Nursing Education, 26*, 266–271.

Johnson, J. H. (1988). Differences in the performances of baccalaureate, associate degree, and diploma nurses: A meta-analysis. *Research in Nursing & Health, 11*, 183–197.

Kelly, L. Y., & Joel, L. A. (1995). *Dimensions of professional nursing* (7th ed.). New York: McGraw-Hill.

Lawler, T. G. (1988). Measuring socialization to the professional nursing role. In O. L. Strickland & C. F. Waltz (Eds.), *Measurement of nursing outcomes: Vol. 2. Measuring nursing performance: Practice, education and research* (pp. 33–49). New York: Springer.

Meleis, A. I. (1988). Doctoral education in nursing: Its present and its future. *Journal of Professional Nursing, 4* (6), 436–446.

Mullinix, C. F. (1990). The next shortage: The nurse educator. *Journal of Professional Nursing, 6,* 133.

Murdock, J. E. (1987). Counseling clears the way for return-to-school decisions. *Nursing & Health Care, 8* (1), 33–36.

National League for Nursing. (1991). *Nursing's agenda for health care reform.* New York: Author.

National League for Nursing. (1992, October). *An agenda for nursing education reform in support of nursing's agenda for health care reform.* New York: Author.

Neighbors, M., Eldred, E., & Sullivan, M. (1991). Nursing skills necessary for competency in the high-tech health care system. *Nursing & Health Care, 12,* 92–97.

Oermann, M. H. (1990). Research on teaching methods. *Annual review of research in nursing education* (pp. 1–31). New York: National League for Nursing.

Oermann, M. H. (1991). Effectiveness of a critical care nursing course: Preparing students for practice in critical care. *Heart & Lung, 20,* 278–283.

Oermann, M. H., Dunn, D., Munro, L., & Monahan, K. (1992). Critical care education at the baccalaureate level. *Nurse Educator, 17* (2), 20–23.

Oermann, M. H., & Jamison, M. T. (1989). Nursing education component in master's programs. *Journal of Nursing Education, 28,* 252–255.

Oermann, M. H., & Provenzano, L. M. (1992). Students' knowledge and perceptions of critical care nursing. *Critical Care Nurse, 12,* 72–77.

Primm, P. L. (1986). Entry into practice: Competency statements for BSNs and ADNs. *Nursing Outlook, 34* (3), 135–137.

Primm, P. L. (1990). Approaches and strategies. In American Organization of Nurse Executives (Ed.), *Current issues and perspectives on differentiated practice* (pp. 17–134). Chicago: American Hospital Association.

Reilly, D. E., & Oermann, M. H. (1990). *Behavioral objectives: Evaluation in nursing* (3rd ed.). New York: National League for Nursing.

Rendon, D. (1988). The registered nurse student: A role congruence perspective. *Journal of Nursing Education, 27,* 172–177.

Rose, M. A. (1988). ADN vs. BSN: The search for differentiation. *Nursing Outlook, 36* (6), 275–279.

Scherer, P. (1988). Hospitals that attract (and keep) nurses. *American Journal of Nursing, 88* (1), 34–40.

Schutzenhofer, K. K. (1988). Measuring professional autonomy in nurses. In O. L. Strickland & C. F. Waltz (Eds.), *Measurement of nursing outcomes: Vol. 2. Measuring nursing performances: Practice, education, and research* (pp. 3–18). New York: Springer.

Sharkey, C. J. (1988). Decide to manage your career. *American Journal of Nursing, 88* (1), 105–106.

Styles, M. M. (1982). *On nursing: Toward a new endowment.* St. Louis: Mosby.

Tagliareni, E., Sherman, S., Waters, V., & Mengel, A. (1991). Participatory clinical education. *Nursing & Health Care, 12,* 248–250, 261–263.

Thurber, F. W. (1988). A comparison of RN students in two types of baccalaureate completion programs. *Journal of Nursing Education, 27,* 266–273.

Van Cleve, L. (1988). Nursing image as reflected in sex role preferences. *Journal of Nursing Education, 27,* 390–393.

Vena, C., & Oldaker, S. (1994). Differentiated practice: The new paradigm using a theoretical approach. *Nursing Administration Quarterly, 19*(1), 66–73.

Warner, S. L., Ross, M. C., & Clark, L. (1988). An analysis of entry into practice arguments. *Image: Journal of Nursing Scholarship, 20,* 212–216.

Watson, J., & Phillips, S. (1992). A call for educational reform: Colorado nursing doctorate model as exemplar. *Nursing Outlook, 40,* 20–26.

Winstead-Fry, P. (1990). *Career planning: A nurse's guide to career advancement.* New York: National League for Nursing.

Witt, B. S. (1991). The homeless shelter: An ideal clinical setting for RN/BSN students. *Nursing & Health Care, 12,* 304–307.

The Historical Evolution of Nursing as a Profession

Linda Kay Tanner Strodtman

As Baer (1990) pointed out,

> Nurses are the prototypically invisible women whose minds, hearts, and hands shaped a huge industry, yet whose story is essentially untold except by themselves—to preserve their memories, celebrate their triumphs, argue their point of view, or win support for their cause. As a result, nursing's historiography is inseparable from its social and cultural context. (p. 459)

As nursing's development as a profession has occurred in the "context of time, place, and contemporaneous social interactions" (Baer, 1987, p. 3) and nursing's contribution to the health care system has largely been ignored by social policy experts and decision makers, it is important that nurses develop an understanding of he discipline's historical roots as they address their current and future roles in shaping the health care system. Society's socioeconomic and technological development, along with changes in the role of women, are factors to be considered when examining the development of nursing's science. As nurses acquire knowledge, skills, and a sense of occupational identity in their profession and internalize nursing's norms and values, it is important that they develop an appreciation of these factors and of nurses who have traveled before them and influenced the development of professional nursing.

This chapter presents a perspective about the historical evolution of nursing that started in earnest with the hallmark leadership of Florence Nightingale in the mid-1800s and traces its progress through successive eras that primarily were influenced by changes in women's rights and roles. Men's roles in nursing and their subsequent plight in being recognized as legitimate members of this female-dominated profession are not to be ignored, but because nursing has remained predominantly a woman's occupation, its professional roots spring from a different social context from that of men within nursing and from that of men in other male-dominated professions (Hiestand, 1986). Along with these gender issues, the contributions of African-American nurses to nursing and their struggles to achieve recognition also are discussed, as they have sought to overcome both racial and gender barriers within the discipline and society.

In the 1990s, as nursing redesigns the nature of its work in a highly competitive, cost-conscious health care system; recruits, educates, and retains high-caliber professionals, especially for leadership positions; and becomes a key leader in reformulating health care policy; it is critical "that nurses have a better sense of their professional identity, their professional values and their professional socialization heritage" (Strodtman, 1994, p. 22). Meleis (1991), a prominent nurse theorist, states that by reconstructing our present reality, "we see shadows of our past as well as visions of our future" (p. 3).

PRE-NIGHTINGALE ERA

Dawn of Civilization

Sir William Osler (1932), distinguished professor of Medicine at Oxford and Johns Hopkins University, credits modern "nursing as an art to be cultivated, as a profession to be followed" but recognized that "nursing as a practice originated in the dim past, when some mother among the cave-dwellers cooled the forehead of her sick child with water from the brook or first yielded to the prompting to leave a well-covered bone and a handful of meal by the side of a wounded man left in the hurried flight before an enemy" (pp. 156–157). Osler's quote typifies two of the most prevalent images of the nurse that have endured throughout the ages—the role of mother who cares for the children, the elders, and other sick and infirm members of the family and neighborhood, and that of "angel of mercy" who cares for wounded soldiers during time of military conflict.

Nursing initially "evolved as an intuitive response to the desire to keep people healthy as well as to provide comfort and assurance to the sick" (Dolan, 1973, p. 2), and the nurse, as part of her maternal role, traditionally assumed responsibility for nursing the sick. The inception of nursing took root in the Christian period in the first century A.D. when it was closely allied to religion. Deaconesses provided care to those who were underprivileged, distributing food and medicines that they carried in a basket, their visiting nurse's bag (Dolan, 1973). In the Roman church, matrons, upper-class Roman women, used their independent positions and great wealth in community work for charity and nursing work (Donahue, 1985).

With the decline of Rome during the Middle Ages, people turned to feudalism, with the noble landlord's wife being in charge of the household's sick, and care of the sick provided by monks within various orders (Dolan, 1973; Donahue, 1985). From these monasteries city hospitals developed with much of the nursing care provided by monks and repentant women and widows called sisters, although they were not members of a religious group (Dolan, 1973, p. 64). Three of these famous medieval hospitals were the Hôtel Dieu in Lyons, Hôtel Dieu in Paris, and Santo Spirito Hospital in Rome.

The Crusades

During the first 1,000 years after Christ there were few attempts to organize nursing, but the Crusades (1096–1291) stimulated a demand for hospitals and providers of health care as a result of the "fatigue, malnutrition, digestive disturbances from food poisoning, poor sanitary conditions and contact with communicable diseases" faced by the Crusaders (Dolan, 1973, p. 68). Three organizations, military, religious, and secular orders, developed to meet these demands. The military orders drew large numbers of men—knights, monks, and brothers. "There is no doubt that the religious zeal that called forth groups of knights to care for the wounded and the sick was important to the organization and structure of European hospitals and to the pattern of nursing service that was established and standardized by them" (Donahue, 1985, p. 147).

The Crusades stimulated the development of military and religious nursing orders with well-known leaders in the care of the sick, building of hospitals, and organization of educational institutions. With urban development, cultural growth, travel, and commerce came an unwitting spread of disease due to a lack of sanitary and hygienic conditions (Dolan, 1973). Besides leprosy, the people of the Middle Ages also endured epidemics of St. Anthony's fire (erysipelas), typhus, and bubonic plague (also called the Black Death), with an estimated death toll of more than 60 million in Europe and Asia. Knowledge about causation was limited to cosmic or atmospheric changes, and once the epidemics occurred, little could be done.

The Renaissance

Between 1500 and 1700, the Renaissance movement resulted in a tremendous societal expansion economically, politically, socially, and intellectually with the development of university centers of learning (Dolan, 1973). With the increased use of textiles, metal, and glass by skilled craftsmen came the construction of microscopes and telescopes and the use of mathematical procedures. These improvements of vision, along with the invention of the printing press, opened up education that was formerly limited to the wealthy. Medical education moved into universities, which spurred the advance of medicine, but the same did not happen for nursing. Medicine benefited by the work of individuals who revised the view of disease being due to imbalances of the four humors (blood/fire, bile/air, phlegm/water, and black bile/earth), including Leonardo da Vinci and Andreas Vesalius, who expanded knowledge of the body's anatomy; Ambrose Paré, an army surgeon, who reintroduced the use of ligatures to tie off hemorrhaging blood vessels; William Harvey, who discovered the process by which the heart keeps the blood circulating; and Anton van Leeuwenhoek, who improved the microscope and used it to identify bacteria that led to the development of the field of bacteriology. Pharmacy became a field separate from medicine, and "by 1498 the first official Pharmacopoeia was published and became the legal guide for all pharmacists" (Dolan, 1973, p. 111).

The Reformation (Protestant Revolt) movement that began in 1517 also made its mark on health care delivery and affected nursing, particularly in Protestant countries where hospitals that had previously been operated by Catholic religious orders were closed, and the monks and nuns were driven out, resulting in a shortage of nurses. With no qualified group to take the place of the nursing religious orders, women of all ranks, including criminals, beggars, and debtors, were recruited, which resulted in a rapid deterioration in the care of the sick and poor. Working conditions for those who did become nurses were dismal, and long work hours and low wages led many to accept bribes. These conditions were aptly portrayed by the Charles Dickens characters of Mrs. Sairey Gamp and Mrs. Betsy Prig in his novel *Martin Chuzzlewit* (1844). This dark hour of nursing persisted past the mid-1800s until public concern resulted in the beginning of significant changes that directed steady reform in nursing (Donahue, 1985).

Colonial America

In Colonial America the status of health care was similar to that in Europe or perhaps worse. Medical education was through apprenticeship with established practicing physicians, with a rare physician receiving medical education in Europe. Except for a few religious orders, nursing was left to women, most often mothers, to care for their families and neighbors, and there was no formal educational program for nurses. In addition, the colonists faced harsh living conditions and several catastrophic epidemics, such as the diphtheria epidemics of 1735 and 1740, in which at one point nearly one half of the children died (Dolan, 1973), and smallpox, which affected about one person in five (Kalisch & Kalisch, 1995).

Hospitals were established in the early 1700s, but most of these were connected with asylums for the poor. The Pennsylvania Hospital in

Philadelphia, founded in 1751; the New York Hospital, which started receiving patients in the 1790s; and Boston's Massachusetts General Hospital that opened in 1821 were not places for members of "prosperous and respectable" families (Rosenberg, 1987). Instead, early hospitals were seen as places for the morally worthy unfortunates who needed care and as a place for teaching clinical medicine to physicians so that they would not have to go abroad for their education. In most cities the early voluntary hospitals were founded by prominent physicians in the community. The hospital staff consisted of servants, attendants, coachmen, and others who may have had some nursing or housekeeping experience but were of a different class from the hospitals' trustees, medical staff, and superintendents:

> Nurses and attendants were few in number . . . they occupied a marginal status somewhere between that of patient and employee. . . . Nursing was a 5:00 A.M. to 9:00 P.M. occupation, and "watchers" were engaged to oversee only the critically ill at night. Convalescent patients normally cared for their more seriously ill brethren after dark. (Rosenberg, 1987, p. 40)

The hospital was seen as a last resort for most respectable people, including the urban working class, all of whom relied on being cared for in one's own home in time of illness with nursing care provided by family members.

With the advent of the Revolutionary War, the colonies were not prepared for giving care to the ill and wounded, and even toward the end of the war when General Washington ordered that women be employed as nurses, they did little more than provide meals. Additionally, the war signaled a change in the progress of medicine, as female practitioners, including midwives, were excluded from practice. "In the male monopoly of medicine, there was no room for the trained nurse: any grandmother, any destitute old woman who could be hired, was requisitioned as nurse, and none other was desired" (Donahue, 1985, p. 285).

NIGHTINGALE ERA AND THE BIRTH OF MODERN NURSING

The Crimean War

Another war, the Crimean War, was the setting for the work of Florence Nightingale, who, with her cadre of nurses, led the way to professional nursing by demonstrating the benefits of an organized, intelligent approach to caring for patients. It is difficult to sort out all of the specific influences that may have contributed to Nightingale's formulation of her concept of nursing as it seems to have been a lifelong process starting from an early age (Appendix 2.A). Undoubtedly the most significant influence was her experience with organizing and providing nursing care for the British military personnel during the Crimean War.

It should be noted that she and her 38 women volunteers were not the only nurses to serve in Crimea. Other nurses included Mary Grant Seacole, a Jamaican nurse who was expert in the care of tropical diseases who financed her own way to Crimea and set up nursing services in a lodging house. Her efforts to become an army nurse were unfruitful. She was refused by Nightingale and others, but she did volunteer nights and served alongside Nightingale after having cared for the sick in her own lodging house (Carnegie, 1986).

The deplorable conditions at Scutari prompted Nightingale and her nurses to initiate many sanitary reforms, including cleaning, laundry services, and a diet kitchen. They met much resistance from the military men, but through her data collection on preventable deaths related to changes in sanitation, Nightingale made compelling arguments for the needed reforms. She and her nurses were able to achieve a reduction in mortality rate at the Barrack Hospital in Scutari from 60% to a fraction over 1%, and for all the British military hospitals, the mortality rate dropped from 42% to 2.2% (Kalisch & Kalisch, 1995). This was all the more remarkable considering the general state of knowledge about infections and their causes and transmission.

On her return to England, the two goals that Nightingale set about accomplishing were to reform army sanitation practices and to establish a school for nurses—both of which she achieved. The publication of her *Notes on Hospitals* in 1859 was viewed as one of the most valuable contributions to sanitary science at the time, and it revolutionized many ideas about hospitals and their construction (Cook, 1914). The publication of her *Notes on Nursing: What It Is and What It Is Not* also in 1859, was the most widely distributed of all her writings. In the first month after publication, 15,000 copies were sold (Cook, 1914). It was translated into German, French, and other European languages, and it was instantly reprinted in America. One measure of its popularity in the United States is that a lengthy editorial, reviewing its merits, appeared in *Godey's Lady's Book*, which had a circulation of 150,000, the largest among the periodicals of the time (Garwood, 1931). The September 1860 editorial by Sarah Josepha Hale, the editor, exclaimed:

> This little volume of eighty pages is one of the most important works ever put forth by a woman; and very few medical books, produced by the most eminent men, equal it in usefulness and in the good it must initiate and produce for the sick and suffering. (p. 269)

Mrs. Hale went on to say that she hoped that every lady who read the editorial would "study the work and practice its precepts" (p. 269).

For decades after its publication, *Notes on Nursing* served as a standard text on nursing, although Miss Nightingale indicated in the first line of the preface that it was not to be considered a textbook or "rule of thought by which nurses can teach themselves to nurse, still less as a manual to teach nurses to nurse" (Nightingale, 1859/1946, preface, p. 3). Instead, the preface outlined a philosophy or "hints for thought" on principles of nursing for every woman. The conditions of health, or "laws of health," were to apply to the care of the well and sick. An 1867 article by Mrs. Hopkinson on "Hygiene" in *Godey's Lady's Magazine* refers to these laws of health as being "good enough to improve everybody" (p. 258), thus indicating that laypeople, and particularly women, found Nightingale's *Notes* of value.

The development of Nightingale's ideas on health and views about nursing and its role occurred in response to societal needs. In the mid-19th century, the time and circumstances were ripe for Nightingale's initiation of health care reforms, and she was at the vanguard of the health reform movement that was occurring in Europe as well as America. The key scientific breakthroughs in bacteriology were yet to come (in the 1860s and 1870s), with the work of Pasteur and Koch (Starr, 1982), but it should be noted that Nightingale "unequivocally spurned the concepts that illness and disease could be the result of specific microorganisms rather than of dampness and dirt" (Palmer, 1977, p. 87).

Her views about health and disease involved visualizing the body in terms of being a dynamic system constantly interacting with its environment. "Disease was no specific entity . . . but rather a general state of disequilibrium. Health, on the other hand, was synonymous with balance in the body's physiological state" (Rosenberg, 1979, p. 117). She was adamantly against the germ theory, as this would indicate "denial of the filth, disorder, and contaminated atmosphere which seemed responsible for hospital fevers and infections" (Rosenberg, 1979, p. 117). Disease was a "reparative process . . . an effort of nature to remedy a process of poisoning or decay" (Nightingale, 1859/1946, p. 5), and the role of nursing was "to put the patient in the best condition for nature to act upon him" (p. 75).

The nurse's goal was to promote the "laws of health or of nursing" to keep a well person well and to put the sick person in the best position to get well (p. 6). This was to be accomplished by initiating some basic principle of domestic hygiene that mainly dealt with manipulating the environment. Her concept of environment included ventilation and warmth; concern in the home for pure air and water, sewage disposal, cleanliness and exposure to sunlight; and regulation of environmental noise, provision of variety in life, and nourishment or food. Miss Nightingale herself was not in good enough health to be in charge of day-to-day operations of the Nightingale Training School for Nurses at St. Thomas Hospital in London, but she did plan the details of its organization and continued in its overall supervision until around 1872 when she retired from active work.

Miss Nightingale was a prolific writer. She remained a heroine to the public not only in Great Britain but around the world. At the turn of the century, she was still being written about in popular magazines in the United States (Gardner, 1895):

> The legend of Florence Nightingale, however, should not be interpreted in the light of the Great Man [Woman] Theory, wherein one individual by genius, power, and manipulation is able to bring about social change. Rather it must be remembered that the society of 19th century Europe itself was in rapid change associated with the industrial revolution and these changes were congruent with the changes occurring in nursing. (Whittaker & Olesen, 1964, p. 126)

The poor sanitation associated with urban crowding and the disorganization with the industrial revolution made society receptive to the actions of Miss Nightingale.

DEVELOPMENT OF NURSING IN THE UNITED STATES

The Civil War

Americans were under their own duress with the advent of the Civil War in April 1861. Sanitation and health care conditions similar to those that Nightingale found in the Crimean War were prevalent in the United States. Another similarity is that, although the work of nurses in the Crimean War stimulated the introduction of professional nursing in Europe, likewise the Civil War served as the impetus for the development of professional nursing in the United States. When the war started, there were no army nurses, organized medical corps, or ambulance or field hospital service, only a few hundred sisters from religious orders who volunteered their services. Wives, mothers, sisters, and men volunteered to nurse soldiers, but the need was great, and in June of 1861 Dorthea Lynde Dix, a New England school teacher who had previously crusaded for humane treatment, was appointed Superintendent of the Female Nurses of the Army with the mission of recruiting and equipping a corps of army nurses.

Among the more famous of the nursing volunteers were: Clara (Clarissa Harlowe) Barton, a frontline nurse independent from Dix's nurses (Hanson, 1995), who operated a large-scale war relief operation to provide supplies to the battlefields and hospitals and who set up a service postwar to find missing soldiers (13,000 men who had perished were eventually identified and buried) (Bullough, Church, & Stein, 1988); Mary Ann Ball Bickerdyke, a widow and self-taught botanic physician, who, because of her interventions on behalf of the well being of soldiers, became known as Mother Bickerdyke. She continued postwar as a combination missionary, social worker, and nurse to address the rehabilitation and counseling needs of war veterans; Louisa May Alcott, popular author, who served as a nurse for 6 weeks before taking ill, and who made a more significant contribution by writing in newspapers and *Hospital Sketches* about the nursing of soldiers; and Walt (Walter) Whitman, a writer who used his talents as war correspondent and nurse to write prose about the war and nursing in *Drum Taps, Sequel to Drum Taps, Memoranda during the War, and Specimen Days and Collect* (Bullough, Church, & Stein, 1988).

In the Confederate states most of the nursing was performed by infantrymen because of widespread public pressure in the South against having women exposed to army contact, but there were women who ignored the opposition, such as Kate Cumming, who served from 1862 to 1865 and kept a diary of her experience. Another nurse, Sally Tompkins, operated a 25-bed hospital out of a donated house, and, in lieu of military pay, she received hospital supplies. Eventually she was appointed as a captain in the Confederate cavalry.

"Colored nurses" (as they were referred to during this era) were employed under the General Orders of the War Department at a salary of $10 a month. The exact number of these contract nurses is unknown, but there are records of 181 such colored nurses (men and women) who served in eleven hospitals in three states (Carnegie, 1986). Among the more famous African American women who made contributions to nursing in the Civil War were: Harriet (Araminta) Ross Tubman, well known for leading slaves to freedom, who was asked by Governor Andrew of Massachusetts to become a hospital nurse. She responded by working throughout the war, moving from camp to camp as she was needed; Sojourner Truth, a famous abolitionist and early feminist, who in 1851 addressed the National Women's Suffrage Convention where she delivered her famous "And [ain't] I a Woman?" speech; and Susie (Baker) King Taylor, who served as a nurse to the first official African American regiment formed to fight in the Civil War as Union Army volunteers. Her retrospective self-published memoirs of this experience "continues to raise relevant, haunting questions about racial prejudice and racial equality in the post–Civil War years in the United States" (Buchinger, 1992, p. 321).

Many nurses as volunteers, particularly women, performed an unprecedented number of services for the sick and wounded soldiers—direct care, the procurement of badly needed supplies, communication between the soldiers to their families on the homefront, and networking activities. The total number who served is unknown, but it is estimated to be from 1,000 to 20,000, largely because there was no agreed-upon definition of what a nurse was (Hanson, 1995). Nursing was unorganized, no formal education or "training" programs existed, and frequently it was not approved of by physicians and military men, but it served not only as a stimulus postwar for the founding of formal nurse training schools in the United States but also on a larger scale as an opportunity for women to move out of the home to pursue more purposeful societal roles. It was natural, then, for many society women from prominent families who had served during the war to turn their energies to better the lot of women, such as establishing formal nursing education programs.

The Formation of Schools of Nursing

As Kalisch and Kalisch (1995) point out, "Intermittently throughout the first 70 years of the 19th century, physicians gave lectures to nurses and midwives at state hospitals in several large Eastern cities of the United States, but these activities could not be construed as formal courses of instruction" (p. 59). During the mid-1800s there were other instances of short courses to train nurses (6 months or less) offered at various hospitals, but the first recognized Training School for Nurses was established at the New England Hospital for Women and Children. Melinda (Linda) Ann Judson Richards received the first diploma on October 1, 1873, and the claim to be America's first trained nurse. The expectations for performance at this school were rigorous, and of the 42 students who entered the school in 1878, only four students graduated. One of these was Mary Eliza Mahoney, who on August 1, 1879, gained the honor of being America's first African American professional nurse. This school was unique in its progressive philosophy on accepting a diversity of students, and by 1899 five other African American nurses had graduated from the program (Davis, 1988). The first schools for African American nurses were at Spelman Seminary in Atlanta, Georgia; Hampton Institute in Virginia; and Tuskegee Institute in Alabama. Many, if not most, schools in the north banned African Americans from entering nursing schools, so separate schools were usually established. In the south the pattern that emerged was a dual system in keeping with the "separate but equal doctrine" (Carnegie, 1986).

Three training schools after the one at New England Hospital for Women and Children opened, and they were all modeled after Nightingale's school: The New York Training School (May 1873) as a part of Bellevue Hospital, The Connecticut Training School for Nurses at New Haven State Hospital (October 1873), and The Boston Training School for Nurses at Massachusetts General Hospital (November 1873). Under the Nightingale plan, the school of nursing was to be an autonomous unit for education, and the hospital was to be used for practical experience in patient care. The school's objective was to educate nurses, but the plan as adopted in the United States had as its primary objective improved care of the patient in the hospital with the education of the nurse taking a secondary role. This premise of service first, education second, proved through the years to be a major, if not a prime, stumbling block in attempts to educate professional nurses. Most early schools then were established by hospitals principally to provide student nurses as staff to care for patients.

A typical student admitted to a school of nursing in the late 1800s and early 1900s was a single woman or a widow (married women were not allowed) between the ages of 20 and 30 years of age, of sound health, and with the physical and mental capacity for the duties of a nurse, which meant that one had to be able to endure long hours (12-hour shifts) of exhausting work. The educational program usually lasted 2 years, and most of this time

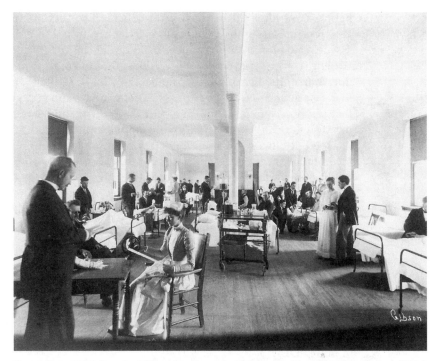

Figure 2–1. 1893 Surgical Dressing Rounds, University Hospital, Ann Arbor, Michigan. Nurse in foreground is operating a bandage winding machine, an early piece of technology used by nurses. Photograph credit: Bentley Historical Library, University of Michigan.

was spent not in classroom work, which frequently consisted of a series of physician lectures on various topics, but cleaning and caring for patients on the hospital wards.

It was typical for the student to have educational sessions in the evening after a long day of caring for patients on the wards. The hospital staff consisted of a superintendent of nurses and a few assistants or supervisors. The rest of the staff was comprised of student nurses who were both in charge of the patient wards and the caregivers. There was minimal use of technology, except for an occasional bandage-winding machine to assist the nurse in caring for the patient. Beds were below waist height and could not be raised or lowered, so the nurses had to bend over to care for the patients. There was no mechanism to elevate the bed's head or foot; if the patient's head needed to be elevated, the nurse would prop the patient up with pillows or use a turned-over straight chair placed at the head of the bed so the pillows could be stacked against the chair's back. Heat often was provided by a wood or coal-burning potbelly stove centered in the middle of the ward that the nurse would have to keep going. Electric lights were available, but the wards were constructed with many windows so that sunlight was used as the primary light source. The thermometer was available for measuring the patient's body temperature, but it may have been a scarce item, and the physician usually did the readings, not the nurse (Dolan, 1973). Later, in the early 1900s, the nurse, especially the private duty nurse, might have a thermometer of her own that she would carry in a case attached to her uniform pocket with a chain and pin. Treatments that the nurse might administer would be turpentine stupes for abdominal distention; the preparation and application of mustard plasters and flaxseed poultices to increase circulation to an area; cupping to increase local circulation and to relieve congested organs such as the lung; the application of leeches for the treatment of inflammation; and the preparation and administration of various types of enemas. The nurse would also frequently be responsible for cooking as well as serving food to the patient.

In spite of these primitive working conditions and the hardships imposed on the nurse, nurses did bring respectability to hospital care and were instrumental in changing the image of the hospital from a place to go to die to a place to receive skilled nursing care. Discoveries in sanitation, medicine, and antiseptic surgery contributed to the more widespread acceptance of hospitals for care of the ill around 1900 (Kalisch & Kalisch, 1995). This led to a demand for more nurses, and schools of nursing grew in number.

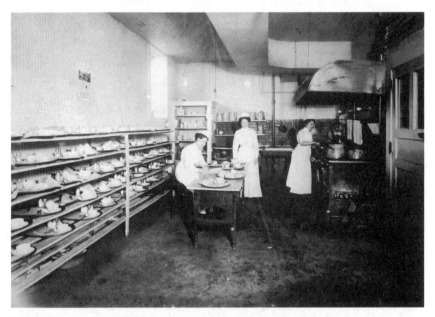

Figure 2–2. Early 1920s University Hospital. Nurses preparing patient meals in dietary kitchen. Photograph credit: The Nursing History Society of the University of Michigan.

Nursing's Professional Development

As the number of schools grew, so did other aspects of nursing's professional development. During the late 1800s nurses began to publish textbooks and teaching materials. In 1878, nurses and physicians at the Connecticut Training School at New Haven Hospital wrote the *Hand-Book of Nursing for Family and General Use*; in 1885 Clara S. Weeks wrote *A Textbook of Nursing*; and Isabel Hampton's 1893 *Nursing: Its Principles and Practice for Hospital and Private Use* continued to be used widely for 20 years or more (Kalisch & Kalisch, 1995). Nursing journals came into existence: first the *Nightingale* in 1886 (until 1891); the *Trained Nurse and Hospital Review* in 1888 (ceased publication in 1960); and finally in 1900, the nurse-managed *American Journal of Nursing* began publication, which continues today.

The next major step in the professionalization of nursing was the founding of the first nursing professional organizations. The 1893 meeting of nursing leaders at the World's Fair and Colombian Exposition in Chicago was the first time nurses met as a unified group. Isabel Hampton, superintendent of nurses at Johns Hopkins Training School for Nurses, presented a paper on the "Educational Standards for Nurses." After the main meeting, about 18 attendees met and established the first national nursing organization, the American Society of Superintendents of Training Schools; in 1912 it became the National League of Nursing Education, and in 1952 it was reorganized into the National League for Nursing (James, 1979). In the late 1800s, schools of nursing began forming alumnae associations, and in 1894 the Nurses' Associated Alumnae of the United States and Canada was formed. In 1911 the American Nurses Association became its successor. Another professional organization formed was the International Council of Nurses (1899) by Mrs. Bedford Fenwick of Great Britain and nursing leaders from many countries. Early presidents from the United States were Miss Annie Goodrich in 1912, Miss Effie Taylor in 1937, and Miss Agnes Ohlson in 1957 (Dolan, 1973).

Because of the need to address discriminatory practices facing African American nurses as well as to foster leadership in the membership, The National Association of Colored Graduate Nurses (NACGN) was organized in 1908 under the leadership of Martha M. Franklin, founder and first president (Carnegie, 1986). This organization was doubly important for African American nurses, as many, especially those from southern states, could not join the American Nurses Association (ANA) from 1916 until the early 1960s because of an association membership policy that required acceptance through one's state organization. Unfortunately, many southern states denied African American nurses membership in their state organizations. The organization dissolved in 1951, and Mabel Keaton Staupers, the first executive director and last president, presided over its merger with the ANA.

Another element in nursing's development as a profession was the writing of the Florence Nightingale Pledge, which is to nursing as the Hippocratic Oath is to medicine (Appendix 2.B). This undertaking was conceived by Mrs. Lystra Eggert Gretter, superintendent of nurses of the Farrand Training School for Nurses at Harper Hospital in Detroit, Michigan. The pledge, written by a small committee of nurses under Gretter's direction, was first administered to the Farrand graduating class of 1893. It was "generally adopted as the climax of 'capping,' or graduating exercises in training schools all over the world" (Woodford & Mason, 1964, p. 312). Ethical issues for the profession were next addressed in an August 1926 editorial of *American Journal of Nursing*, when a proposed Code of Ethics was presented for reader consideration. A formal Code of Ethics was not adopted by the profession until 1950 (Viens, 1989).

A number of significant nursing leaders emerged at this time. As the first president of the ANA, Isabel Hampton Robb also was the initiator of the grading policy for nursing students (Bullough, Church, & Stein, 1988); Lystra Gretter revised the work day of the student nurse from 12 hours to 8 in order to improve the student's education (Woodford & Mason, 1964); and Mabel Keaton Staupers was a successful leader in the campaign to integrate African American nurses in the segregated Army and Navy Nurse Corps in World War II.

There were other noteworthy nurse leaders during the late 1800s and early 1900s. Lavinia Lloyd Dock was editor of the *American Journal of Nursing*; a coauthor with her physician brother George Dock of the nursing text *Materia Medica for Nurses* and with Mary Adelaide Nutting of *A History of Nursing*; a labor leader who encouraged nurses to organize; a feminist who worked to promote women's suffrage; and a public health nurse at the Henry Street Settlement. Mary Adelaide Nutting was an educator and principal of Johns Hopkins Training School; the discipline's first professor of nursing (1907 at Teachers College, Columbia University); an author of textbooks and articles; an education innovator who initiated tuition fees and scholarships and introduced social subjects into the curriculum; and one of the founders of the American Home Economics Association and its Journal of Home Economics (Donahue, 1988). Her book, *A Sound Economic Basis for Schools of Nursing*, raised the need for a different pattern of education in which she encouraged the separation of schools for nursing from hospital control.

The turn of the century saw the beginning of graduate education for nurses. In 1899, an 8-month course in hospital economics was initiated at Teachers College. During the first 10 years after schools of nursing started, there was a change in terminology to signify the change in status that nursing leaders hoped to attain for nursing. "Training" was slowly changed to "education," "superintendent" to director, and "training school" to "school of nursing" (Dolan, 1973). Several schools established nursing programs in university settings. In 1893, a diploma school of nursing for African American nurses was started under the aegis of Howard University (Carnegie, 1986). In 1909, the University of Minnesota offered a 3-year diploma program, and by 1916, 16 colleges and universities "maintained schools, departments, or courses in nursing education" (Kalisch & Kalisch, 1995, p. 246). The first autonomous collegiate school of nursing was established at Yale University in 1924.

Two other events in the closing years of the nineteenth century helped to shape the development of professional nursing. One was the Settlement House Movement, a response to the needs of people in the tenement slums and poor sanitation associated with the rapid growth in American cities. In 1893, Lillian D. Wald, a New York Hospital graduate, and Mary Brewster, a classmate, opened the Henry Street Settlement in the lower East Side in New York City to care for the sick poor. This led the expansion of visiting nursing to the development of public health nursing. Lillian Wald coined the phrase "public health nursing" by creating "a system whereby patients had direct access to nurses and nurses had direct access to patients" (Donahue, 1985, p. 346). She also initiated the first public school nursing program in the United States. With the changes associated with society's move from an agricultural to an industrial society and urbanization with immigration of peoples of many nationalities, public health issues came to the forefront. Communicable disease management, such as for tuberculosis (the leading killer among infectious disease), typhus, scarlet fever, and smallpox, and high infant mortality related to infectious diseases provided ample opportunity for nurses to demonstrate the value of their services.

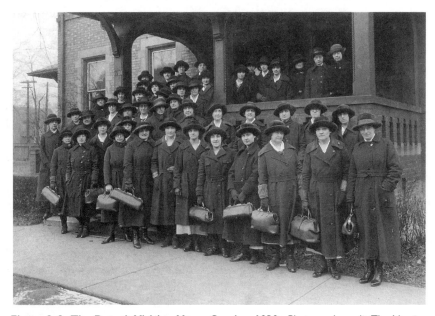

Figure 2–3. The Detroit Visiting Nurse Service, 1930s. Photograph credit: The Nursing History Society of the University of Michigan.

Another event at the close of the century was the Spanish-American War, which at its start in 1898 found no organized army nurse corps and no system to provide nurses for service in the war. As nurses were recruited under Dr. Anita Newcomb McGee, Acting Assistant Surgeon General, they found similar conditions as faced in society—casualties from communicable diseases. As the war was in a tropical climate and there was poor sanitation, typhoid fever, yellow fever, malaria, and dysentery claimed more lives than did gunfire. Clara Louise Maass became a legendary heroine for volunteering in a yellow fever experiment that claimed her life. The merits of "trained nurses" during this war led to the establishment of a permanent Army Nurse Corps in 1901 and the Navy Nurse Corps in 1908.

At the beginning of the 20th century, the nursing discipline continued to emphasize the need to address the social conditions and related health needs of people. In rural areas, such as the Appalachian Mountains of Kentucky, Mary Breckinridge instituted the Frontier Nursing Service to provide midwifery and health services to isolated people in the region. Visiting nursing expanded with the Metropolitan Life Insurance Company contracting with community visiting nurse services to provide health care to their company policyholders. In 1912 a small group of visiting nurses (Lillian Wald, Ella Crandall, Mary Beard, Mary Lent, Edna Foley, Lystra Gretter, and Elizabeth Fox) who favored the term *public health nurse* formed the National Organization for Public Health Nursing (NOPHN) in an effort to organize and standardize the requirements for becoming a public health nurse. Lillian Wald was the first NOPHN president (Kalisch & Kalisch, 1995).

This effort to address the competence of practicing nurses continued with the introduction of legislation for registration to practice. In 1903, North Carolina, New Jersey, New York, and Virginia passed the first laws for establishing a legal system of registration (Dolan, 1973), and eventually every state passed registration laws. In 1950, states began using identical state board examinations from a test pool regulated by the National League for Nursing, making nursing the first profession to use the same licensing examination throughout the 48 states, the District of Columbia, and Hawaii (Kalisch & Kalisch, 1995).

Just as medicine addressed in the 1910 Flexner Report their admission and curriculum standards, nursing hoped to do likewise through several initiatives. The National League for Nursing developed a series of curriculum guides in 1917, 1927, and 1937 that identified minimum curriculum standards. A Committee for the Study of Nursing Education facilitated by the Rockefeller Foundation published its results in the 1923 Goldmark Report. The report recommended that more schools of nursing should be independent units in universities and that all nursing schools should be supported independently of hospitals. Unlike the Flexner report, this report did not cause much change to occur until the 1950s when associate degree educational programs began and diploma nursing schools started to phase out

(Moloney, 1992). Through the next four decades, various studies conducted by nursing leaders advocating that nursing education be based in collegiate settings culminated in the 1965 ANA position paper on educational preparation that recommended the baccalaureate degree as minimum preparation for professional nursing practice and associate degree for technical practice. This two-level preparation for practice was recommended again by the ANA House of Delegates in 1978 with implementation by 1985. But as of 1989, 49% of the registered nurses practicing in the United States received their basic education in diploma programs, and as late as 1992, 34% of all nurses had a diploma in nursing as their highest educational level (Moses, 1992, p.6; NLN Nursing Data Review, 1991).

World War I and the 1920s

The image of nurses as angels of mercy was never more prevalent than during World War I. With the start of the war, both the Army and Navy Nursing Corps grew dramatically. Besides creating a demand for nurses, the war opened new fields of specialization, such as anesthesiology, and for the first time in history, an adequate number of nurses were available with more than 20,000 trained nurse volunteers (Kalisch & Kalisch, 1995). Over 50,000 American men were killed in battle, and another 62,000 died from disease, primarily from influenza, which was pandemic between 1918 and 1919 (Norman, 1995). The war made the military leadership and public aware of their need for well-trained nurses, and as a result, the Army School of Nursing was organized in 1918 with Annie W. Goodrich as the first dean.

With women proving during war that they could take the place of men in many occupations, in the 1920s the role of women changed. The number of women working outside of the home was nearly twice what it had been at the turn of the century, but in nursing there was a shortage. Many women who had entered nursing for the duration of World War I and the subsequent influenza epidemic dropped out. Hospitals in need of nurses increased their number of training schools, but the schools had difficulty recruiting enough students. Hospital care was improving, including the amount of technology available, but hospitals still preferred using students over graduate nurses for meeting their labor needs.

Public health nurses continued to take care of the indigent poor who could not afford hospital care, and federal legislation, the Sheppard-Towner Act of 1921, infused a massive amount of federal money into infant and maternal care. The public health nurse was actively involved in efforts to promote the health and welfare of children and their mothers through health education, home visits, and health screening. By the time the Shepard-Towner Act expired in 1929, 45 states and Hawaii had established child health agencies. Public health nurses had made more than three million home visits to mothers and babies, and almost 20,000 classes for high schools girls, moth-

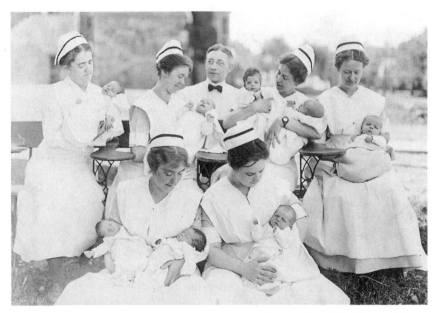

Figure 2–4. Elba L. Morse, Maternity Instructor at University of Michigan, with Dr. Loomis and nursing students about 1915. Photograph credit: The Nursing History Society of the University of Michigan.

ers, and midwives had been conducted (Kalisch & Kalisch, 1995, p. 286). Public health nurses were clearly instrumental in the conduct of this program, and in nine of the states, the programs were directed by nurses (physicians directed the others). The benefits of the programs included a fall in the infant morality rate to 69 per 1,000 births in 1928 as compared to a 1914 rate of 100 per 1,000 births. The greatest decrease was in deaths from gastrointestinal illness, a direct effect of maternal education about caring for and feeding their infants (Kalisch & Kalisch, p. 286). The birth control movement spearheaded by Margaret Sanger, a New York public health nurse, contributed to the decline in maternal and infant mortality as well.

Because of the opposing efforts of the American Medical Association, the Sheppard-Towner Act was not renewed in 1929, and public health nursing lost a valuable support system for their education and care of mothers and their infants. According to Rothman (1978), this also represented "the end of female expertise in the field of health care and at the same time . . . women trained in hygiene working in state-supported clinics gave way to physicians engaged in private practice" (p. 142). With the massive unemployment that resulted from the Great Depression and stock market crash in 1929, nursing was left in a disastrous state, and many nurses worked in hospitals in return for room and board. The public could not afford private-duty nurses, and there was little funding for public health programs. When

Congress responded with the Civil Works Administration (CWA) program in 1933, more than 10,000 unemployed nurses were put to work. To illustrate how destitute nursing was, some nurses in the state of Washington had to be given clothing and shoes before they could accept work (Kalisch & Kalisch, 1995, p. 306).

World War II and Its Effect on Nursing

Nursing was at one of its lowest points in the 1920s and 1930s, and a dramatic change resulted with the advent of World War II. This war not only had a profound effect on society but also brought revolutionary changes to nursing with the first infusion of federal dollars into nursing education. Fifty thousand more nurses were needed than were available. To increase the number of nurses as rapidly as possible, the U.S. Cadet Nurse Corps was created, and scholarships were given to qualified young women. The quality of nursing education increased as standards were developed that participating schools of nursing had to meet to be a part of the cadet program. In exchange for military or civilian service, the nursing student received funding for her or his education and a living stipend. About 95% of all nursing students were enrolled in the Cadet Corps (Dolan, 1973).

Ironically, in spite of the shortage of nurses, the Army Nurse Corps had no provisions "for the appointment of colored nurses in the Corps," but after pressure from African American nurses, a quota of 56 African American nurses were allowed to serve in the Army, but were to serve only in hospitals or wards "devoted exclusively to the treatment of Negro soldiers" (Carnegie, 1986, p. 169). After an intense media campaign by the National Association of Colored Graduate Nurses in 1945, African American nurses were finally accepted into the Army Nurse Corps without regard to race.

Nearly 69,000 nurses were in the Army and Navy Nurse Corps at their peak strength (Donahue, 1985). Among the professions, there were more war-service volunteers from nursing than from any other profession. By the end of the war, nurses had been stationed in approximately 50 nations in all types of settings, from the battle zones to stateside hospitals, again demonstrating their contribution to the recovery of the sick and wounded. The "angel of mercy" image of the nurse prevailed in society, and nurses were portrayed in popular Hollywood produced films as heroines and featured on popular magazine covers of *Life* and *Ladies' Home Journal*.

The Post-War Through the 1960s

It had been expected that after the war the nursing shortage would be relieved by the return of the military nurses to civilian service, but this did not happen. Largely as a result of a massive government campaign to get women out of the work force to make employment available for the returning soldiers, women were forced out of positions that had been held traditionally by men. Most women chose marriage and childbearing, resulting in a baby boom of 40 million babies in the 1950s, overemployment outside the home, and nurses were no exception. The hospital industry found itself in a postwar building surge thanks largely to the availability of federal funding under the Hill-Burton Act of 1946 and to the increased affordability of hospital care for families who had health insurance. These factors contributed to a need for nurses.

Along with the shortage of nurses, other issues facing the profession were increased use of nurse aides and practical nurses, and factions within and outside the profession, especially medicine, were questioning the value of collegiate education for nurses. Associate degree programs in nursing were initiated in the gradual move of nursing education into institutions of higher education, and the debate grew about the best type of basic educational preparation for nurses. Nevertheless, the change in mix of educational programs for nurses continued in the 1960s, and toward the end of the decade, 64% of nursing students received their education in diploma programs, down from 83% in 1956. The number of associate degree and baccalaureate nursing programs rose sharply (Kalisch & Kalisch, 1995).

As intensive care units and the introduction of technology developed in the 1960s, the need for specialty practice nurses heightened. The Vietnam War created an additional demand for highly skilled nurses, as did the growth in the number of the elderly patients and introduction of Medicare. All of these factors generated additional and more complex work for nurses. The passage of the Nursing Training Act of 1964 helped many nurses to pursue graduate nursing education in preparation for specialty practice and roles as clinical nurse specialists. Nursing research, which started in earnest in the early 1950s, continued along with the growth of graduate nursing education—first at the master's level (the 1960s) and then at the doctoral level (the 1970s). Nursing's knowledge base also expanded through the work of nurse theorists.

1970s to the Present

During the 1970s and 1980s, the professionalization of nursing continued with: (1) revisions in nurse practice acts to recognize nursing as an autonomous profession; (2) expansion of clinical nurse specialists, nurse practitioners (starting in 1965), and nurse midwives; (3) further evolution of the knowledge base of nursing; (4) development of nursing information systems (nursing informatics) and the definition of a minimum data set for nursing (Werley, Lang, & Westlake, 1986); (5) attention by the profession to economic issues and a focus on collective bargaining resulting in many work stoppage actions; and (6) political activism with the founding of the Nurses Coalition for Action in Politics (N-CAP), a forerunner to political action committees of the ANA.

This latter activity resulted in nurses lobbying effectively for the creation of a National Center for Nursing Research, which in the 1990s became established as the National Institute for Nursing Research, an independent institute within the National Institutes of Health. As educational opportunities increased, nurses developed new viewpoints and began to value the integration of nursing research and theory development (Mason, Talbott, & Leavitt, 1993).

In the 1990s, as society addresses health care reform in the framework of rising costs of health care and an increased number of people who have no or minimal health insurance, nurses again find themselves in difficult situations. In the mid-1990s, after another round of nurse shortage, the American Medical Association tried unsuccessfully, after intense opposition from the ANA, to introduce a Registered Care Technologist role to address the inadequate supply of nurses. At the same time, more health care was being delivered in managed care environments, which resulted in a shift of location for health care. The focus now is on providing care in outpatient settings and on limiting expensive inpatient hospitalization for the sickest of patients. This has resulted in a shortage of primary care and generalist physicians but an opportunity for nursing to demonstrate the potential for advanced practice nurses such as nurse practitioners and nurse midwives. Studies indicate that 60% to 80% of "primary-care services traditionally rendered by physicians could be provided by nurse practitioners and nurse-midwives" (Kalisch & Kalisch, 1995, p. 484).

As the nation addresses issues of health care reform, it is apparent that the current illness-based health care system must be refocused on disease prevention, health maintenance, and health promotion. Nurses are prepared to deliver the types of services needed, "health (not disease) risk assessment based on environmental and family factors, as well as individual factors; health promotion and disease prevention strategies; counseling and health education; and the knowledge to craft a care regimen using community and family resources" (Mundinger, 1995, p. 255). This area is distinct from the knowledge of disease detection and treatment that is the primary focus of physicians. As the realization that "comprehensive health care today requires the broad spectrum of knowledge that no one practitioner can provide" and that "nurses and physicians are not in competition for the patient," much more collaboration will, and must, occur between the disciplines of nursing and medicine (Fagin, 1992, p. 297).

SUMMARY

Nursing has followed a long road to professional maturity since Nightingale first introduced a broadened scope for nursing. As nursing enters the twenty-first century, there is much to be hopeful for. The uniqueness of nursing and its purpose and scope are coming into sharper focus. Being able to identify, label, and define the work of nursing along with the productivity of nursing's researchers, scholars, practitioners, and leaders puts nursing in a much better position for influencing policymaking as the health care system is overhauled in a competitive arena of shrinking resources. The values that have led people—women and men of diverse ethnic backgrounds—into nursing over the centuries, "values like caring for the sick, the infirm, the young, and those who cannot care for themselves," and nursing's focus on "helping people help themselves stay well or return to health," or experience a peaceful death, have remained strong throughout nursing's history. It is now up to "nurses to ensure shrinking resources are best utilized for the health of the nation" (Noel, 1993, p. 46).

REFERENCES

Baer, E. D. (1987). Nursing's social history: New insights, new solutions. *Journal of Nursing History, 2*, 3–5.

Baer, E. D. (1990). Nurses. In R. Apple (Ed.), *Women, health and medicine in America: A historical handbook* (pp. 459–475). New York: Rutgers University Press.

Buchinger, K. L. (1992). Susie (Baker) King Taylor. In V. L. Bullough, L. Sentz, & A. P. Stein (Eds.), *American nursing: A biographical dictionary* (Vol. II, pp. 319–321). New York: Garland.

Bullough, V. L., Church, O. M., & Stein, A. P. (Eds.) (1988). *American nursing: A biographical dictionary* (Vol. I). New York: Garland.

Carnegie, M. E. (1986). *The path we tread: Blacks in nursing, 1854–1984.* Philadelphia: Lippincott.

Cook, D. E. (1914). *The life of Florence Nightingale* (Vols. I–II). London: Macmillan.

Davis, A. J., & Aroskar, M. A. (1983). *Ethical dilemmas and nursing practice* (2nd ed.). Norwalk, CT: Appleton-Century-Crofts.

Davis, A. T. (1988). Mary Eliza Mahoney. In V. L. Bullough, O. M. Church, & A. P. Stein (Eds.), *American nursing: A biographical dictionary* (Vol. I, pp. 226–228). New York: Garland.

Dolan, J. A. (1973). *Nursing in society: A historical perspective* (13th ed.). Philadelphia: Saunders.

Donahue, M. P. (1985). *Nursing the finest art: An illustrated history.* St. Louis: Mosby.

Donahue, M. P. (1988). Mary Adelaide Nutting. In V. L. Bullough, O. M. Church, & A. P. Stein (Eds.), *American nursing: A biographical dictionary* (Vol. I, pp. 244–247). New York: Garland.

Fagin, C. M. (1992). Collaboration between nursing and physicians: No longer a choice. *Academic Medicine, 67*(5), 295–303.

Gardner, F. R. (1895, May). Florence Nightingale at seventy-five. *The Ladies' Home Journal, 13*(6), 7.

Garwood, I. (1931). *American periodicals from 1850 to 1860.* Monmouth, IL: Commercial Art Press.

Hale, S. J. (1860, September). Florence Nightingale's book. *Godey's Lady's Book and Magazine, 62*, 269–270.

Hanson, K. S. (1995). A network of service: Female nurses in the Civil War. *Caduceus, 11*(1), 11–22.

Hiestand, W. C. (1986). Conceptualizing historical research. In P. Moccia (Ed.), *New approaches to theory development* (pp. 105–117). New York: National League for Nursing.

Hopkinson, M. (1867). Hygiene. *Godey's Lady's Book and Magazine, 74,* 258–260.

James, J. W. (1979). Isabel Hampton and the professionalization of nursing in the 1890s. In M. J. Vogel, & C. E. Rosenberg (Eds.), *The therapeutic revolution: Essays in the social history of American medicine* (pp. 201–244). Philadelphia: University of Pennsylvania Press.

Kalisch, P. A., & Kalisch, B. J. (1995). *The advance of American nursing* (3rd ed.). Philadelphia: Lippincott.

Mason, D. J., Talbott, S. W., & Leavitt, J. K. (1993). *Policy and politics for nurses: Action and chance in the workplace, government, organizations and community* (2nd ed.). Philadelphia: Saunders.

Meleis, A. I. (1991). *Theoretical nursing: Development and progress* (2nd ed.). Philadelphia: Lippincott.

Moloney, M. M. (1992). *Professionalization of nursing: Current issues and trends* (2nd ed.). Philadelphia: Lippincott.

Moses, E. B. (1992, March). *1992 Registered Nurse Population: Findings from the national sample survey of registered nurses.* Washington, DC: U.S. Department of Health and Human Services.

Mundinger, M. O. (1995). Advanced practice nursing is the answer. . . . What is the question? *Nursing & Health Care, 16*(5), 254–259.

National League for Nursing. (1991). *Nursing Data Review 1991.* New York: Author.

Nightingale, F. (1946). *Notes on nursing: What it is, and what it is not* (Facsimile of 1859 ed.). Philadelphia: Lippincott.

Noel, N. L. (1993). Historical overview: Policy, politics, and nursing. In D. J. Mason, S. W. Talbott, & J. K. Leavitt (Eds.), *Policy and politics for nurses: Action and change in the workplace, government, organizations and community* (2nd ed., pp. 36–46). Philadelphia: Saunders.

Norman, E. M. (1995). American military nurses in wartime and the impact of their experiences on peacetime practice. *Caduceus, 11* (1), 23–34.

Osler, Sir William. (1932). *Aequanimitas: With other addresses to medical students, nurses and practitioners of medicine* (3rd ed.). Philadelphia: P. Blakiston's Son & Co.

Palmer. I. S. (1977). Florence Nightingale: Reformer, reactionary, researcher. *Nursing Research, 26*(2), 84–89.

Rothman, S. M. (1978). *Woman's proper place.* New York: Basic Books.

Rosenberg, C. E. (1979). Florence Nightingale on contagion. In *Healing and history* (pp. 116–136). New York: Science History.

Rosenberg, C. E. (1987). *The care of strangers: The rise of America's hospital system.* New York: Basic Books.

Seymer, L. R. (1932). *A general history of nursing.* London: Faber & Faber.

Starr, P. (1982). *The social transformation of American medicine.* New York: Basic Books.

Strodtman, L. K. T. (1994). Becoming a "real woman": Historical analysis of the characteristics, ethos and professional socialization of diploma nursing students in two midwestern schools of nursing from 1941 to 1980 (Doctoral dissertation, Wayne State University, 1994). *Dissertation Abstracts International,* 9519970.

Viens, D. C. (1989). A history of nursing's Code of Ethics. *Nursing Outlook, 37*(1), 45–49.

Werley, H. H., Lang, N. M., & Westlake, S. K. (1986). Brief summary of the Nursing Minimum Data Set Conference. Use and costs of nursing resources. *Nursing Management, 17*, 42–45.

Whittaker, E., & Olesen, V. (1964). The faces of Florence Nightingale: Functions of the heroine legend in an occupational sub-culture. *Human Organization, 23*(48), 123–130.

Woodford, F. B., & Mason, P. P. (1964). *Harper of Detroit: The Origin and Growth of a Great Metropolitan Hospital.* Detroit: Wayne State University Press.

BIBLIOGRAPHY

Apple, R. (Ed.). (1990). *Women, health and medicine in America: A historical handbook.* New York: Rutgers University Press.

Bullough, V. L., Sentz, L., & Stein, A. P. (1992). *American nursing: A biographical dictionary* (Vol. II). New York: Garland.

Carnegie, M. E. (1995). *The path we tread: Blacks in nursing. 1854–1984* (3rd ed.). Philadelphia: Lippincott.

Donahue, M. P. (1996). *Nursing the finest art: An illustrated history* (2nd ed.). St. Louis: Mosby.

Hine, D. C. (1989). *Black women in white: Racial conflict and cooperation in the nursing profession, 1890–1950.* Bloomington: Indiana University Press.

Jones, A. H. (1988). *Images of nurses: Perspectives from history, art, and literature.* Philadelphia: University of Pennsylvania Press.

Jones, K. W. (1983, Fall). Sentiment and science: The late nineteenth century pediatrician as mother's advisor. *Journal of Social History, 17*, 79–96.

Kalisch, P. A., & Kalisch, B. J. (1987). *The changing image of the nurse.* Menlo Park, CA: Addison-Wesley.

Lagemann, E. C. (1983). *Nursing history: New perspectives, new possibilities.* New York: Teachers College.

Reverby, S. M. (1987). *Ordered to care: The dilemma of American nursing, 1850–1945.* Cambridge: Cambridge University Press.

Florence Nightingale: Biographical Sketch

Florence Nightingale, who was born May 12, 1820, to William Edward and Frances Nightingale, was named after her birthplace of Florence, Italy. She had a sister, Frances Parthenope, who was 1 year older. Florence Nightingale was born into the worldly wealth of British upper-class society, and from the age of 5 years, she and her family lived between two country estates, Lea Hurst and Embley Park. Part of the time each year also was spent in London.

Florence's father was well educated and held a view far in advance of his time about the intellectual development of women. He supervised the home education of both daughters, which included music, philosophy, grammar, composition, modern languages, Latin, Greek, mathematics, and history (Cook, 1914). Florence became quite proficient in Latin and Greek.

Florence's mother introduced her to the woman's role that was typical of upper-class Victorian England: visiting poor neighbors, arranging school treats for a local school, and other charitable acts. Another aspect of education for Florence was the family's frequent travels to France, Italy, and Switzerland, which included mixing with the elite.

Florence's commitment to becoming a nurse was strong, and her family struggled with her over her desires because it was not an acceptable role for gentlewomen of 19th-century England. To distract her from this persistent calling, her family sent her on many foreign travels, but each trip reaffirmed her desire to pursue nursing. Finally, at the age of 31, she was able to persuade her family to allow her to go to Kaiserswerth for training at the Institution for Deaconesses. Without telling anyone outside of the immediate family, Florence spent 3 months in 1851 learning about nursing from the deaconesses. After returning home, she was finally able to convince her family to acquiesce to her desire to enter nursing. In 1853, she became the

Superintendent of an "Establishment for Gentlewomen during Illness," also known as the Upper Harley Street Nursing Home, in London. This first independent position in nursing paved the way to her illustrious career. Along with her accomplishments in the Crimean War and her establishment of the Nightingale school, she is known for her writings *Notes on Nursing* and *Notes on Hospitals* and for reforming the British military health care system. She died August 13, 1910, at 90.

The Florence Nightingale Pledge

I solemnly pledge myself before God and in the presence of this assembly;

To pass my life in purity and to practice my profession faithfully; I will abstain from whatever is deleterious and mischievous and will not take or knowingly administer any harmful drug;

I will do all in my power to maintain and elevate the standard of my profession and will hold in confidence all personal matters committed to my keeping and family affairs coming to my knowledge in the practice of my calling;

With loyalty I will endeavor to aid the physician in this work, and devote myself to the welfare of those committed to my care. (Davis & Aroskar, 1983, p. 11)

three **3**

Nursing Models
and Their Use
in Practice

Marjorie A. Isenberg

The importance of explicating a body of substantive knowledge that can be called nursing science has been a dominant theme in the nursing literature since the mid-1950s. This concern for the development of nursing knowledge has paralleled nursing's quest for professional status. Implicit in the term *profession* is the expectation that a body of knowledge exists to serve as the fundamental rationale for practice (Greenwood, 1957). Thus, to be recognized as a profession, nursing must establish a knowledge base for nursing practice. As Johnson (1959) pointed out, no profession can exist without making explicit its theoretical basis for practice. Moreover, nursing, like all professions, has a societal mandate to use its specialized knowledge and skills for human betterment. This mandate assumes that the body of knowledge will undergo continual refinement to ensure an adequate basis for nurses to meet the ever-changing health needs of society. Thus, concern for the development of nursing knowledge is of considerable significance for nursing's development as a recognized profession.

This chapter provides a historical perspective on the development of nursing knowledge and explores reasons for the need for theory development in nursing. The relationship between nursing's evolution as a profession and the quest for nursing knowledge is explained. The chapter also explores the conceptual models of selected nurse scholars. An attempt is made to differentiate between theories and conceptual models, and the purposes of each structure are explained. Finally, by examining the models of

Orem, Roy, and Neuman, the chapter explores the relevance of nursing models to nursing practice.

DEVELOPMENT OF NURSING AS A SCIENCE

The 1950s and early 1960s marked a period of intense effort to develop nursing knowledge. These early attempts at knowledge development, however, were often stymied by an uncertainty about what phenomena to study and what research questions to ask. Frequently during this phase, nurses and the tasks performed by nurses served as the subject matter of research efforts. It soon became apparent that the study of nurses and their duties is not the study of nursing. Consequently, the research conducted during this period contributed little to nursing knowledge and offered limited direction in terms of decision making about patient care.

Since this early phase of knowledge development, nursing science has advanced considerably. In reviewing the nursing research literature since 1960, numerous changes are evident. One of the most significant developments is a transition from essentially atheoretical studies to research designed to test nursing theories that specifically address phenomena of concern to nursing. Nursing research has progressed from studies focused on the duties of nurses to studies focused on patients in need of nursing care.

THE NURSING PERSPECTIVE

Clarification of the nursing perspective is a pivotal step in the process of explicating the structure of the body of knowledge that constitutes the discipline of nursing. As pointed out by Donaldson and Crowley (1978) in their seminal article on the discipline of nursing, it is the perspective of a discipline that determines what phenomena are to be viewed. It is the nursing perspective that eliminates uncertainty about what nurses should study and what type of research questions nurse scientists should ask. Moreover, the nursing perspective provides clarification for what constitutes and does not constitute nursing research.

The nursing perspective is intricately linked with practice. As a professional discipline, the nursing perspective is derived from its practical aim of enhancing the health and well being of human beings. That is, research that is conceptualized within the nursing perspective should reveal knowledge relevant to the practical aim of nursing, the enhancement of the health and well being of clients with various health problems. Several nurse scholars have analyzed the nursing literature in search of the themes or topics of major importance to nursing (Fawcett, 1978; Walker, 1971; Yura & Torres, 1975).

Based on her analysis of the literature, Newman (1983) concluded that, historically, nursing has been concerned with the client, nurse, health care situation in which the nurse and client find themselves, and the purpose of their being together, which is the health and well being of the patient. Furthermore, she noted that most of the current nursing theories address the concepts of patient–client, environment, health, and nursing action. Differences do exist, however, among the nursing theories with respect to the following: the emphasis each theorist places on one or more of the components, the world-views within which the components are described, and the interrelationships depicted among the components.

More recently, Newman, Sime, and Corcoran-Perry (1991) concluded that the focus of nursing as a professional discipline is *caring in the human health experience*. Clarification of nursing's focus serves to delimit the boundaries of our discipline and to reaffirm our long-standing social mandate. Similarly, in 1859, Nightingale stated that the laws of nursing were the same as the laws of health. At that time, she described nursing practice in terms of putting patients in the best possible environment so that nature could heal them. Thus, the nursing profession's long-established concern with human beings, their health, the world in which they live, and the caring nature of our practice continue to be reflected in descriptions of the nursing perspective.

CONCEPTUAL MODELS AND THEORIES

As a professional discipline, nursing is deeply involved in identifying the conceptual base for building and refining nursing knowledge. Several nurse scholars have contributed significantly to this process by proposing nursing conceptual models and nursing theories. Norris (1982) defines a *concept* as an abstraction of concrete events that represent ways of perceiving phenomena. That is, concepts are mental pictures that each person uses as he or she tries to understand and make sense out of experiences in the world. Pain and anxiety are common concepts that nurses encounter in their care of patients. Nurses cannot see "pain" as such, but by carefully observing clients, they pick up cues that fit their mental picture of "pain." Thus, concepts can be described as labels or words used to classify events, objects, or behaviors that are observed in the world. Concepts differ from one another with respect to their breadth. For instance, the concept of stressor is broader than the concept of pain; the concept of "headache" is narrower than the concept of pain. Broad concepts such as stressors tend to be abstract, and narrow concepts such as headache tend to be more concrete.

Concepts are the building blocks of theories and conceptual models. Both theories and conceptual models are conceptual structures designed to provide a vision or way of viewing sets of phenomena. Although both theories and conceptual models are composed of concepts, differences do exist between them. In differentiating between these structures, Ellis (1982) describes a scientific *theory* as comprising a set of propositional statements that expresses relationships between the concepts of the theory. The relationships between the concepts in a theory are more clearly stated than those in a model. These sets of relational statements serve to describe, explain, and predict phenomena and to provide a basis for deriving hypotheses for research purposes. Thus, theories comprise concepts that can be linked to the real world.

In contrast, Ellis (1982) defines a *conceptual model* as comprising abstract concepts that have no counterpart or link in the real world. Thus, concepts in a model tend to be broader and more abstract than those in a theory. Furthermore, in a conceptual model, the relationships between concepts are seldom clearly stated and often are missing. Conceptual models are types of pretheoretical structures.

In the past, nursing theories and conceptual models have contributed significantly to nursing practice and nursing education. Nursing theories offer specific direction to nursing practice. Theories provide nurses with a way of viewing their practice and organizing clinical knowledge. Nursing theory provides a view of the client and defines the substantive focus of the nursing process. A theory provides structure and guidelines for collecting relevant nursing data. It designates categories of data for patient assessment. Given the endless numbers and types of observations that could be included in the nursing assessment, a theory offers a rationale for making decisions about what observations to include in the assessment and which ones to exclude. A theory contributes further to the assessment phase of the nursing process by providing a schema for categorizing patient data and thereby helping nurses to organize clinical knowledge. Examples of assessment forms based on selected nursing theories are found in Appendices A–D. Clearly, theories define all phases of the nursing process and give direction for clinical decision making. Theoretical knowledge provides the basis for rationalizing nursing actions in practice situations. Thus, the development of theoretical knowledge is vital to professional nursing practice.

Not only have theories and conceptual models given direction to nursing practice, but they also have contributed to educational programs designed to prepare nurses. Many of the nursing conceptual models were developed initially to organize the curricula of nursing programs. A conceptual model provides a central focus for an educational program and a way of organizing content. It determines the nature of courses, course objectives, and sequencing of content and learning experience in the program. A conceptual model provides a unifying component for an educational program.

NURSING CONCEPTUAL MODELS

The 1970s marked the introduction of several conceptual models by nurse scholars, including Rogers' (1970) Model of Unitary Human Beings, King's (1971) General Systems Model, Orem's (1971) Self-Care Model, Roy's (1976) Adaptation Model, and Neuman's (1974) Systems Model. Since their introduction, these conceptual models have offered significant direction to nursing education, practice, and research. Each of the models has contributed to the process of identifying the conceptual structure for developing nursing knowledge. An overview of selected theorists' works is included in this section. In Chapter 5, specific examples of the use of nursing models in terms of the nursing process are described.

Rogers' Model of Unitary Human Beings

With the intention of offering direction to nursing in establishing its specific body of abstract knowledge, Martha Rogers (1970) introduced her conceptual Model of Unitary Human Beings. She offered a fresh look at nursing through a view of the world that was in keeping with the most progressive knowledge available. Rogers' model focuses on the irreducible nature of human beings, the integrality of human beings and their environments, a universe of open systems, and the pandimensional nature of reality (Rogers, 1992). Human beings are viewed as unified wholes, not as parts. Rather than looking at parts of human beings, such as the mind or psyche, or the body or spirit, the model emphasizes that human beings can be understood only in their wholeness. The model also emphasizes the integral nature of human beings and their environments; human beings and their environments are seen as mutual and continuous. No spatial (space) or temporal (time) boundaries exist between them. Furthermore, the model proposes a continuous flow of energy through human beings and their environments. In this context, then, clients can be understood only when they are studied in their wholeness and in relation to their environments.

Rogers' model emphasizes an optimistic view of life's potentials and highlights the human capacity to participate knowingly in the process of change. Change, according to Rogers, is a fundamental characteristic of the life process. Change is viewed as continuously innovative and creative (Rogers, 1992). Moreover, nursing practice aims to help people to participate in change knowingly. One example of how nurses can help clients to participate in change knowingly is through empowerment. Empowerment of clients involves recognizing them as partners in health care and sharing knowledge and skills with them (Malinski, 1986). This process enables clients to make informed decisions as they explore options and ultimately make choices. Thus, as clients experience changes in their health, nurses empower them to exercise their choices in making decisions about their health and health care.

Although the relevance of Rogers' conceptual model for practice is apparent, her prime intention in offering the model is to provide the basis for the development of nursing science. Rogers contends that the scientific knowledge derived from her conceptual model provides direction for nursing practice. She views the practice of nursing as the use of scientific nursing knowledge for human betterment (Rogers, 1994). This confirms the idea that the practice of nursing is rooted in the science of nursing. By specifying the body of scientific knowledge basic to nursing, Rogers has contributed significantly to the evolution of nursing as a professional discipline.

King's General Systems Model

In the interest of describing the transactional process that occurs between nurse and patient, Imogene King (1971) introduced her general systems framework of nursing. King's (1989) nursing conceptual system focuses generally on human beings interacting with their environments and, more specifically, on the interpersonal process between the recipient of care (the client) and the caregiver (the nurse). This framework is based on the premise that human beings are open systems that interact with the environment. According to King (1981), this framework (Figure 3–1) comprises three interacting systems:

1. Personal systems
2. Interpersonal systems
3. Social systems

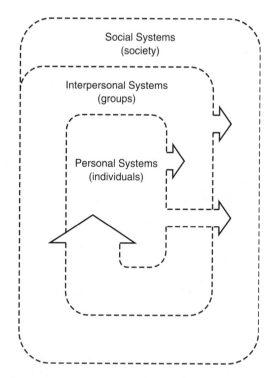

Figure 3–1. A Conceptual Framework for Nursing: Dynamic Interacting Systems *(Reprinted from King, I. M. (1981). A theory for nursing: Systems, concepts, processes. New York: Wiley J., p. 11, with permission from the author.)*

Personal systems refer to individuals; each individual is viewed as a personal system. *Interpersonal systems* encompass dyads (two interacting individuals, such as nurse and client); triads (three interacting individuals, such as nurse, client, and the spouse of a client); and groups (small and large). *Social systems* are concerned with society in general and with health care systems in particular. Examples of social systems relevant to nurse–client interactions are family systems, school systems, work systems, hospitals, and community health agencies. According to King (1995), this framework describes environments within which human beings grow, develop, and perform daily activities. Furthermore, she identifies the goal of nursing as helping individuals to attain, maintain, or regain health or live with a chronic illness or disability (King, 1989).

From this systems framework, King (1981) derived the theory of goal attainment. The focus of the theory is the process of transaction between nurse and client and the nature of those interactions that lead to goal attainment for both the client and nurse. The theory of goal attainment is based on the following beliefs about the rights of clients:

- The right to know about themselves
- The right to participate in decisions that influence their health and life
- The right to accept or reject health care
- The right to information that will help them to make informed decisions about their health care

Inherent to this theory is a basic respect for the capacity of human beings to think, acquire, and use knowledge, make choices, and select courses of action (King, 1986). This theory proposes the following key elements that must be present in nurse–client interactions to achieve goals:

- Perceptual congruence between nurse and client
- Effective communication between nurse and client
- Mutual goal setting between nurse and client

In this theory, then, nursing is described as a process of human interactions between nurse and client in which each assesses the other and the situation. Then, by means of communication, they explore and set goals together and mutually agree on means to achieve those goals (King, 1981). The theory also proposes the consequences or outcomes of goal attainment. King contends that goal attainment in nurse–client interactions leads to both nurse and client satisfaction and effective nursing care.

Thus, the theory of goal attainment has a high degree of relevance to nursing practice. It offers direction by describing the essential components of an effective nurse–client transaction, that is, perceptual congruence, communication, and mutual goal setting. The theory identifies the latter as an important factor in achieving effective nursing care and satisfaction on the part of both the nurse and client.

Orem's Self-Care Model

Dorothea Orem (1971, 1980, 1985, 1991, 1995) pursued her theoretical endeavors out of a need to define the domain and boundaries of nursing as a field of study and of practice. She sought answers to the question: What condition characterizes people when judgments are made that nursing is required? She identifies the condition that constitutes the need for nursing as health-related limitations for engaging in self-care (Orem, 1980). Thus, Orem's conceptual model focuses on individuals' self-care needs and their capabilities for meeting these needs. In this perspective the goal of nursing is to help people to meet their needs for self-care at a therapeutic level and on a continual basis. Furthermore, people are considered legitimately in need of nursing care when they experience an actual or potential health-related limitation in performing self-care. Orem's major concepts are *self-care, therapeutic self-care demand, self-care agency, nursing agency*, and *nursing systems*.

Orem (1985) defines *self-care* as "the practice of activities that individuals initiate and perform on their own behalf in maintaining life, health and well-being" (p. 84). Self-care is viewed as a form of deliberate action that is learned in a sociocultural context. As such, self-care is affected by culturally determined goals and practices (Orem, 1995, p. 106). In conceptualizing self-care, Orem uses the word *self* in the sense of one's whole being. Self-care is conceptualized as purposeful in that it contributes in specific ways to human structural integrity, functioning, and development. Orem (1980) describes the purposes to be attained through self-care actions as self-care requisites. She identifies the following three types of self-care requisites:

1. *Universal self-care requisites* are common to all human beings during all stages of the life cycle. They are associated with life processes, the maintenance of the integrity of human structure and functioning, and general well being.
2. *Developmental self-care requisites* are associated with human developmental processes, with conditions and events occurring during various stages of the life cycle (e.g., prematurity and pregnancy), and with events that can adversely affect development.
3. *Health-deviation self-care requisites* are associated with genetic and constitutional defects and human structural and functional deviations, with their effects, and with medical diagnostic and treatment measures. (Orem, 1995, pp. 108–109)

Self-care requisites represent the types of purposeful self-care that persons require in order to sustain life and promote health and general well being. Orem (1995) expresses them as general sets of actions, such as "maintenance of a balance between activity and rest" (p. 193). The maintenance of a balance between activity and rest controls voluntary energy expenditure, regulates environmental stimuli, and provides outlets for interests and talents, all of which are vital to a sense of well being. When clients effectively perform sets of actions for meeting the universal self-care

TABLE 3–1. GENERAL ACTIONS FOR MEETING UNIVERSAL SELF-CARE REQUISITES

A. Maintenance of Sufficient Intakes of Air, Water, Food
1. Taking in that quantity required for normal functioning with adjustments for internal and external factors that can affect the requirement or, under conditions of scarcity, adjusting consumption to bring the most advantageous return to integrated functioning
2. Preserving the integrity of associated anatomical structures and physiological processes
3. Enjoying the pleasurable experience of breathing, drinking, and eating without abuses

B. Provision of Care Associated With Eliminative Processes and Excrements
1. Bringing about and maintaining internal and external conditions necessary for the regulation of eliminative processes
2. Managing the processes of elimination (including protection of the structures and processes involved) and disposal of excrements
3. Providing subsequent hygienic care of body surfaces and parts
4. Caring for the environment as needed to maintain sanitary conditions

C. Maintenance of a Balance Between Activity and Rest
1. Selecting activities that stimulate, engage, and keep in balance physical movement, affective responses, intellectual effort, and social interaction
2. Recognizing and attending to manifestations of needs for rest and activity
3. Using personal capabilities, interests, and values as well as culturally prescribed norms as bases for development of a rest-activity pattern

D. Maintenance of a Balance Between Solitude and Social Interaction
1. Maintaining that quality and balance necessary for the development of personal autonomy and enduring social relations that foster effective functioning of individuals
2. Fostering bonds of affection, love, and friendship; effectively managing impulses to use others for selfish purposes, disregarding their individuality, integrity, and rights
3. Providing conditions of social warmth and closeness essential for continuing development and adjustment
4. Promoting individual autonomy as well as group membership

E. Prevention of Hazards to Life, Functioning, and Well Being
1. Being alert to types of hazards that are likely to occur
2. Taking action to prevent the occurrence of events that may lead to the development of hazardous situations
3. Removing or protecting oneself from hazardous situations when a hazard cannot be eliminated
4. Controlling hazardous situations to eliminate danger to life or well being

F. Promotion of Normalcy
1. Developing and maintaining a realistic self-concept
2. Taking action to foster specific human developments
3. Taking action to maintain and promote the integrity of one's human structure and functioning
4. Identifying and attending to deviations from one's structural and functional norms

Reprinted from Orem, D. E. (1995). Nursing: Concepts of practice (5th ed.). St. Louis: Mosby, p. 193.

requisites, they are acting in ways that promote their health and general well-being. The universal self-care requisites and general actions for meeting them are summarized in Table 3–1.

The developmental self-care requisites acknowledge that individuals develop as unique entities in society, and that within societies, community and family conditions and resources that promote development vary (Orem, 1995). With this premise in mind, three sets of developmental requisites are identified:

1. Provision of conditions that promote development
2. Engagement in self-development
3. Prevention of or overcoming effects of human conditions and life situations that can adversely affect human development (p. 197)

An example of a requisite that involves self in the process of development (set 2) is to form habits of introspection and reflection so as to acquire insights about self, one's perception of others, relationships to others, and attitudes toward them (p. 198).

Health-deviation self-care requisites exist for people with known or potential health problems. Six categories of health-deviation self-care requisites are identified:

1. Seeking and securing appropriate medical assistance in the event of exposure to specific physical or biological agents or environmental conditions associated with human pathological events and states, or when there is evidence of genetic, physiological, or psychological conditions known to produce or be associated with human pathology
2. Being aware of and attending to the effects and results of pathological conditions and states, including effects on development
3. Effectively carrying out medically prescribed diagnostic, therapeutic, and rehabilitative measures directed to prevent specific types of pathology, to the pathology itself, to regulate human functioning, to correct deformities or abnormalities, or to compensate for disabilities
4. Being aware of and attending to the discomforting or deleterious effects of medical care measures, including effects on development
5. Modifying self-concept (and self-image) and accepting oneself as being in a particular state of health and in need of specific forms of health care
6. Learning to live with the effects of pathological conditions and states and the effects of medical diagnostic and treatment measures in a lifestyle that promotes continued personal development (Orem, 1995, p. 202)

Orem (1995) contends that when the three types of self-care requisites are effectively met, they provide human and environmental conditions that support life processes, maintain human structure and functioning, support development, prevent injury and pathological states, contribute to the cure or regulation of pathology, and promote general well being (p. 109).

Therapeutic self-care demand, a major concept in the Self-Care Model, is closely linked with the self-care requisites. The actions needed to meet the three categories of self-care requisites are what constitutes the therapeutic self-care demands of clients. To formulate a therapeutic self-care demand, one must assess and analyze which self-care requisites exist and then decide which self-care practices need to be carried out to meet them (Orem, 1995, p. 111). For example, the therapeutic self-care demand for a client with a recent diagnosis of diabetes mellitus might include some of the following needs:

- To learn to live with a chronic health problem such as diabetes mellitus
- To alter dietary intake in keeping with a diabetic diet
- To master self-administration of insulin

As this example illustrates, the nature of the therapeutic self-care demand is determined by the self-care requisite from which it was made. In this case, the therapeutic self-care demand is linked to a health-deviation self-care requisite. Thus, the therapeutic self-care demand can be expected to vary according to the self-care requisites from which it was derived.

Another concept of considerable consequence in Orem's model is that of *self-care agency*, the human capability for engaging in self-care (Orem, 1995, p. 212). *Agency* in this context is used in the sense of a power that can be acquired. Thus, self-care agency refers to the complex sets of acquired capabilities that are specific to the performance of self-care at a therapeutic level. Note that Orem (1980, 1985) uses the term *therapeutic* to describe those self-care actions that: (1) are supportive of life processes, (2) are remedial or curative when related to disease processes, and (3) contribute to personal development and maturation. Self-care agency varies according to the developmental level of individuals from childhood through old age. Other factors such as health state, life experiences, and sociocultural orientation also have been described as factors that influence the self-care agency of individuals. Orem (1985) indicates that self-care agency can be examined in relation to the capabilities individuals have for engaging in self-care, including their skill repertoires and the kinds of knowledge they have and use.

Self-care agency can be described with respect to its development, operability, and adequacy (Orem, 1979). Development of self-care agency is defined in terms of the kinds of self-care actions individuals *can* perform. Operability is described in terms of the types of self-care actions that people *do* perform on a consistent and effective level. The adequacy of self-care agency is determined by comparing the number and types of self-care actions people *can* engage in with the number and kinds of self-care actions *required* to meet the existing or projected therapeutic self-care demand. The adequacy of self-care agency is crucial in nursing situations.

This process of assessing the adequacy of self-care agency is viewed by Orem (1995) as essential in judging the presence or absence of self-care deficits. The term *self-care deficits* refers to the relationship between self-care agency and therapeutic self-care demand in which self-care agency is inadequate in meeting the therapeutic self-care demand. This relationship is depicted in Figure 3–2.

According to Orem (1995), it is the presence of an existing or projected self-care deficit that identifies those people with a legitimate need for nurs-

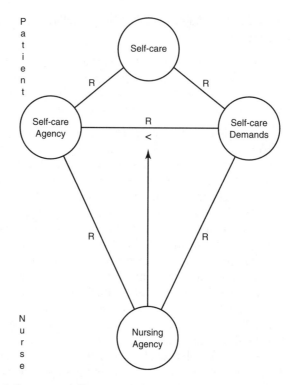

Figure 3–2. A Conceptual Framework for Nursing Note: (R) relationship: (<) Less than (deficit relationship). (Reprinted from Orem, D. E. (1995). Nursing: Concepts of practice (5th ed.). St. Louis: Mosby, p. 435.)

ing. The complex capability required for nursing actions is conceptualized by Orem as *nursing agency*. More specifically, *nursing agency* refers to those specialized abilities that enable nurses to provide care that compensates for or aids in overcoming health-related self-care deficits (Orem, 1985). Nurses exercise or use these specialized abilities to produce nursing actions that can benefit others.

In using Orem's model in practice situations, the major foci of the nursing assessment are the individual's self-care needs or requisites, the individual's self-care agency or capabilities, and those factors that influence (enhance or hinder) the individual's self-care agency. The three categories of self-care requisites are included in self-care assessment: (1) universal self-care requisites, which consist of those needs supportive of the life processes (e.g., intake of nutrients, balance of activity, and rest patterns); (2) developmental self-care requisites, which consist of those conditions that promote developmental processes at each period of the life cycle (e.g., adolescence, childbearing, and child rearing); and (3) health deviation self-care requisites, which exist for people who are ill, are injured, and have or are predisposed to specific health problems. These three sets of self-care requisites designate categories of patient data for inclusion in the nursing assessment.

The concept of self-care agency identifies subsequent categories of data for the patient assessment. With regard to self-care agency, the nurse seeks data to determine whether the individual's capabilities for self-care are developed (e.g., have the necessary knowledge and skills been acquired?); whether the capabilities are operable (e.g., are the acquired knowledge and skills being used?); and whether an individual's capabilities are adequate for meeting the requirements for self-care. Those people whose self-care capabilities are assessed as being less than their demands for self-care are viewed as experiencing a self-care deficit and are designated as needing nursing (Orem, 1980). Within Orem's perspective, then, a nursing diagnosis is expressed as an existing (actual) or emerging (potential) self-care deficit.

Continuing with this application of Orem's conceptual model to nursing practice, once nursing judgments are made about existing or emerging self-care deficits, the nurse designs a system of nursing for the patient. The goal of a nursing system is to contribute to the patient's performance of therapeutic self-care. Orem (1995) defines *nursing system* as a helping system that is structured according to the patient's limitations for engaging in self-care. There are three basic variations of nursing systems:

1. A *wholly compensatory system* that is intended for patients who cannot or should not engage in any form of deliberate action
2. A *partly compensatory system* that is intended for situations in which the patient can perform some but not all of the care measures required
3. A *supportive-educative system* that is intended for situations in which the patient is able to perform or can and should learn to perform self-care measures but cannot do so without assistance (Orem, 1995, p. 310)

As depicted in Figure 3–3, the role of the nurse and role of the patient are identified for each of the three nursing systems. The helping actions performed by the nurse vary depending on the patient's limitations for engaging in self-care. Six methods of helping in a nurse–patient situation are described in Table 3–2. As can be seen in the table, the methods of helping prescribe general roles for the helper and the helped.

In this model, outcomes for evaluation of nursing care relate to whether the patient's self-care needs are being met and whether the patient can realize self-management and perform therapeutic self-care. Orem (1985) views self-care as essential for life itself, for health, and for well-being. Thus, within this perspective, nurses help people to attain their health goals by assisting them to perform therapeutic self-care. Orem's theory offers direction to the practice and study of nursing.

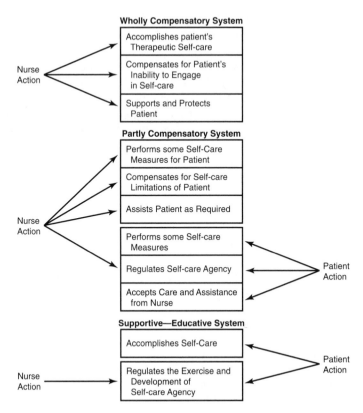

Figure 3–3. Basic Nursing Systems *(Reprinted from Orem, D. E. (1995) Nursing Concepts of Practice (5th ed.). St. Louis: Mosby, p. 307.)*

Roy's Adaptation Model

Another conceptual model that has relevance to nursing is Roy's Adaptation Model (1970, 1976; Roy & Andrews, 1991; Roy & Roberts, 1981). Sister Callista Roy's model views persons as adaptive systems in constant interaction with changing environments. In this model, persons are said to cope with the changing environment by means of *adaptive or coping mechanisms* (Roy & Andrews, 1991). Some of these mechanisms are innate or inborn and others are acquired or learned. The innate mechanisms that Roy categorizes as *regulators* refer primarily to coping mechanisms of a physiological nature. The reflex response of people as they touch potentially injurious items, such as a hot iron or broken glass, is an example of regulator activity. When contact is made with the hot iron or broken glass, a person immediately withdraws his or her hand from the item. This action reflects the functioning of an innate mechanism that does not require learning or thought.

TABLE 3–2. NURSE AND PATIENT ROLES IN NURSING SITUATIONS AS SPECIFIED BY METHODS OF HELPING

Method of Helping	Nurse Role	Patient Role
Doing for or action for another	A person who acts in place of and for the patient	Recipient of care to meet the therapeutic self-care demand and to compensate for self-care limitations Recipient of services relevant to environment control and resources
Guiding and directing another	Provider of factual or technological information relevant to the regulation of self-care agency or the meeting of self-care requisites	Receiver, processor, and user of information as self-care agent or as regulator of self-care agency
Providing physical support	A partner cooperating in performing self-care actions to regulate the exercise of or the value of self-care agency by patient	Performer of actions to meet self-care requisites or regulator of the exercise of or the value of self-care agency in cooperation with a nurse
Providing psychological support	An "understanding presence,"* a listener, a person who can institute the use of other methods of helping if necessary	A person confronting, resolving, and solving difficult problems or living through difficult situations
Providing an environment that supports development	Supplier and regulator of essential environmental conditions and a significant other in a patient's environment	A person who is confronted with living and caring for himself or herself in a way and in an environment that supports and promotes personal development
Teaching	Teacher of: Knowledge, describing and explaining self-care requisites and the therapeutic self-care demand Methods and course of actions to meet self-care requisites Methods of calculating the therapeutic self-care demand Methods of overcoming or compensating for self-care action limitations Methods of managing self-care	Learner engaged in the development of knowledge and skills requisite for continuous and effective self-care

*van Kaam, S. (1966). *The art of existential counseling.* Wilkes-Barre, PA: Dimension Books. The term *understanding presence* is from van Kaam.

Reprinted from Orem, D. E. (1995). Nursing: Concepts of practice (5th ed.). St. Louis: Mosby, p. 305.

In contrast to the innate mechanisms, the acquired mechanisms that Roy categorizes as *cognators* require learning and involve cognitive and emotional processes. Situations in which people use relaxation techniques such as yoga and other forms of meditation as a way of coping with stress in life illustrate cognator activity. Coping mechanisms such as yoga must be acquired or learned. Furthermore, recognizing the need for such mechanisms involves a number of cognitive and emotional processes. It is through the functioning of both regulator and cognator mechanisms, then, that the processes of adaptation occur.

The responses evoked by the cognator and regulator mechanisms are manifested in the subsystems of the person. Roy and Roberts (1981) refer to these subsystems as the *adaptive modes* and categorize them as:

- Physiological mode
- Self-concept mode
- Role function mode
- Interdependence mode

The *physiological mode* involves those responses that are associated with physiological functioning and reflects the way the person responds as a physical being to stimuli from the environment (Roy & Andrews, 1991, p. 15). Five needs have been identified in relation to adaptation in the physiological mode:

1. Oxygenation
2. Nutrition
3. Elimination
4. Activity and rest
5. Protection

The *self-concept mode* is one of the three psychosocial modes and involves responses of a psychological and spiritual nature (Roy & Andrews, 1991, p. 16). Adaptation in this mode is geared toward maintaining psychic integrity—the need to know who one is so that one can exist with a sense of wholeness (Andrews & Roy, 1986). Two subareas have been identified for the self-concept mode:

1. Physical self that includes body sensation and body image
2. Personal self that involves self-consistency, self-ideal, and moral-ethical-spiritual self (Andrews & Roy, 1986)

The statement, "I look ugly," can be categorized as related to body image, whereas the statement, "I'm going to get an 'A' on my nursing exam," is more reflective of the notion of self-ideal.

The *role function mode* (social mode) focuses on the roles people assume in society and the way these roles are fulfilled. Adaptation in this mode is directed toward meeting individuals' needs for knowing who they are in relation to others so that they can act accordingly (Andrews & Roy, 1986). Roles people might assume in society include child, parent, spouse, patient, nurse, and chair of an organization.

The *interdependence mode* focuses on interaction related to the giving and receiving of love, respect, and value (Roy & Andrews, 1991). Adaptation in this mode relates to meeting the need of individuals for the feeling of security in nurturing relationships. Two specific relationships are identified as the major foci of the interdependence mode:

1. *Significant others*, people who are important to the individual
2. *Support systems*, other people who contribute to meet interdependence needs (Andrews & Roy, 1986)

In Roy's model, individuals are viewed as adaptive systems coping with change by means of innate and acquired mechanisms. These adaptive mechanisms function to maintain adaptation in each of the four modes. This concept of the person as an adaptive system is illustrated in Figure 3–4.

In Roy's perspective, then, the goal of nursing is to bring about the person's adaptation in the four adaptive modes, which, in turn, contributes to the person's health, quality of life, and dying with dignity (Roy & Andrews, 1991, p. 20). According to this model, the environment includes all conditions, circumstances, and influences that surround and affect the development and behavior of the person. These environmental influences are described as *focal, contextual,* and *residual stimuli.*

The *focal stimulus* is a stimulus that is immediately confronting the person (Roy & Roberts, 1981). It is the focal stimulus that necessitates a response or action from the person so that he or she can deal or cope with it. For example, when a person experiences a headache (the focal stimulus), it consumes his or her attention and energy until some action is taken to ease the pain.

Contextual stimuli encompass all other stimuli present in the environment that contribute to the influence of the focal stimulus (Roy & Roberts, 1981). In contrast to the focal stimulus, these stimuli are not the main concern of the person. Furthermore, contextual stimuli include factors that are both internal and external to the person. For instance, the person with a headache may be more upset by the pain if he or she en-

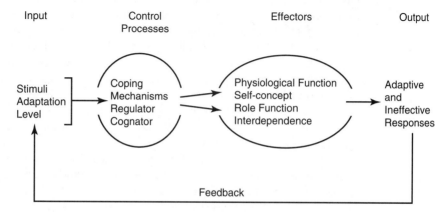

Figure 3–4. Person as an Adaptive System *(Reprinted from Roy, C. (1984). Introduction to nursing: An adaptation model (2nd ed.). Englewood Cliffs, NJ: Prentice-Hall, p. 30, with permission.)*

counters a traffic jam while driving to an important business meeting. This is an example of contextual stimuli from outside the person. If the person is worried about the outcome of the business meeting, his or her headache may be intensified further. This is an example of contextual stimuli from within the person.

Residual stimuli are environmental factors whose effect in the situation are unclear (Roy & Roberts, 1981). These stimuli cannot be validated in that the person may be unaware of the factors. For example, a person with a headache may be unaware of a previous unpleasant experience such as an injury that resulted in head pain. Hence, residual stimuli are possible or potential factors in the situation that may influence the confronting focal stimulus.

Roy's model has been and is used currently to direct nursing practice. Roy has described the nursing process in the context of her model. According to her, nursing assessment involves a two-level process. A first-level assessment involves the identification of patient responses in each of the four modes—(1) physiological, (2) self-concept, (3) role function, and (4) interdependence—and the categorization of the responses as adaptive or ineffective. Behaviors are judged as adaptive to the extent that they promote the integrity of the person (Roy & Andrews, 1991, p. 12). In contrast, ineffective responses are viewed as those behaviors that do not contribute to the goal of adaptation and thus disrupt integrity (Roy & Andrews, 1991). This process of judging behaviors and categorizing them as adaptive or ineffective responses can be viewed in Roy's model as a way of identifying people who need nursing care. Thus, for nurses practicing from Roy's model, the primary concern is behavior that is disrupting the person's integrity rather than promoting adaptation. In the second-level assessment, the nurse looks for the stimuli (focal, contextual, and residual) that influence these responses. Consequently, ineffective behaviors and the most relevant influencing stimuli provide the basis for a nursing diagnosis.

The general goal of nursing intervention is to change ineffective behavior to adaptive behavior and to maintain and enhance adaptive behavior (Andrews & Roy, 1986). Nursing interventions in this model involve the management of stimuli. Nursing interventions can take the form of altering, increasing, decreasing, removing, or maintaining environmental stimuli (Andrews & Roy, 1986). The nurse manipulates the stimuli so that the patient can adapt. For example, if the nursing diagnosis is that the client is eating a nutrient-deficient diet as a result of his or her lack of understanding about the basic food groups, then the nursing intervention would be directed to altering the client's level of understanding of proper nutrition through booklets and classes on good nutrition.

Interventions are evaluated in terms of whether or not ineffective responses have been changed to adaptive responses and whether adaptive responses have been maintained. Figure 3–5 illustrates Roy's nursing process. In Roy's perspective, then, nurses help patients to achieve health by promoting adaptive responses to environmental changes.

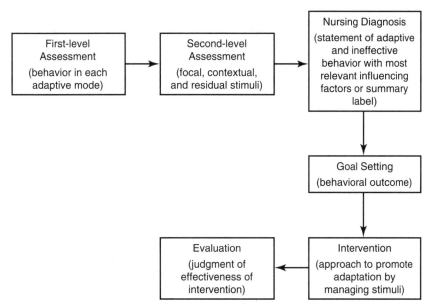

Figure 3–5. Roy's Nursing Process Flow Chart *(Reprinted from Roy, C. (1984).* Introduction to nursing: An adaptation model *(2nd ed.). Englewood Cliffs, NJ: Prentice-Hall, p. 62, with permission.)*

Neuman's Systems Model

With the intent of helping nurses to develop nursing as a field of practice, Betty Neuman (1974) introduced a comprehensive conceptual framework for nursing that is based on a systems point of view. In Neuman's Systems Model (1974, 1989, 1995), the client is viewed as a system functioning harmoniously in relation to environmental influences. The client system comprises five interacting variables:

1. Physiological, which refers to bodily structure and function
2. Psychological, which refers to mental processes and relationships
3. Sociocultural, which refers to combined social and cultural functions
4. Developmental, which refers to life developmental processes
5. Spiritual, which refers to spiritual beliefs (Neuman, 1995, p. 28)

The model is concerned with the stability of the client system as it encounters internal and external stressors in the environment. *Stressors* are tension-producing forces present in both the internal and external environment of the client system. Neuman (1995) proposes an environmental typology that consists of three classes of environmental stressors:

1. *Internal environment*—intrapersonal in nature
2. *External environment*—inter- and extrapersonal in nature
3. *Created environment*—intra-, inter-, and extrapersonal in nature

In essence, the model is based on concepts of stress and reaction, or possible reaction, to stressors in the total environment of the client system and is intended to explain how client system stability is achieved in relation to stressors imposed on it.

Neuman (1989) contends that the process of interaction and adjustment between the client system and environmental stressors results in varying degrees of harmony, stability, or balance between the client and environment. She equates the health of clients to optimal system stability and refers to it as "the best possible wellness state at any given time" (Neuman, 1995, p. 32).

To illustrate her ideas about the client system, Neuman uses a series of concentric circles surrounding a central core structure (Figure 3–6). She refers to the core as the *basic structure* and indicates that it comprises basic survival factors, such as organ strength and ego structure, that are common to the species. The concentric circles identified in Figure 3–6 as *flexible line of defense, normal line of defense,* and *lines of resistance* represent protective mechanisms for the *basic structure*. Although unique in their specific functions, each line of defense and resistance possesses similar properties related to the physiological, psychological, developmental, sociocultural, and spiritual variables (Neuman, 1989).

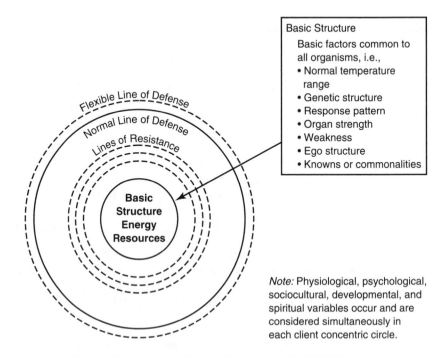

Figure 3–6. Client–Client System *(Reprinted from Neuman, B. (1995). The Neuman systems model (3rd ed.). Norwalk, CT: Appleton & Lange, p. 26, with permission.)*

The *flexible line of defense* forms the outer boundary of the client system and serves to protect the normal line of defense. In ideal situations, the flexible line of defense is thought to prevent invasion of the system by stressors. Neuman (1995) describes the function of the flexible line of defense as accordionlike. "As it expands away from the normal line of defense, greater protection is provided; and as it draws closer, less protection is available" (p. 27). The flexible line of defense is dynamic and can be altered rather quickly by such conditions as sleep loss or loss of body fluids.

The *normal line of defense*, the second protective mechanism, is represented in Figure 3–6 by the solid line next to the flexible line of defense. Neuman (1995) defines this concept as "the state to which the client has evolved over time, or the usual wellness level" (p. 30). She views the normal line of defense as a standard against which changes from the usual wellness state can be determined. Thus, it reflects the effectiveness of previous client system functioning. The normal line of defense also is described as dynamic or being able to expand or contract. Factors that influence the normal line of defense are coping patterns and lifestyle. According to the model, when the normal line of defense has been invaded by a stressor, the client presents symptoms of illness or instability (Neuman, 1989). Invasion of the normal line of defense by stressors activates the third protective mechanism, the lines of resistance.

The *lines of resistance* are represented in Figure 3–6 by the broken circles surrounding the basic structure. The lines of resistance involve known and unknown internal and external resources that support the basic structure and normal line of defense (Neuman, 1995, p. 30). An example of this protective mechanism is the shunting of blood to organs in need of it. According to the model, when the lines of resistance are effective in reversing the reaction to stressors, the client system is able to stabilize, and wellness is achieved. However, ineffective lines of resistance lead to failure of the client system and ultimately to death (p. 30).

The three protective mechanisms function in relation to one another to retain, maintain, or attain stability of the client system. The flexible line of defense protects the normal line of defense, and the lines of resistance protect the basic structure. When the client system is confronted with a stressor, the flexible line of defense is the first mechanism to respond. If the flexible line of defense is effective, stability is maintained and no stressor reaction occurs. However, if the flexible line of defense is ineffective, then the stressor crosses the normal line of defense and stressor reaction ensues. This also is the point at which the lines of resistance are activated. When effective, the lines of resistance enhance stabilization and wellness.

In Neuman's model, the main goal of nursing is to facilitate optimum wellness of the client through retention, attainment, or maintenance of client system stability. The major concern for nursing, then, is to keep the client system stable. This task requires that nurses make a careful and accurate assessment of actual and potential stressors, as well as their effects, and provide assistance to clients in their adjustment to stressors. To facilitate use of the Neuman Systems Model in nursing practice, a Neuman nursing process format has been designed. This format describes the nursing process in the context of Neuman's System Model (1995). The Neuman nursing process format designates the following seven categories of data about the client system as the major areas of nursing assessment:

1. Potential and actual stressors
2. Condition and strength of basic structure factors and energy resources
3. Characteristics of the flexible and normal lines of defense, lines of resistance, degree of reaction, and potential for reconstitution
4. Interactions between the client and environment
5. Life processes and coping patterns (past, present, and possible future)
6. Actual and potential resources (internal and external) for optimal wellness
7. Perceptual differences between caregiver (nurse) and client (Neuman, 1989)

This database in intended to help the nurse to assess the impact or possible impact of environmental stressors on the client system and to determine any variances from wellness. The data are then interpreted through the use of relevant theories to explain the client's condition and formulate a nursing diagnosis.

In the Neuman nursing process format, the goal of keeping the client system stable is achieved through nursing actions derived from the following three modes of prevention:

1. *Primary prevention*: actions taken to retain stability
2. *Secondary prevention*: actions taken to attain stability
3. *Tertiary prevention*: actions taken to maintain stability (Neuman, 1995, p. 33)

The *primary prevention mode* is geared toward retention of wellness and toward health promotion through stress prevention and the reduction of risk factors. Interventions derived from this mode should strengthen the flexible line of defense and should focus on health promotion. The *secondary prevention mode* is appropriate for clients with symptoms when the goal is to attain stability or wellness. Interventions are designed to protect the basic structure by strengthening the internal lines of resistance and may take the form of symptom management and energy conservation. The *tertiary prevention mode* is directed toward wellness maintenance. Interventions derived from this mode are conceptualized as supporting existing strengths and conserving client system energy (Neuman, 1995). These three modes of prevention can provide direction for nursing interventions with diverse client groups.

NURSING THEORIES OF CARE

In addition to the models of Rogers, King, Orem, Roy, and Neuman, two care theories currently offer direction to nursing practice, research, and education. These theories are (1) Leininger's Theory of Cultural Care Diversity and Universality and (2) Watson's Theory of Human Caring. Both Leininger and Watson view care as central to nursing, yet their approaches to the study of care differ.

Leininger's Theory of Cultural Care Diversity and Universality

In the interest of discovering the differences and similarities of care among diverse cultures, Madeleine Leininger introduced her Theory of Cultural Care Diversity and Universality. The central focus of the theory is human care. Leininger (1988) contends that care is the essence of nursing. According to her theory, care is viewed as a universal phenomenon that exists in all cultures; yet, diverse expressions, meanings, and forms of care practices exist in different cultures (Leininger, 1985). That is, care as a phenomenon is common across all cultures, but the way in which care is expressed varies from culture to culture.

According to the theory, when there are differences between the cultural values, beliefs, and practices of the client and those of the nurse, undesired outcomes can occur in nurse–client situations (Leininger, 1988). In situations in which the nurse and client are from different cultures, acts that are viewed by one person as expressions of caring behavior may not be viewed in the same way by the other person. This difference in cultural views about what is and what is not considered caring behavior can lead to dissatisfaction in the nurse–client situation. Moreover, Leininger (1988) contends that nursing care must be congruent with the client's culture if nursing intends to promote client health and client satisfaction. Thus, the theory places high importance on the study of the values, meanings, and expressions of care among diverse cultures. Leininger (1991) also contends that studies of this type will provide the knowledge needed for nursing to achieve the goal of providing care that fits with the cultural beliefs and practices of clients. The theory proposes that nursing can contribute to the health of clients by providing nursing care that is congruent with their culture.

In the Culture Care Theory, Leininger has conceptualized three major modalities to guide nursing decisions or actions. By using these modalities in nursing practice, nurses are able to provide culturally congruent care that is beneficial, satisfying, and meaningful to the people they serve (Leininger, 1988). The three modes are: (1) *cultural care preservation or maintenance,* (2) *cultural care accommodation or negotiation,* and (3) *cultural care repatterning or restructuring* (Leininger, 1991).

Culture care preservation refers to those supportive or enabling professional actions that help clients to maintain their culturally learned lifeways in a health care situation (Leininger, 1988). Wenger's study (1991) of the meanings and expressions of care in the culture of the Old Order Amish throws some light on culture care preservation. She found that care had the same meanings over generations for people of this culture. Knowledge about culture care is carefully communicated from generation to generation. Moreover, culture care is the core of the Amish worldview. The findings of this study emphasized the importance of culture care preservation in providing congruent care to Old Order Amish. Wenger (1991) concluded that the care actions of the extended family, neighborhood, and church district must be understood and encouraged by nurses caring for Amish clients.

Culture care accommodation refers to those supportive or enabling professional actions that help clients to adapt specific cultural care practices to a health care situation. In Stasiak's (1991) study of the meanings, values, and practices of folk care among Mexican-Americans in an urban context, "obtaining and giving respecto [respect]" emerged as a dominant care value. This finding offers important direction to nurses in terms of culture care accommodation. According to Stasiak's findings, respect may be expressed by talking directly to Mexican-American clients, maintaining casual but not intense direct eye contact with them, and addressing clients in a formal fashion. To address a Mexican-American client by his or her first name without permission is considered disrespectful. These findings offer direction to nurses as to ways in which culture care accommodation can be promoted.

Cultural care repatterning refers to those supportive or enabling professional actions that help clients to change their lifeways for new or different patterns that are culturally meaningful and satisfying (Leininger, 1988). Changing lifeways and adopting new or different care patterns is difficult in any culture. Therefore, this mode offers the biggest challenge to nurses and clients. When planning change, it is important to move slowly and to process the change through the appropriate cultural structures. It is vital that the new care pattern be congruent with the client's culture. This mode requires the nurse to have extensive knowledge and understanding of the client's culture and to use the knowledge in a creative and sensitive way (Leininger, 1991).

Leininger's Culture Care Theory has tremendous implications for the study and practice of nursing. Study findings, such as those of Wenger (1991) and Stasiak (1991), can help nurses to understand that different cultures tend to have specific meanings and expressions of care. Furthermore, the three care modalities can guide nurses in making decisions and plans of action that are satisfying to clients. The theory offers direction to nurses in discovering and using culture care knowledge in promoting the well being of diverse peoples. It is important for nurses to plan and implement culturally sensitive and competent care and to advance the knowledge base of how best to promote the health and well being of diverse peoples (Meleis, Isenberg, Kaerner, Lacey, & Stern, 1995).

Watson's Theory of Human Caring

In contrast to Leininger's transcultural view of care, Jean Watson, in her theory of human caring, emphasizes the moral and ethical dimensions of care. Watson (1989) views human caring as "the moral ideal of nursing" (p. 220). She describes caring as consisting of transpersonal processes designed to help a person find meaning in illness, suffering, pain, and existence and to help an individual gain self-knowledge, self-control, self-care, self-healing, and, in turn, inner harmony (Watson, 1985).

Watson's (1989) theory of human caring is based on a value system associated with respect for life, acknowledging a spiritual dimension to life, and recognizing the internal power of the human caring process. Accordingly, the theory proposes that individuals engaged in caring for others must possess a high regard for people and human life and respect for autonomy and freedom of choice.

In Watson's perspective, the goal of nursing is to help clients to gain a greater degree of harmony in the mind, body, and soul (Watson, 1985). This goal is achieved through the transpersonal caring process in which the nurse and client are co-participants. As a co-participant in the caring process, the nurse should aim for mental-spiritual growth for self, as well as discovery of inner power and self-control (Watson, 1989). This theory proposes that it is through the human caring process that healing, health, and transcendence are achieved for the client and nurse.

SUMMARY

The development of nursing knowledge has been a major concern of the nursing profession. This concern has been intricately linked with nursing's quest for professional status. Nurse leaders realized that for nursing to be recognized as a profession, the scientific knowledge base for nursing practice had to be established. Efforts to develop this knowledge base marked the emergence of nursing science.

The theoretical works of such noted nurse scholars as Rogers, King, Orem, Roy, Neuman, Leininger, and Watson have contributed significantly to the clarification of the nature of nursing knowledge. In addition, their models have given direction to nursing practice and to the curricula of nursing programs. These models offer a view of the client in relation to his or her health and environment. Furthermore, they define nursing as a caring process and offer direction for clinical decision making and throughout all phases of the nursing process.

The development of nursing knowledge is as important today as it was in 1950. In her appraisal of the future of the nursing profession, Aydelotte (1987) identified strategies that must be followed if nursing is to attain its desired future. First and foremost on her list of strategies is the need to delineate the nursing profession's unique body of knowledge. She prompts the profession to recall that as a professional discipline, the first responsibility is the development of knowledge that will enhance the fulfillment of nursing's practical aims. To meet nursing's social mandate, Aydelotte proposes that the profession must garner knowledge, refine it, and identify that knowledge that belongs exclusively to the nursing profession.

The discipline of nursing has reached a new milestone in its development. The focus of nursing as a professional discipline has been characterized as *caring in the human health experience* (Newman et al., 1991). The major phenomena of current concern to nursing include self-care, adaptation, mutual goal attainment, culture care, and human becoming. These care phenomena are being used to guide research and practice and to further expand nursing knowledge. Furthermore, nursing as a discipline has moved from debates about whether we should have one or more nursing theories to an acceptance of a pluralistic approach to theory development and utilization. Consequently, a rich array of diverse nursing theories are currently being used to direct professional practice, formulate research questions, and guide the design of nursing curricula.

REFERENCES

Andrews, H., & Roy, C. (1986). *Essentials of the Roy adaptation model.* Norwalk, CT: Appleton-Century-Crofts.

Aydelotte, M. K. (1987). Nursing's preferred future. *Nursing Outlook, 35,* 114–120.

Donaldson, S., & Crowley, D. (1978). The discipline of nursing. *Nursing Outlook, 26,* 113–120.

Ellis, R. (1982). Conceptual issues in nursing. *Nursing Outlook, 30,* 406–420.

Fawcett, J. (1978). The "what" of theory development. In National League for Nursing, *Theory development: What, why, how?* (pp. 17–33). New York: National League for Nursing.

Greenwood, E. (1957). Attributes of a profession. *Social Work, 2,* 44–46.

Johnson, D. (1959). The nature of a science of nursing. *Nursing Outlook, 7,* 291–294.

King, I. M. (1971). *Toward a theory for nursing.* New York: Wiley.

King, I. M. (1981). *A theory for nursing: Systems, concepts, processes.* New York: Wiley.

King, I. M. (1986). *Curriculum and instruction in nursing.* Norwalk, CT: Appleton-Century-Crofts.

King, I. M. (1989). King's general systems framework and theory. In J. Riehl-Sisca (Ed.), *Conceptual models for nursing practice* (pp. 149–158). Norwalk, CT: Appleton & Lange.

King, I. M. (1995). A systems framework for nursing. In M. A. Frey & C. L. Sieloff (Eds.), *Advancing King's systems framework and theory of nursing* (pp. 14–22). Thousand Oaks, CA: Sage.

Leininger, M. M. (1985). Transcultural care diversity and universality: A theory of nursing. *Nursing & Health Care, 6,* 209–212.

Leininger, M. M. (1988). Leininger's theory of nursing: Cultural care diversity and universality. *Nursing Science Quarterly, 1*(4), 152–160.

Leininger, M. M. (Ed.). (1991). *Culture care diversity and universality: A theory of nursing.* New York: National League for Nursing.

Malinski, V. (Ed.). (1986). *Explorations on Martha Rogers' science of unitary human beings.* Norwalk, CT: Appleton-Century-Crofts.

Meleis, A., Isenberg, M., Kaerner, J., Lacey, B., & Stern, P. (1995). *Diversity, marginalization, and culturally competent health care: Issues in Knowledge Development.* Washington, DC: American Academy of Nursing.

Neuman, B. (1974). The Betty Neuman health-care systems model: A total person approach to patient problems. In J. Riehl & C. Roy (Eds.), *Conceptual models for nursing practice,* (pp. 99–114). New York: Appleton-Century-Crofts.

Neuman, B. (1989). *The Neuman systems model* (2nd ed.). Norwalk, CT: Appleton-Century-Crofts.

Neuman, B. (1995). *The Neuman systems model* (3rd ed.). Norwalk, CT: Appleton & Lange.

Newman, M. (1983). The continuing revolution: A history of nursing science. In. N. Chaska (Ed.), *The nursing profession: A time to speak* (pp. 385–393). New York: McGraw-Hill.

Newman, M. A., Sime, A. M., Corcoran-Perry, S. A. (1991). The focus of the discipline of nursing. *Advances in Nursing Science, 14,* 1–6.

Nightingale, F. (1859). *Notes on nursing: What it is and what it is not.* London: Harrison and Sons. (Facsimile edition, J. B. Lippincott, 1946).

Norris, C. (1982). *Concept clarification in nursing.* Rockville, MD: Aspen.

Orem, D. E. (1971). *Nursing: Concept of practice.* New York: McGraw-Hill.

Orem, D. E. (1979). *Concept formalization in nursing: Process and product* (2nd ed.). Boston: Little, Brown.

Orem, D. E. (1980). *Nursing concepts of practice* (2nd ed.). New York: McGraw-Hill.

Orem, D. E. (1985). *Nursing concepts of practice* (3rd ed.). New York: McGraw-Hill.

Orem, D. E. (1991). *Nursing concepts of practice* (4th ed.). St. Louis: Mosby.

Orem, D. E. (1995). *Nursing concepts of practice* (5th ed.). St. Louis: Mosby.

Rogers, M. (1970). *An introduction to the theoretical basis of nursing.* Philadelphia: Davis.

Rogers, M. (1992). Nursing science and the space age. *Nursing Science Quarterly, 5*(1), 27–34.

Rogers, M. (1994). The science of unitary human being: Current perspectives. *Nursing Science Quarterly, 7*(1), 33–35.

Roy, C. (1970). Adaptation: A conceptual framework for nursing. *Nursing Outlook, 18*(3), 42–45.

Roy, C. (1976). *Introduction to nursing: An adaptation model.* Englewood Cliffs, NJ: Prentice-Hall.

Roy, C., & Andrews, H. A. (1991). *The Roy adaptation model: The definitive statement.* Norwalk, CT: Appleton & Lange.

Roy, C., & Roberts, S. (1981). *Theory construction in nursing: An adaptation model.* Englewood Cliffs, NJ: Prentice-Hall.

Stasiak, D. B. (1991). Culture care theory with Mexican-Americans. In M. M. Leininger (Ed.), *Culture care diversity and universality: A theory of nursing* (pp. 179–203). New York: National League for Nursing.

Walker, L. O. (1971). Toward a clearer understanding of the concept of nursing theory. *Nursing Research, 20,* 428–435.

Watson, J. (1985). *Nursing: Human science and human care.* Norwalk, CT: Appleton-Century-Crofts.

Watson, J. (1989). Watson's philosophy and theory of human caring in nursing. In J. Riehl-Sisca (Ed.), *Conceptual models for nursing practice* (pp. 219–236). Norwalk, CT: Appleton & Lange.

Wenger, A. F. (1991). The culture care theory and the old order Amish. In M. M. Leininger (Ed.), *Culture care diversity and universality: A theory of nursing* (pp. 147–178). New York: National League for Nursing.

Yura, H., & Torres, G. (1975). Today's conceptual frameworks within baccalaureate nursing programs. In National League for Nursing, *Faculty-curriculum development. Part III. Conceptual framework—Its meaning and function* (pp. 17–25). New York: National League for Nursing.

BIBLIOGRAPHY

Barret, E. A. M. (1990). *Visions of Rogers' science based nursing*. New York: National League for Nursing.

Benner, P. (1984). *From novice to expert*. Menlo Park, CA: Addison-Wesley.

Fawcett, J. (1989). *Analysis and evaluation of conceptual models of nursing* (2nd ed.). Philadelphia: Davis.

Frederickson, K. (1991). Nursing theories—A basis for differentiated practice: Application of the Roy adaptation model in nursing practice. In I. M. Goertzen (Ed.), *Differentiating nursing practice: Into the twenty-first century* (pp. 41–44). Kansas City, MO: American Academy of Nursing.

Frey, M. A. (1989). Social support and health: A theoretical formulation derived from King's conceptual framework. *Nursing Science Quarterly, 2,* 138–148.

Frey, M. A., & Sieloff, C. L. (Eds.). (1995). *Advancing King's systems framework and theory of nursing*. Thousand Oaks, CA: Sage.

Gaut, D. (1983). Development of a theoretically adequate description of caring. *Western Journal of Nursing Research, 5,* 313–324.

Gaut, D. (1986). Evaluating caring competencies in nursing practice. *Topics in Clinical Nursing, 8*(2), 77–83.

George, J. B. (Ed.). (1995). *Nursing theories: The base for a professional nursing practice* (4th ed.). Norwalk, CT: Appleton & Lange.

Henderson, V. (1966). *The nature of nursing: A definition and its implications for practice, research, and education*. New York: Macmillan

Isenberg, M. A. (1991). Insights from Orem's nursing theory on differentiating nursing practice. In I. E. Goertzen (Ed.), *Differentiating nursing practice: Into the twenty-first century* (pp. 45–49). Kansas City, MO: American Academy of Nursing.

Leininger, M. M. (1981a). *Care: An essential human need*. Thorofare, NJ: Slack.

Leininger, M. M. (1981b). *Care: The essence of nursing and health*. Thorofare, NJ: Slack.

Leininger, M. M. (1986). Care facilitation and resistance factors in the culture of nursing. *Topics in Clinical Nursing, 8*(2), 1–12.

Meleis, A. I. (1991). *Theoretical Nursing: Development and progress* (2nd ed.). New York: Lippincott.

Newman, M. (1986). *Health as expanding consciousness*. St. Louis: Mosby.

Nicole, L. H. (Ed.). (1992). *Perspectives in nursing theory* (2nd ed.). Philadelphia: Lippincott.

Orem, D. E. (1988). The form of nursing science. *Nursing Science Quarterly, 1*(2), 75–79.

Riehl-Sisca, J. (Ed.). (1989). *Conceptual models for nursing practice*. Norwalk, CT: Appleton & Lange.

Rogers, M. (1986). Science of unitary human beings. In V. Malinski (Ed.), *Explorations on Martha Rogers' science of unitary human beings* (pp. 3–8). Norwalk, CT: Appleton-Century-Crofts.

Rogers, M. (1989). Nursing: A science of unitary human beings. In J. Riehl-Sisca (Ed.), *Conceptual models for nursing practice* (pp. 181–188). Norwalk, CT: Appleton & Lange.

Rosenbaum, J. N. (1991). The health meanings and practices of older Greek-Canadian widows. *Journal of Advanced Nursing, 16*, 320–327.

Spangler, S. (1991). Culture care of Philippine and Anglo-American nurses in a hospital context. In M. M. Leininger (Ed.), *Culture care diversity and universality: A theory of nursing* (pp. 119–146). New York: National League for Nursing.

Villarrel, A. M., & Ortiz de Montellano, B. (1992). Culture and pain: A Mesoamerican view. *Advances in Nursing Science, 15*(1), 21–32.

Walker, I. O., & Avant, K. C. (1988). *Strategies for theory construction in nursing* (2nd ed.). Norwalk, CT: Appleton-Century-Crofts.

Individual, Family, and Community as Client

Marilyn H. Oermann and Nancy T. Artinian

Nursing clients may be singular, as in the individual, or may be plural, as in the family or community. When the client is an individual, the focus is on the health state, problems, or needs of a single person. When the client is a family, the focus is on the needs and health states of individual family members and their reciprocal effects on each other or on the needs and health state of the family unit as a whole. The focus may be at either the individual family member level or the family unit level. When the client is a community, the focus is on promoting and preserving the health of population groups.

Although the nurse may plan and deliver care to individuals, families, and communities, the family is a critical intervening variable between the individual and the community. Individuals are members of a family unit, and family members and the family unit are part of a community. Because the family occupies a critical position between the individual and community and because the family constitutes an important context in which wellness and illness occur, the family as client is a major focus of this chapter, although the individual and community also are discussed. This chapter centers on family for another important reason, to meet the needs of registered nurses (RNs) who are advancing their education and obtaining baccalaureate and higher degrees. Nursing education at the associate degree and diploma levels emphasizes primarily assessing individual needs and providing nursing interventions to individuals; thus, the nurse prepared at these levels already has acquired a significant amount of knowledge about *individuals* as clients of nursing services. The *family* as client is an area in which the nurse needs to be more knowledgeable. Furthermore, planning and delivering comprehensive health care to communities are a major focus of baccalaureate programs, which generally devote an entire course or courses to community health nursing.

INDIVIDUAL AS CLIENT

Professional nursing practice involves the care of individual clients, families, and communities. In care of the individual, the emphasis is on the particular client's health problems. A nursing assessment of an individual would include the individual's health history, physical and psychosocial development, and family and social history. Nursing interventions for the individual would include coordinating his or her care; patient teaching; delivering physical care and emotional support; counseling; and acting as the person's advocate. Many theoretical perspectives focus on the individual and assist nurses in assessing and planning care for individual clients. The nursing theories discussed in Chapter 3 provide a framework for understanding the health needs of the client and providing care in a nursing perspective. Other theories, such as ones dealing with stress and coping, growth and development, and pain, to name a few, contribute to the nurse's understanding of the individual client and his or her health problems. These theories and other concepts about health, responses to illness, and nursing management enable the nurse to make decisions about assessment, plan care for the client, develop relevant interventions, and evaluate the outcomes of care.

FAMILY AS CLIENT

Family clients of nursing care may be either individual family members or entire family units. An understanding of the family unit may be enhanced by assessing the family members, just as an understanding of each family member can be gained from assessing the family unit. Family nursing care is directed at both the family as a unit and individual members within the family (Smith & Maurer, 1995, p. 218). Friedman (1992) views the focus of family nursing as "nursing practice where the family is seen and treated as the client or recipient of care" (p. 23).

What actually constitutes a family is no longer easy to define. Traditionally, the family has been defined in various ways. Burgess, Locke, and Thomas (1963) cite the following characteristics that are common to families and distinguish them from other social groups:

- The family comprises people united by bonds of marriage, blood, or adoption.
- The members of a family usually live together under one roof and constitute a single household; or, if they live separately, consider the household their home.
- Family members interact and communicate with each other in family social roles such as husband and wife, mother and father, son and daughter, and brother and sister.
- The family maintains a common culture. It is derived mainly from the general culture, but each family has some distinctive features. (p. 7)

Traditional definitions, however, are no longer adequate for understanding the needs of families. Friedman (1992) defines the family in a broader sense as a unit comprising two or more people who are emotionally involved with each other and identify themselves as being part of the family (p. 9). Currently, several family structural forms exist in the United States that lead to various nontraditional definitions of family:

- *Nuclear family*—Husband, wife, and children living in same household (including first marriage and blended families)
- *Nuclear dyad family*—Childless husband and wife
- *Single-parent family*—One parent, as a consequence of divorce, abandonment, or separation
- *Single adult*—Living alone
- *Three-generation family*—Three generations or more living in a common household
- *Unmarried parent and child family*—Usually mother and child
- *Unmarried couple and child family*—Usually a commonlaw marriage
- *Gay/lesbian family*—Persons of same sex living together with or without children
- *Cohabitating couple*—Unmarried couple living together
- *Commune family*—Household of more than one monogamous couple with children, sharing common facilities, resources, and experience*

Several implications for nurses arise from the various definitions of family. It is important for nurses to remember that the family, however it is defined, is an important group in which people find a sense of membership and identity. Nurses also need to remain flexible in their interpretation of the word *family*. All types of families need nursing care. Nurses' personal preferences about a particular mode of living should not influence their clinical judgments when intervening with families. Assumptions about a family should not be made on the basis of family structure.

---

* Adapted from Friedman, M. M. (1992). Family nursing: Theory and practice (3rd ed., p. 12.) Norwalk, CT: Appleton & Lange, with permission. Adapted by Friedman from Sussman, M.B. (1974). Family systems in the 1970s: Analysis, policies, and programs. In A. Skolnick & J.H. Skolnick (Eds.). Intimacy, family and society (pp. 579–598). Boston: Little, Brown; and from Macklin, E. D. (1988). Nontraditional family forms. In M. B. Sussman & S. K. Steinmetz (Eds.). Handbook of marriage and the family (pp. 317–353). New York: Plenum.

Family Theoretical Perspectives

Many family theoretical perspectives exist. An understanding of the most widely used frames of reference can enable nurses to study and analyze family behavior in an organized and logical manner. The following seven family perspectives are discussed in this section: (1) structural-functional, (2) systems, (3) developmental, (4) interactionist, (5) ecological, (6) social exchange, and (7) stress.

Structural-Functional Perspective

The structural-functional perspective centers on the relation between a family whole and its individual members. It looks at the way in which the family members are arranged, the relationship between the members, and the relationships of the members to the whole. The main concern is the family structure and how well the family structure performs its functions. Assumptions of the structural-functional perspective include the following:

- A family is a social system with functional requirements.
- A family is a small group possessing certain generic features common to all small groups.
- Social systems such as the family accomplish functions that serve the individuals in addition to those that serve society.
- Individuals act in accordance with norms and values that are learned in the family through socialization. (Friedman, 1992, p. 74)

The structure of the family means the way the family is organized, the manner in which units are arranged, and how these units relate to each other. One way to view family structure is to look at it according to the aforementioned different family forms. The structural components of a family are those variables that provide organization for the family. Other structural dimensions of the family are role structure, value systems, communication patterns, and power structure (Friedman, 1992).

The family's structure serves to facilitate the achievement of family functions, which are the outcomes of family structure or what the family does. Friedman (1992) identifies five family functions:

1. Affective function (meeting the psychological needs of family members)
2. Socialization and social placement function (socializing children and making them productive members of society)
3. Reproduction function (producing new members for society)
4. Economic function (providing sufficient economic resources and allocating resources effectively)
5. Health care function (providing food, clothing, shelter, and health care) (p. 75)

The structural-functional perspective provides a useful framework for assessing families in any setting because it enables the nurse to explore the interrelationship between the whole and its parts. A nurse in an acute care setting can use the structural-functional approach to guide care of seriously ill patients and their families. Serious illness of a family member results in alteration of the family structure. Serious illness may have an impact on family role relations, thus resulting in stress. The illness may prevent the family member from carrying out usual roles, and another member may have to take on additional responsibilities to compensate. For example, if the father is ill, he may not be able to carry out the breadwinner role. The mother may have to seek employment so that the family can meet their economic needs. If the mother is the one who is ill, child care functions in the family may be altered. Illness may incapacitate the family if the power structure in the family is patriarchal and it is the father who is ill. Communication may cease if the mother is the person in the family through whom all communication passes and she is the one who is ill.

A nurse grounded in the structural-functional approach interested in the impact of illness on the family might ask several questions: Does family size affect the impact of illness on family functioning? What is the impact of illness on specific role relationships among family members? Does alteration of family structure by illness have a debilitating effect or enhancing effect on family cohesion? Nursing interventions would differ based on the answers to each of these questions.

Family Systems Perspective

The family systems perspective is closely related to the structural-functional perspective. In a systems perspective, however, the focus is on the interaction of the various parts of the systems rather than on a description of the functions of the parts themselves (Friedman, 1992).

A *system* is a set of interacting and interrelated elements (von Bertalanffy, 1968). Activities of a system are goal directed; to achieve a goal, the system interacts continuously and adaptively with its environment, moving from a lesser to a more defined state. Systems may be open or closed. An *open system* promotes the exchange of matter, energy, and information with other systems and the environment and strives to maintain a steady state. All living systems are open systems. A *closed system* does not interact with other systems nor with the environment, and matter, energy, and information do not flow into or out of a closed system.

The structure of the system is the static arrangement of the system's parts. In a system that is hierarchical, there are three levels: (1) target system, (2) subsystem, and (3) suprasystem. If the focal or target system is the individual, then the subsystems, for instance, would be the biological systems, such as the gastrointestinal, lymphatic, and reproductive systems. The suprasystem of the person would be the family. If, however, the family is the target system, then the individual family members would be considered the subsystem and the community would be considered the suprasystem. The community, as the target system, implies the family or other groups as the subsystems and the state/region/nation as the suprasystem.

The family is a small group of interrelated and interdependent individuals; thus, the family is a system. A change in one member of the family system inevitably results in changes in the entire system. Illness represents a change in one part of the family system that is followed by compensatory changes in the other parts. Assumptions of the systems perspective include the following:

- There are subsystems within the family, such as the spouse subsystem, parent–child subsystem, and sibling subsystem. There is a logical relationship between the subsystems. The subsystems interact with one another, and the whole family system interacts with other systems, such as the educational, health care, and political systems.
- The family is distinguishable from the community; a boundary exists. Boundaries regulate the input from and the output to the environment. Family systems may be open, closed, or random. A family system that isolates itself from the community is viewed as a *closed system*. A family system that exchanges energy and resources with the community is an *open system*. In the *random system*, family territorial guidelines are not organized. (Mercer, 1989, pp. 21–22)

The family systems perspective encourages the nurse to expand his or her own concept of the patient from that of an individual in a bed to that of a participating member in a family. The following example depicts the systemic qualities of a family.

John and Kathy Jones experienced the birth of baby Sally, who had congenital heart defects. Sally was ill for 2 years, and John and Kathy constantly took her to doctors and hospitals. Almost all their attention was focused on Sally. During this time, the three older boys had to adjust to a different lifestyle, and they each responded in a different way. Jim went crazy in school. He got into fights and never did his work. Bob, who was quiet to begin with, withdrew further. Jack tried to help in any way he could to get extra attention from his parents. After Sally started getting stronger, John and Kathy could focus on the whole family again, and life started to shift back to the way it originally had been.

This example depicts the effects of a crisis on a system; everyone was affected. According to family systems theory, a nurse caring for baby Sally at the hospital would assess the whole family rather than just Sally. The parent–baby subsystem interacted with the other sibling subsystems to cause change in the whole family system. Therefore, nursing interventions would be directed toward family members as well as baby Sally.

Family Developmental Perspective

The developmental perspective attempts to account for change over time in the family system. The developmental approach is based on the observation that families are long-lived groups with a natural history, or life cycle, that must be assessed if the dynamics of the group are to be fully and accurately interpreted (Duvall, 1977). Although this framework seems to have a middle-class bias and neglects the diversity of family patterns, it can be helpful in providing insight into family dynamics.

There are predictable stages within the life cycle of every family. Just as individuals go through stages of growth and development, so do families go through stages of development. Table 4–1 presents the widely used formulation of family developmental stages. Duvall (1977) used the age and school placement of the oldest child as a guidepost for the life cycle intervals. Family developmental tasks are associated with each phase of the family life cycle, just as individuals have developmental tasks.

Carter and McGoldrick (1988) describe six stages of the family life cycle and associated tasks to be accomplished for successful transition from one stage to another (Table 4–2). They also describe the shifts that occur in the family life cycle during divorce and for the reconstituted family making this model more timely for contemporary society (Danielson, Hamel-Bissell, & Winstead-Fry, 1993). Danielson et al. emphasize that the diversity of family life today precludes establishing any stages and accompanying tasks as norms for families to follow.

A nurse interacting with family members of ill patients could use the developmental framework to direct care. The time in life during which a

TABLE 4–1. EIGHT STAGES OF THE FAMILY LIFE CYCLE

Stage	Period
1. Married couple (beginning families)	From time of marriage until birth of first child
2. Childbearing	Begins with birth of first baby and continues until firstborn is in preschool
3. Preschool age	When first child is between 2½ years and 5 years old
4. School age	When first child is between 6 and 12 years old
5. Teenage	When first child turns 13 years old until first child departs from home
6. Launching young adults	Begins with first child leaving as a young adult until the last child leaves home
7. Middle-aged parents	Begins with departure of last child from home (empty nest) and continues through retirement
8. Aging family members	Begins with retirement and ends with death of both parents

Adapted from Duvall, E. M., & Miller, B. C. (1985). Marriage and family development (6th ed.). New York: Harper & Row, with permission.

TABLE 4–2. STAGES OF FAMILY LIFE CYCLE, DURING DIVORCE, AND FOR RECONSTITUTED FAMILY

Family Life Cycle Stage	Family Life Cycle With Divorce	Life Cycle for Reconstituted Family
1. Leaving home: Single young adults	1. Decision to divorce	1. Entering new relationship
2. Joining of families through marriage	2. Planning breakup of system	2. Planning new marriage and family
3. Families with young children	3. Separation	3. Remarriage and reconstitution of family
4. Families with adolescents	4. Divorce	
5. Launching children and moving on	5. Postdivorce family	
6. Families in later life		

Adapted from Carter, B., & McGoldrick, M. (1988). The changing family life cycle (2nd ed.). New York: Gardner Press, pp. 15, 22, 24. Copyright (1989) by Allyn and Bacon, adapted by permission.

member may be incapacitated by a serious illness may affect the kind of problems created for the family as well as the family's financial, social, and psychological resources for resolving those problems. For example, if a man enters the hospital for a myocardial infarction (MI) and states he is single with two teenage children, the nurse may have some understanding of what the family was dealing with before the illness. During the teenage years, the school and peer groups may be powerful and pervading forces in the socialization of the adolescent. Parent and adolescent value conflict may arise, exhausting the emotional or psychological resources of the parent. When a crisis such as an MI strikes the family during this stage, psychological resources for dealing with stress may be depleted and may serve to explain anxious and demanding behavior of family members in the hospital.

The nurse operating according to the developmental perspective might ask the following questions: Does the impact of serious illness on the family differ according to family stage? Do coping mechanisms used by families differ according to family stage? Because problems and resources for dealing with the problems may differ according to family stage, nursing interventions need to be designed accordingly.

Interactionist Perspective

The interactionist or symbolic interaction perspective focuses on the meanings that acts and symbols have for people in the process of interaction. Before people can act, they must define the situation for themselves. Communication and sustained interaction are possible when people possess a system of shared meanings.

Symbolic interaction addresses a set of interrelated issues. The first issue is socialization, that is, how human beings acquire ways of behaving, values, norms, and attitudes of the social unit of which they are a part. The focus of the second issue is personality, that is, an organization of persistent behavior patterns that depend on social relationships. When symbolic interactionists wish to understand an individual's or group's behavior, they will try to see the world from these people's points of view. Symbolic interactionists are primarily interested in social processes between people: "Family phenomena viewed from the symbolic interactionist approach include internal processes within families such as roles/role conflict, statuses, communication, responses to stress, decision making and socialization" (Mercer, 1989, p. 12).

The symbolic interactionist framework has several implications for nurses who care for families. When caring for families with an ill member, a nurse cannot assume that he or she knows how the illness affects the family. A nurse needs to determine the family's definition of the situation. For example, a wife of a patient who had an MI may perceive her husband's "heart attack" as her fault and may feel guilty that she did not give her husband the right diet or did not care that he smoked cigarettes and did not exercise regularly. A nurse may try desperately to calm the anxious wife by telling her that her husband's "vital signs are good" or tell her it is unnecessary to stay at the hospital 24 hours a day because her "husband is stable." Without knowing the wife's perceptions, however, nursing interventions will not be effective. A nurse who understands the wife's perceptions of guilt will try to relieve that guilt by clarifying with the wife issues such as heredity as an uncontrollable risk factor for coronary artery disease, caring versus caretaking, or her husband's own responsibility for self-care.

Family Ecological Perspective

The ecological perspective or family ecosystem framework examines the family in relationship to its environment. The ecosystem approach focuses on relationships between a changing environment and changing family. This perspective is broader than the family system perspective because the system includes the family and the environment.

An ecosystem has three main organizing concepts: (1) environed unit, (2) environment, and (3) the patterning of interactions and transactions between them (Andrews, Bubolz, & Paolucci, 1980, p. 32). In the family ecosystem, the environed unit is the group of people who constitute the family; that is, a bonded unit of interacting people who have some common goals and resources and, for a part of their life, share living space. The environment provides the resources necessary for family life. The organization of the family ecosystem is also derived from patterns of interactions and transactions between the family and the environment. A nurse who uses this approach to guide assessment would focus on the family and its environment and the transactional relationships between the family and the environment. An ecological assessment could be carried out in the form of an ecomap (Figure 4–1).

Social Exchange Perspective

The major focus of social exchange theory is that human beings maintain involvement in relationships on the basis of rewards and costs. Rewarding

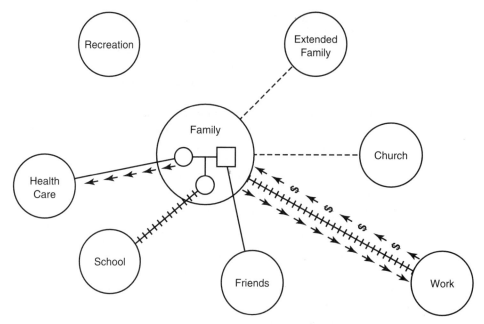

Figure 4–1. Family Ecomap. The larger inner circle depicts the family. The surrounding circles are the family's environment. Family units or family members can be asked to indicate where the connections with their environment exist. The nature of the connections can be indicated by drawing different kinds of lines: solid line indicates strong; dashed line, tenuous; cross-marked line, stressful. Arrows drawn along the lines indicate the direction of the flow of energy or resources. Names of significant people can be filled in the circles as needed. (Reprinted from Hartman, A. (1979). Finding families: An ecological approach to family assessment in adoption. Beverly Hills, CA: Sage, with permission.)

situations are maintained; costly situations are avoided. Marital quality often has been studied from the social exchange perspective. The benefits of a marriage often are the result of rewards minus costs. With the aid of social exchange theory, nurses may understand better why certain patterns of behavior have developed between family members. Nurses interested in fostering family adherence with medical regimens might ask what are the costs of adherence for the family versus its rewards (Mercer, 1989).

Family Stress Perspective

Hill (1949), the father of family stress, conducted research on war-induced separation and reunion within families. From his research, two important theoretical perspectives emerged. First, Hill conceptualizes that families encountering a crisis event experience a roller coaster profile of adjustment, the parts being crisis leading to disorganization leading to recovery leading to family reorganization. Second, Hill identifies variables that are present in a situation that determine whether or not a crisis is created. These variables constitute the *ABCX* Model that explains variability in family response to stress, where A = the hardships of the event, B = resources of the family to meet the event, C = the family's definition of the event, and X = the crisis.

This original model has been advanced by other researchers. McCubbin and McCubbin (1993) describe their Resiliency Model of Family Stress, Adjustment, and Adaptation based on the early work of Hill (1949) and their own and other research over the years. This model is applicable to understanding the effects of illness as a stressor on family life, the family's appraisal of the illness as a stressor, the use of resistance resources to manage the stressor and the demands of it, the family's coping patterns and problem-solving abilities to maintain family functioning while dealing with the stressor, and family adaptation (McCubbin & McCubbin, 1993). The Resiliency Model emphasizes family *adaptation*, which is needed most frequently in response to illness (p. 22).

The Resiliency Model and other models of family stress provide a framework for nursing assessment. The models guide the nurse to view an individual's illness in terms of the stressors and hardships it has placed on the family, as well as to evaluate the number of changes the illness has introduced into the family system. In addition, the nurse should assess for factors that contribute to the pileup of stress, such as expected developmental transitions, prior strains, and consequences of family efforts to cope. The nurse should know about available resources and how the family can access them. A nurse's understanding of the family definition of the stressful event and the meaning the family gives to the situation at hand can lead to empathetic and individualized care.

Several family theoretical perspectives exist. Each of them has relevance for nursing and can be used either alone or in combination to assess, plan, and guide delivery of nursing services to family clients.

Culture and Families

Culture refers to patterned behavioral responses that develop over time. Values, beliefs, norms, and practices are shared among members of the same cultural group (Giger & Davidhizar, 1995). To understand an ethnic group and be able to work efficaciously with families, as well as individuals and communities, from different cultures, one must be aware of that culture's unique distinctive qualities and the variety of lifestyles, values, and beliefs found within that group. Successful nursing care of clients from various ethnic backgrounds depends on knowledge and sensitivity to the client's culture (Browning & Woods, 1993).

Health care personnel share their own cultural system. Nurses have obtained beliefs about health, illness, and health care practices through professional socialization. Nurses' beliefs about health and illness may differ from those of the client. When clients of one belief system encounter nurses who have other beliefs regarding health and illness, there is a potential for misunderstanding between the two. Nurses need to gather cultural data about the family to facilitate delivery of culturally congruent or culturally acceptable care. They also need to be aware of their own culture and be willing to explore its influence on their thinking and decision making (Drew, 1996, p. 151).

The following areas are suggested to provide cultural data about the family (Friedman, 1992, pp. 138–139):

- Family's ethnic background
- Family's degree of acculturation. Some behavioral clues that may indicate the degree to which the family maintains traditional/ethnic practices include the following:

  - Recent migration from another country
  - Native culture very different from American culture
  - Family's friends of same ethnic group
  - Family lives in ethnically homogenous neighborhood
  - Religious, social, cultural, recreational, or educational activities within family's cultural group
  - Traditional family roles carried out
  - Home decorations, art, and other visual representations as evidence of cultural background
  - Native language spoken exclusively or frequently in home
  - Traditional dietary habits and dress
  - Wider community family frequents primarily within ethnic community
  - Use of folk medicine or traditional healers by family
  - Community discrimination against identified ethnic group of family
  - Family members nonwhite (creating obvious racial differences and making acculturation more difficult)

- Family's religious preferences and practices

It is important to assess a family's basic value system and whether family members have any particular beliefs about health and specific types of illnesses and treatments. Moreover, it is important to realize the family's involvement in a family member's illness varies according to their culture.

Culture affects client use of and access to health care. It also may affect patient and family behavior and communication during illness. Thus, cultural assessment is vital to nurses who care for families. Nurses sensitive to family culture can plan and deliver culturally relevant care.

Family Health

Nurses may conduct a family health assessment to obtain pertinent data about the functioning of individual family members and of the family system. The individual family member health assessment might include information about current health status; impact of the patient's illness on his or her physical, psychological, and social life; past health history and strategies for coping; access to resources and social support; and the family members' perceptions of the event.

Thomas, Barnard, and Sumner (1993) present a framework for assessing the family as a unit. Five areas of family functioning are assessed:

1. *Family processes.* Assessment in this area addresses basic functional patterns of the family, including relationships among members of the family, how members communicate with each other, how they solve problems, how they adjust to changes associated with health problems, and the family's relationships with others.
2. *Family coping.* In this area of assessment, the nurse examines how the family copes with the health care problem and situation.
3. *Parenting.* Assessment of parenting relates to the care provided for children within the family. Data collected in this area pertain to "physical, emotional and social growth-enhancing activities" provided by the parents (p. 129).
4. *Health maintenance and management.* In this area of assessment, the nurse examines the family's knowledge of and health practices to maintain health, such as nutrition, as well as the family's understanding of the current health problems and treatments.
5. *Home maintenance and management.* In this final area of family assessment, the nurse focuses on the environment in which the family lives and the family's economic and other resources to meet family needs. (pp. 128–130)

These five areas of family functioning provide direction to nurses in assessing families with whom they work as a basis for providing family-centered care.

Assessment and care that nurses provide for families vary according to the stage of the health–illness cycle that families are experiencing. Doherty and Campbell (1988) constructed a health and illness cycle that depicts a series of temporal phases that families may experience relative to health and illness (Figure 4–2). The cycle can be used to guide the assessment and delivery of care to families. The cycle begins with the family health promotion and risk reduction phases that encompass the family beliefs and activities that help family members to maintain good health. A balanced diet, regular exercise, and abstinence from smoking are examples of lifestyle patterns believed to promote the health of family members. Nurses interacting with families during this phase should assess health promotion activities; the family may need assistance to understand how to carry out such activities.

The second phase of the cycle, family vulnerability and illness onset, refers to family life events or experiences that may make family members susceptible to illness or to having a relapse of chronic illness (Doherty & Campbell, 1988). Family stress may predispose some family members to illness.

The third phase in the family health cycle is the family illness appraisal

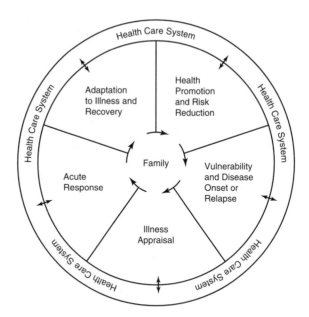

Figure 4–2. Family Health and Illness Cycle *(Reprinted from Doherty, W.J., & Campbell, T. L. (1988). Families and health. Beverly Hills, CA: Sage Inc., with permission.)*

phase, which involves the family's efforts to give meaning to the family member's symptoms of illness and to family decisions about how to deal with the illness. "In appraising the illness episode, the family gives its own meaning to the situation, a meaning that may be close to or distant from the professional consensus" (Doherty & Campbell, 1988, p. 24). It is important for nurses interacting with families during this phase to learn the family's perceptions of the situation and plan care accordingly.

The fourth phase of the family health cycle is the acute response phase, which refers to the immediate adjustments a family must make to accommodate the ill member (Doherty & Campbell, 1988). Nurses interacting with families during this phase need to assess the impact of the illness on the family. Artinian (1989) conducted a qualitative study with 14 family members of coronary artery bypass graft patients. Families were affected by the surgery in various ways. Findings reveal that the spouses experience feelings of fear, numbness, and panic at the time of surgery. Other family member problems and concerns are insensitivity and impersonalization from hospital staff, disrupted family relations, and waiting. Spouses report hardships such as taking on additional responsibilities, having more demands on their time, experiencing fatigue, and having to handle an increased number of phone calls at home.

The final phase of the cycle is family adaptation to illness and recovery, which refers to how the family reorganizes itself around a chronic illness or disability of a family member and the ways in which a family adapts after the recovery of a family member (Doherty & Campbell, 1988). Problems or concerns to nurses during this phase are family coping strategies, family and community resources, and the family's adherence to medical regimens.

Families in the Hospital

The family's experiences in the hospital have recently become an area of concern for health care providers (Leavitt, 1989, p. 263). Families experience many stressors during the hospitalization of a family member. These include the hospital environment itself, a lack of understanding about the illness and treatments, separation from the ill person, waiting for information from health providers, and dealing with emotions such as fear, guilt, and anger (Artinian, 1996). Stress and anxiety related to hospitalization may be even greater for a family member than for the patient.

Several barriers to family-centered care in hospitals are limited time, lack of a systematic approach to the family as a unit of care, and lack of knowledge and skills of how to deal with families (Artinian, 1996). However, family involvement in hospital care may have economic and therapeutic outcomes and may increase the chances for enhanced recovery after discharge.

Based on qualitative data, Thorne and Robinson (1988) describe family relationships with health care professionals as an evolving three-stage process. The first stage is naive trusting, which refers to family members' trusting that all health care professionals will act in the sick member's best interests; family members wait passively for this to happen while they familiarize themselves with the professional care setting. Later, family members discover their trust was founded on naive assumptions, as discrepancies arise between family members' views and the professional's view regarding the best interests of the sick member. "Family members learned that the long-term nature of their experience was often disregarded as was their involvement and expertise in illness management" (p. 297).

The second phase is the disenchantment phase, characterized by dissatisfaction with care, frustration, and fear. Families learn that they are expected to leave care of their ill member in the hands of the professionals and that involvement in care is hindered by difficulty in obtaining information. "Health care relationships often became adversarial and the family members came to view their sick member as vulnerable and in need of protection" (Thorne & Robinson, 1988, p. 297). Families face a dilemma, knowing that if they remain passive, the sick member might suffer a negative experience and if they actively seek involvement, they may alienate the health care professionals, thus placing the sick member in greater jeopardy.

The third phase is guarded alliance, in which involved families renegotiate trust with health care professionals. "In this phase, families actively sought the information they needed, demonstrated understanding of the differences in perspective, stated their own perspective and expectations more clearly, and promoted negotiation of mutually satisfying care" (Thorne & Robinson, 1988, p. 298). However, families still experience the frustration of waiting, fear of not knowing the right questions to ask to get the information they need, and anger of recognizing that their own expertise is devalued.

Thorne and Robinson's stages provide insight for nurses into the dynamics of their relationships with families. Nurses able to locate which stage families are at can intervene more appropriately, using strategies such as assessing family perceptions or arranging regular nurse–family conferences to prevent disenchantment and promote cooperative caring that can occur in guarded alliance.

Because families experience many stressors when a family member is hospitalized, nurses need to be sensitive to families' problems and demands and to demonstrate concern for them. Families should know by name the nurse who is responsible for caring for them and their ill member. Families with hospitalized members can be helped by teaching them about the illness and treatments, providing information in words they can understand, and encouraging the family to express their feelings.

Family members who are informed about and participate in the care of a patient will be better prepared to provide care after the individual is discharged from the hospital. The stress of illness is not confined to hospitalization but continues after discharge, highlighting the importance of discharge planning. Discharge planning consists of a series of actions that occur after a person is admitted to a hospital and other types of health care settings to facilitate care throughout hospitalization and provide for continuity of care at home. To be effective planners, nurses must learn as much as possible about the range of resources within the community and how to assess them as well as to anticipate problems for both the patient and family after discharge. Specific content relative to what family members can expect at home and how family members can participate in care at home needs to be included in discharge teaching.

COMMUNITY AS CLIENT

The purpose of community health nursing is to improve the health of the entire community. Although the community health nurse works with both individuals and families, individuals and families are not considered separately but in relationship to the community. Nurses who care for communities assess the entire community to discover possible groups of people with a common health need, such as expectant mothers or child abuse victims.

Community health nursing is concerned with promoting the health of populations and of communities as a whole. Smith (1995) views community health nursing as the care provided by nurses directed toward "promoting, restoring, and preserving the health of the total population or community" (p. 7).

More and more nurses are working in community health, a trend predicted to continue (Oermann, 1994a, b). Most community health nurses work in home health and hospice care; others are in state and local health departments, community health centers, schools, and worksites. Between 1988 and 1992, nurses employed in home health nearly doubled (U.S. Department of Health and Human Services, 1993). The number of nurses in other community settings also has increased significantly. Smith (1995) emphasizes that the employment setting does not determine whether the nurse is a community health nurse. Instead, the distinguishing factors are educational preparation for practice in the community and "the community focus of their practice" (p. 5).

There are several reasons for assessing a community: (1) identifying health risks of a community, (2) identifying vulnerable population groups, (3) collecting data for health planning for the community, and (4) identifying community resources. Community nursing diagnoses are different from individual and family diagnoses. Community nursing diagnoses are summary statements of the health status of the community in addition to an identification of the high-risk groups whose problems need to be addressed through intervention. A community nursing diagnosis includes a summary of the health status of the community, high-risk groups in the community, and the community's health resources. Interventions directed toward community health problems are usually broadly directed toward the community system. These include, for instance, health education; screening programs; establishing health services to meet the needs of a particular population, such as school health clinics, day care centers, and community nursing centers, to name a few; policy setting; and interventions that involve the community in solving their own health-related problems (Trotter, Smith, & Maurer, 1995b). Evaluation of nursing care for communities involves evaluating programs that deal with care of populations.

Nurses who care for communities use epidemiological information and approaches to promote health. Epidemiology is the study of factors that influence the health status of populations. Populations at risk and rates of occurrence are two central epidemiological concepts. The population at risk becomes the target group for interventions designed to prevent or control the problem. Rates of occurrence also are of concern in epidemiology. Rates provide statistical data necessary for making comparisons among populations (Neal, 1995, p. 270). Rates provide insight into the occurrence of a particular problem in relation to the size of the group. For example, a community with a population of 1000 may report two cases of acquired immunodeficiency syndrome (AIDS) this year, which is a rate of 0.2%.

Mortality and morbidity rates are examples of rates that are of concern in epidemiology.

Several frameworks guide the assessment and planning of community care. One framework is the epidemiological triangle (Figure 4–3). The host is the susceptible person; causative agents include the presence or absence of factors that may influence the health of the person; and the environment includes anything external to the person or agent. "A change in any of these factors (the person, the causative agent, or the environment) has the potential to change the balance of health" (Neal, 1995, p. 274). With an epidemiological perspective, the community health nurse focuses on the health of populations, identifying people at greater risk for developing health problems so interventions can be targeted to reduce this risk.

Another approach to the study of the community is the structural-functional approach. In the structural-functional approach, the concern lies with the ability of the community to carry out its functions to attain community goals (Trotter, Smith, & Maurer, 1995a). The nurse who uses this approach will evaluate the community's ability to carry out its functions.

Still another approach to studying the community is the systems approach. In a systems framework the focus is on identifying the community system and its component parts and the system's capacity to meet the goals of the community. Trotter, Smith, and Maurer (1995a) identify seven components of the community to assess when using a systems approach:

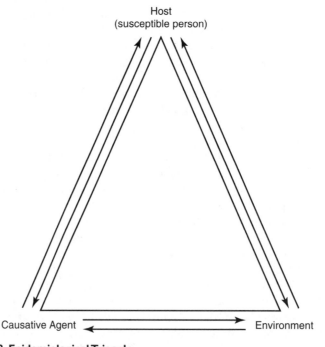

Figure 4–3. Epidemiological Triangle

1. *Boundaries.* Factors that separate a community from its environment
2. *Goals.* Purposes of the community, such as promoting the well being of its members and meeting their needs
3. *Set factors.* The physical and psychosocial characteristics of the community, its demographics
4. *Inputs.* External influences on the community that affect its functioning, such as economic status, facilities, human services, health information, legislation, and values
5. *Throughputs.* Internal functioning of the community
6. *Outputs.* Health status of the community
7. *Feedback.* Information that is returned to the system regarding its functioning (pp. 308–319)

SUMMARY

Individuals, families, and communities may be the recipients of nursing care. Nurses who care for individuals assess the health state, problems, or needs of a single person. There are many theoretical perspectives that assist nurses in planning care for individuals.

Family as client refers to individual family members and the family unit as the focus of nursing care. Structural-functional, systems, developmental, interactionist, ecological, social exchange, and stress theoretical perspectives provide ways of looking at and understanding family phenomena.

Family health may be assessed at the individual member or family unit levels. Nurses may deliver care to families during any one of the family health–illness cycles: family health promotion and risk reduction, family vulnerability and illness onset, family illness appraisal, acute response, and family adaptation to illness and recovery.

Families in the hospital recently have become an issue of concern for nurses. Studies indicate that the stress related to hospitalization may be greater for a family member than for the patient. The research literature has suggested several family nursing interventions, such as providing information about patient care or information about the hospital, helping family members to clarify their goals and needs and to identify resources, explaining visiting policies and arranging flexible visiting hours, and demonstrating sensitivity to families' problems and demands.

When the community is the client of nursing services, the focus of care is on the personal and environmental health of population groups. The aim of community health nursing is to improve the health of the entire community. Community assessment includes identifying the health risks of a community and high-risk groups within the community and collecting data for program planning within the community. The epidemiological, structural-functional, and systems approaches are possible frameworks to guide nurses in their assessment and planning of community care.

REFERENCES

Andrews, M. P., Bubolz, M. M., & Paolucci, B. (1980). An ecological approach to study of the family. *Marriage & Family Review, 3*(1/2), 29–49.

Artinian, N. T. (1989). Family member perceptions of a cardiac surgery event. *Focus on Critical Care, 16,* 301–308.

Artinian, N. (1996). Family nursing in medical-surgical settings. In S. H. Hanson & S. T. Boyd (Eds.), *Family health care nursing: Theory, practice and research* (pp. 269–300). Philadelphia: Davis.

Browning, M. A., & Woods, J. H. (1993). Cross-cultural family-nurse partnerships. In S. L. Feetham, S. B. Meister, J. M. Bell, & C. L. Gilliss (Eds.), *The nursing of families* (pp. 177–187). Newbury Park, CA: Sage.

Burgess, E. W., Locke, H. J., & Thomas, M. M. (1963). *The family* (3rd ed.). New York: American Book.

Carter, B., & McGoldrick, M. (1988). *The changing family life cycle* (2nd ed.). New York: Gardner Press.

Danielson, C. B., Hamel-Bissell, B., & Winstead-Fry, P. (1993). *Families, health, & illness.* St. Louis: Mosby.

Doherty, W. J., & Campbell, T. L. (1988). *Families and health.* Beverly Hills, CA: Sage.

Drew, J. C. (1996). Cultural competence in partnerships with communities. In E. T. Anderson & J. M. McFarlane, *Community as partner: Theory and practice in nursing* (pp. 138–161). Philadelphia: Lippincott.

Duvall, E. M. (1977). *Marriage and family development* (5th ed.). Philadelphia: Lippincott.

Friedman, M. M. (1992). *Family nursing: Theory and practice* (3rd ed.). Norwalk, CT: Appleton & Lange.

Giger, J. N., & Davidhizar, R. E. (1995). *Transcultural nursing: Assessment and intervention* (2nd ed.). St. Louis: Mosby.

Hartman, A. (1979). *Finding families: An ecological approach to family assessment in adoption.* Beverly Hills, CA: Sage.

Hill, R. (1949). *Families under stress.* New York: Harper & Row.

Leavitt, M. B. (1989). Transition to illness: The family in the hospital. In C. L. Gilless, B. L. Highley, B. M. Roberts, & I. M. Martinson (Eds.), *Toward a science of family nursing* (pp. 262–283). Menlo Park, CA: Addison-Wesley.

McCubbin, M. A., & McCubbin, H. I. (1993). Families coping with illness: The Resiliency Model of Family Stress, Adjustment, and Adaptation. In C. B. Danielson, B. Hamel-Bissell, & P. Winstead-Fry (Eds.), *Families, health, & illness* (pp. 21–63). St. Louis: Mosby.

Mercer, R. T. (1989). Theoretical perspectives on family. In C. L. Gilliss, B. L. Highley, B. M. Roberts, & I. M. Martinson (Eds.), *Toward a science of family nursing* (pp. 9–36). Menlo Park, CA: Addison-Wesley.

Neal, M. T. (1995). Epidemiology: Unraveling the mysteries of disease and health. In C. M. Smith & F. A. Maurer (Eds.), *Community health nursing: Theory and practice* (pp. 269–298). Philadelphia: Saunders.

Oermann, M. H. (1994a). Professional nursing education in the future: Changes and challenges. *Journal of Obstetric, Gynecologic, and Neonatal Nursing, 23,* 153–159.

Oermann, M. H. (1994b). Reforming nursing education for future practice. *Journal of Nursing Education, 33,* 215–219.

Smith, C. M. (1995). Responsibilities for care in community health nursing. In C. M. Smith & F. A. Maurer (Eds.), *Community health nursing: Theory and practice* (pp. 3–29). Philadelphia: Saunders.

Smith, C. M., & Maurer, F. A. (1995). *Community health nursing: Theory and practice*. Philadelphia: Saunders.

Thomas, R. B., Barnard, K. E., & Sumner, G. A. (1993). Family nursing diagnoses as a framework for family assessment. In S. L. Feetham, S. B. Meister, J. M. Bell, & C. L. Gilliss (Eds.), *The nursing of families* (pp. 127–136). Newbury Park, CA: Sage.

Thorne, S. E., & Robinson, C. A. (1988). Health care relationships: The chronic illness perspective. *Research in Nursing & Health, 11,* 293–300.

Trotter, J. O., Smith, C. M., & Maurer, F. A. (1995a). Community assessment. In C. M. Smith & F. A. Maurer (Eds.), *Community health nursing: Theory and practice* (pp. 299–339). Philadelphia: Saunders.

Trotter, J. O., Smith, C. M., & Maurer, F. A. (1995b). Community planning and intervention. In C. M. Smith & F. A. Maurer (Eds.), *Community health nursing: Theory and practice* (pp. 340–364). Philadelphia: Saunders.

U.S. Department of Health and Human Services. (1993). *Registered nurse population 1992: Findings from the national sample survey of registered nurses.* Washington, DC: Division of Nursing, Bureau of Health Professions, Health Resources and Services Administration.

von Bertalanffy, L. U. (1968). *General system theory.* New York: Braziller.

BIBLIOGRAPHY

Anderson, E. T., & McFarlane, J. M. (1996). *Community as partner: Theory and practice in nursing.* Philadelphia: Lippincott.

Anderson, E. T., McFarlane, J.M., & Helton, A. (1986). Community-as-client: A model for practice. *Nursing Outlook, 34,* 220–224.

Artinian, N. T. (1989). Family member perceptions of a cardiac surgery event. *Focus on Critical Care, 16,* 301–308.

Artinian, N. T. (1994). Selecting a model to guide family assessment. *Dimensions of Critical Care Nursing, 13,* 3–12.

Bellack, J. P. (1995). Educating for the community. *Journal of Nursing Education, 34,* 342–343.

Berkey, K. M., & Hanson, S. M. H. (1991). *Pocket guide to family assessment and intervention.* St. Louis: Mosby.

Biegel, D. E., Sales, E., & Schulz, R. (1991). *Family caregiving in chronic illness.* Newbury Park, CA: Sage.

Craft, M. J., & Willadsen, J. A. (1992). Interventions related to family. *Nursing Clinics of North America, 27,* 517–540.

Eshleman, J. R. (1991). *The family: An introduction* (6th ed.). Boston: Allyn & Bacon.

Friedemann, M. L. (1995). *The framework of systemic organization.* Thousand Oaks, CA: Sage.

Gilliss, C. L., Roberts, B. M., Highley, B. L., & Martinson, I. M. (1989). What is family nursing? In C. L. Gilliss, B. L. Highley, B. M. Roberts, & I. M. Martinson (Eds.), *Toward a science of family nursing* (pp. 64–73). Menlo Park, CA: Addison-Wesley.

Gortner, S. R., Gilliss, C. L., Shinn, J. A., Sparacino, P. A., Rankin, S., Leavitt, M., Price, M., & Hudes, M. (1988). Improving recovery following cardiac surgery: A randomized clinical trial. *Journal of Advanced Nursing, 13*(5), 649–661.

Hanchett, E. S. (1988). *Nursing frameworks & community as client: Bridging the gap.* Norwalk, CT: Appleton & Lange.

Hanson, S. M. H., & Heims, M. L. (1992). Family nursing curricula in U.S. schools of nursing. *Journal of Nursing Education, 31*, 303–308.

Hanson, S. M. H., Heims, M. L., & Julian, D. (1992). Education for family health care professionals: Nursing as a paradigm. *Family Relations, 41*, 49–53.

Hathaway, D., Boswell, B., Stanford, D., Schneider, S., Mocrief, A. (1987). Health promotion and disease prevention for the hospitalized patient's family. *Nursing Administration Quarterly, 11*(3), 1–7.

Henneman, E. A., McKenzie, J. B., & Dewa, C. S. (1992). An evaluation of interventions for meeting the information needs of families of critically ill patients. *American Journal of Critical Care, 1*(3), 85–93.

Hickey, M. (1985). What are the needs of families of critically ill patients? *Focus on Critical Care, 12*(1), 41–43.

Hickey, M. L. (Ed.). (1992). Family issues in critical care. *Critical Care Nursing Clinics of North America, 4*, 549–649.

Holloway, N. M. (1988). *Nursing the critically ill adult* (3rd ed.). Menlo Park, CA: Addison-Wesley.

Leahey, M., & Wright, L. M. (1987). Families and chronic illness: Assumptions, assessment, and intervention. In L. M. Wright & M. Leahey (Eds.), *Families & chronic illness* (pp. 55–76). Springhouse, PA: Springhouse.

Leininger, M. M. (1990). *Transcultural nursing: Concept, theory, and practice* (2nd ed.). New York: Wiley.

Leske, J. S. (1986). Needs of relatives of critically ill patients: A follow-up. *Heart & Lung, 15*, 189–193.

Leske, J. S. (1991). Internal psychometric properties of the Critical Care Family Needs Inventory. *Heart & Lung, 20*, 236–344.

Leske, J. S. (1992). Needs of adult family members after critical illness. *Critical Care Nursing Clinics of North America, 4*, 587–596.

Lynn-McHale, D. J., & Bellinger, A. (1988). Need satisfaction levels of family members of critical care patients and accuracy of nurses' perceptions. *Heart & Lung, 17*, 447–453.

MacPhee, M. (1995). The family systems approach and pediatric nursing care. *Pediatric Nursing, 21*, 417–423, 432–433, 437.

McClowry, S. G. (1992). Family functioning during a critical illness: A systems theory perspective. *Critical Care Nursing Clinics of North America, 4*, 559–564.

McCubbin, M. A., & McCubbin, H. I. (1987). Family stress theory and assessment: The T-Double ABCX Model of family adjustment and adaptation. In H. I. McCubbin & A. I. Thompson (Eds.), *Family assessment inventories for research and practice* (pp. 4–32). Madison, WI: University of Wisconsin-Madison.

McCubbin, H. I., & Patterson, J. M. (1987). FILE: Family inventory of life events and changes. In H. I. McCubbin & A. I. Thompson (Eds.), *Family assessment inventories for research and practice* (pp. 80–98). Madison, WI: University of Wisconsin-Madison.

McCubbin, H. I., & Thompson, A. H. (Eds.). (1987). *Family assessment inventories for research and practice.* Madison, WI: University of Wisconsin-Madison.

McShane, R. E. (1991). Family theoretical perspectives and implications for nursing practice. *AACN Clinical Issues in Critical Care Nursing, 2*, 210–219.

Norris, L. O., & Grove, S. K. (1986). Investigation of selected psychosocial needs of family members of critically ill adult patients. *Heart & Lung, 15*, 194–199.

Ray, D. W. (1986). Epidemiology. In B. B. Logan & C. E. Dawkins (Eds.), *Family-centered nursing in the community* (pp. 131–181). Reading, MA: Addison-Wesley.

Reutter, L. (1984). Family health assessment: An integrated approach. *Journal of Advanced Nursing, 9*, 391–399.

Robinson, P. D., Roe, H., & Boys, L. J. (1987). The focus of hospitals on family care. *Health Values, 11*(2), 19–24.

Rolland, J. S. (1988). A conceptual model of chronic and life-threatening illness and its impact on families. In C. S. Chilman, E. W. Nunnally, & F. M. Cox (Eds.), *Chronic illness and disability: Families in trouble series* (Vol. 2, pp. 17–68). Beverly Hills, CA: Sage.

Ross, B., & Cobb, K. L. (1990). *Family nursing: A nursing process approach*. Redwood City, CA: Addison-Wesley.

Sawa, R. J. (Ed.). (1992). *Family health care*. Newbury Park, CA: Sage.

Schultz, P. R. (1987). When client means more than one: Extending the foundational concept of person. *Advances in Nursing Science, 10*(1), 71–86.

Silva, M. C. (1987). Needs of spouses of surgical patients: A conceptualization within the Roy adaptation model. *Scholarly Inquiry for Nursing Practice: An International Journal, 1*(1), 29–44.

Steinglass, P. (1992). Family systems theory and medical illness. In R. J. Sawa (Ed.), *Family health care* (pp. 18–29). Newbury Park, CA: Sage.

Tringali, C. A. (1986). The needs of family members of cancer patients. *Oncology Nursing Forum, 13*(4), 65–70.

Whall, A. L. (1986). The family as the unit of care in nursing: A historical review. *Public Health Nursing, 3*, 240–249.

Whall, A. L., & Fawcett, J. (1991). The family as a focal phenomenon in nursing. In A. L. Whall & J. Fawcett (Eds.), *Family theory development in nursing: State of the science and art*. Philadelphia: Davis.

Whyte, D. A. (1994). *Family nursing: The case of cystic fibrosis*. Brookfield, VT: Ashgate.

Wright, L. M., & Leahey, M. (1987). Families & life-threatening illness: Assumptions, assessment, and intervention. In M. Leahey & L. M. Wright (Eds.), *Families & life-threatening illness* (pp. 45–67). Springhouse, PA: Springhouse.

Nursing Process

Marilyn H. Oermann

Nursing process is the methodology of nursing practice. Reflecting critical thinking and other cognitive skills, the nursing process enables the nurse to meet the client's health care needs. The client may be an individual, family, or community. Nursing process has been conceptualized as a systematic series of independent nursing actions directed toward promoting an optimum level of wellness for the client (Reilly & Oermann, 1992).

A major emphasis in the literature and of research in nursing today focuses on the nursing diagnosis component of the process in terms of the nature of nursing diagnoses, evolving diagnostic categories, and their use in practice. In addition, research is under way on the cognitive skills required for the nurse to make a diagnosis and decide on nursing management. Various theoretical perspectives have been proposed for describing clinical judgment in nursing. Through this process, the nurse decides on data to be collected about the client, makes an interpretation of the data (inference) to arrive at a diagnosis, and identifies and evaluates the effectiveness of nursing actions. Intuition and experience of the nurse play a role in the clinical judgment process.

This chapter examines the concept of nursing process and its relationship to critical thinking. It discusses the evolving nature of nursing diagnoses and the cognitive processes through which the nurse arrives at a diagnosis and plan of care.

CONCEPT OF NURSING PROCESS

The nursing process is described generally as a four- or five-step process. Some experts describe four steps: (1) assessment, (2) plan, (3) implementation, and (4) evaluation (Reilly & Oermann, 1992; Yura & Walsh, 1988). Others identify five steps: (1) assessment, (2) diagnosis, (3) plan, (4) implementation, and (5) evaluation (Alfaro-LeFevre, 1995; Carpenito, 1995; Do-enges, Moorhouse, & Burley, 1995). In conceptualizing nursing process as a four-step process, diagnosis is considered to be the final component of assessment. As five or more steps, nursing diagnosis becomes a separate phase of the process, distinct from the other phases. Regardless of whether nursing diagnosis is viewed as a separate step, it is an essential phase of the nursing process from which the plan and interventions are generated. The five phases of the nursing process are:

1. *Assessment.* Problem recognition and collection of data
2. *Diagnoses.* Data analysis and statement of nursing diagnoses
3. *Plan.* Setting of priorities, establishment of goals, and selection of interventions
4. *Implementation.* Carrying out planned nursing actions
5. *Evaluation.* Evaluation of outcomes of care

Irrespective of whether the nurse subscribes to four or five phases, the nursing process is a systematic process for meeting the client's health needs and promoting an optimal degree of health. The client served may be an individual, family, group, or community.

Although sometimes viewed in the literature as a linear process, the phases of the nursing process are interrelated and are not carried out in a step-by-step fashion. In assessing a client, for instance, comprehensive and accurate data are collected to arrive at a nursing diagnosis that then provides a basis for planning care, intervening, and evaluating the effectiveness of the care. Assessment, however, also occurs during the other phases of the nursing process. The nurse may decide to collect additional data after identifying the nursing diagnoses and developing the plan because of a continuing unmet client need.

The nursing process is primarily a cognitive or intellectual process that requires critical thinking and skill in clinical judgment. It also requires psychomotor skills for data collection and in terms of interventions to be carried out. The nurse's values influence the nursing process in that they are reflected in the nurse's interaction with the client, decision making regarding care, and the way in which the nurse carries out treatments and other interventions.

In addition to the necessary cognitive skills, three types of nursing knowledge guide the nursing process: (1) scientific knowledge, which includes nursing models and theories, concepts and theories from other disciplines that are applied to nursing, and research findings; (2) ethics of practice; and (3) "practice wisdom," or knowledge based on intuition, tradition, and experience (Ziegler, Vaughan-Wrobel, & Erlen, 1986, pp. 35–36). Nursing models, non-nursing concepts and theories, and research provide a basis for understanding client problems and needed interventions. Such knowledge provides guidelines for the nurse to determine data to collect, ascribe meaning to the data, make a judgment regarding the nursing diagnosis, and formulate a plan. Theory and research also direct the nurse in selecting nursing measures and evaluating care. Ethics of practice refer to the "oughts" and "shoulds" of nursing practice. Another type of knowledge used by nurses is practice wisdom, which is derived from the nurse's experience in practice, intuition, and other sources. The nurse's experience influences decisions in the practice setting. Competency in nursing practice improves as the nurse acquires experience with similar clinical situations. This experience enables the nurse to approach a client with an expectation of the typical problems and nursing approaches for this particular patient, thereby providing a framework for decision making.

Benner (1984) acknowledges the role of intuition in solving clinical problems and making judgments. Intuition reflects an understanding that has occurred about which the nurse is unaware (Reilly & Oermann, 1992). The nurse's intuition, developed through knowledge and experience in nursing, may lead to a judgment regarding client care.

Nursing models provide guidelines for use in the nursing process. They contribute knowledge about nursing through their descriptions of what constitutes nursing practice. The model helps the nurse to choose which data to collect from the client and how to organize the data. The model focuses data collection on patient health problems for which the nurse is concerned (Doenges et al., 1995, p. 14). Nursing models also are reflected in other phases of the nursing process.

Assessment

Assessment is the first phase of the nursing process, on which the other phases are based. Through assessment the nurse collects essential data for making nursing diagnoses and arriving at judgments about the client. Assessment is an interactive process in that the nurse, through interaction with the client, family, and others, collects data to identify health problems. The two steps in the assessment phase are: (1) problem recognition and (2) data collection.

Problem Recognition

The first step in the assessment process begins with problem recognition, in which the nurse identifies a possible health problem that then provides direction in data gathering. Data are collected in terms of the health problems for which the client is seeking nursing care and health promotion. Initial problem recognition focuses subsequent data gathering on these actual or potential health problems and assists the nurse in collecting the most relevant data needed for diagnosis and planning care. Studies in clinical judgment indicate that practitioners generate possible diagnoses about the patient early in an assessment (Elstein, Kagan, Shulman, Jason, & Loupe, 1972; Elstein, Shulman, & Sprafka, 1978). Data are then collected in relation to the possible diagnoses, which provides a way of limiting the data to be gathered. These possible diagnoses guide data collection so the nurse can emphasize in an assessment the health status areas of greatest concern.

Carnevali, Mitchell, Woods, and Tanner (1984) indicate that generating these possible problems early in an assessment reduces cognitive stress by limiting the kinds of information to be collected and making data gathering more manageable (p. 41). It may be the nurse who initially recognizes actual and potential problems, or the client, the family, or other health care professionals may communicate those problems to the practitioner.

Data Collection

The second step in the assessment process involves the actual collection of data. Doenges et al. (1995) identify the nursing history (interview), physical examination, and results of diagnostic tests as major sources of data for establishing the patient database. Both subjective (described by the patient, family, and others) and objective (observable) data are gathered in the assessment process.

The data to be collected and the organization of the data vary with the conceptual model of nursing used and other frameworks for organizing nursing data, such as functional health patterns (Gordon, 1995). The 11 functional health patterns identified by Gordon are common to all clients and represent assessment areas. They are:

1. Health perception–health management
2. Nutritional–metabolic
3. Elimination
4. Activity–exercise
5. Sleep–rest
6. Cognitive–perceptual
7. Self-perception–self-concept
8. Role–relationship
9. Sexuality–reproductive
10. Coping–stress tolerance
11. Value–belief

Appendix A provides an example of an assessment form based on Gordon's functional patterns. Similar instruments are available for family and community assessment. Institutions also use assessment forms developed specifically for the health care agency and organized according to needs and problems particular to their clients. An assessment form, regardless of the framework on which it is based, provides for consistency in the type of data collected in the setting.

Diagnosis

The second step of the nursing process begins with an analysis of data obtained in assessment and results in the statement of nursing diagnoses about the client. The diagnoses are the critical step in the process because they provide the basis for planning care and selecting interventions. Independent nursing actions involving the client arise from these diagnoses.

Data Analysis

When the nurse has collected information from the client that suggests an actual or potential health problem, the process of clinical judgment is initiated. *Clinical judgment* is the cognitive or thinking process used by the nurse for analyzing data, deriving a nursing diagnosis from the information, and deciding on appropriate interventions. In terms of diagnosing, this represents the cognitive process used to interpret the data and arrive at a judgment of the problem and possible cause. The actual nursing diagnosis, the statement of the client's health problem, is the end product of this thinking. The data analysis step, therefore, depends on the nurse's critical thinking skills and ability to recall relevant knowledge for interpreting the data. Clinical knowledge provides a basis for deciding on data to be collected, being sensitive to cues in the data, and understanding the information and how it relates to the whole picture of the client. Data analysis is more than interpreting individual pieces of data; the nurse must see relationships among the data to identify the health problems.

In the diagnostic process, the nurse: (1) collects information (i.e., assessment); (2) interprets the data and identifies cues suggesting patient problems; (3) clusters the cues; and (4) determines the nursing diagnosis. Interpreting and clustering the data and then naming the cluster represent the diagnostic phase of the nursing process. Cues include signs and symptoms suggesting patient problems that can be described by nursing diagnoses (Doenges et al., 1995, p. 45).

Once cues are recognized, the nurse makes an inference or judgment about the meaning of the data. For example, a cue might be 5'3", weight of 200 pounds, which will lead the nurse to infer obesity. An inference of anxiety or fear might be drawn from the following cues: increased pulse and respiratory rate, elevated blood pressure, voice tremors, rapid speech, and dry mouth. The nurse clusters data cues with common properties into groups and then decides how the data fit together. The nurse uses the diagnostic categories as possible explanations of the meaning of cues and clusters of cues (Gordon, 1995, p. 34).

Nursing Diagnosis

Nursing diagnoses are actual or potential health problems of an individual, family, group, or community for which the nurse can intervene. An actual problem is an existing health deficit. Potential problems are situations and conditions predisposing an individual, a family, and a community to health problems. The American Nurses Association's social policy statement (ANA, 1995) describes the merits of using nursing diagnoses. Nursing diagnoses facilitate communication between health care providers and clients and provide a basis for choosing interventions and evaluating the outcomes of care (p. 9). The registered nurse is responsible for identifying nursing diagnoses for clients.

Support for implementing diagnoses in clinical practice also is derived from the ANA's standards of nursing practice (1991). Both generic and specialty standards, which provide a means for determining the quality of nursing practice, refer to the need for nursing diagnoses in practice. Standard II indicates that the nurse analyzes assessment data to determine the nursing diagnoses. Carpenito (1995) suggests that nursing diagnoses provide nurses with a common language to direct assessment, identify client problems, and describe those problems. Nursing diagnoses also facilitate written and oral communication about patient problems, are appropriate for inclusion in a computerized client database, and provide a mechanism for reimbursement of nursing activities (p. 4). Nursing diagnoses, when used in direct patient care, also are reflected in documentation, patient–family education, discharge planning, quality assurance, and staffing.

In addition to nursing diagnoses, in many health care settings nurses also identify *collaborative problems*, which are actual or potential problems resulting from complications of diseases, treatments, or diagnostic studies requiring nurse-prescribed and physician-prescribed interventions (Alfaro-LeFevre, 1995, p. 177; Carpenito, 1995, p. 29). Whereas nursing diagnoses represent health problems that require independent nursing interventions, collaborative problems necessitate interventions by nurses and other health professionals. Collaborative problems cannot be resolved by nursing care alone. Carpenito refers to these problems as "certain physiologic complications that nurses monitor to detect onset or changes in status" (p. 29). Collaborative problems focus on the physiological needs of the patient and require both nursing and medical interventions. In critical care and other acute care settings, these needs often are paramount. Collaborative problems begin with the diagnostic label *potential complications*, for example, potential for sepsis.

PES Format. In the early development of nursing diagnoses, Gordon (1987) identified three essential components of a nursing diagnosis and referred to these components as the *PES format*:

- **P:** Health *p*roblem of the individual, family, or community
- **E:** *E*tiological or related factors
- **S:** *S*igns and *s*ymptoms

The PES format provides a structure for writing nursing diagnoses for clients and for communicating to other practitioners the type of health problem, the contributing factors, and a cluster of signs and symptoms often found with that particular problem.

The problem (*P*) represents a description of the health status of the client (individual, family, or community). The health problem may be an actual health deficit or a potential problem based on the presence of risk factors identified by the nurse. The health problem should be stated clearly and concisely, preferably in two or three words. For example, activity intolerance, ineffective breathing patterns, and pain are concise descriptions of the health problem. The North American Nursing Diagnosis Association (NANDA), the national group responsible for generating nursing diagnoses, provides a list of diagnoses for use by nurses organized according to nine patterns of human responses (Table 5–1). Each of the diagnoses on the list represents a health problem of a client that may be incorporated into a nursing diagnosis. Although many of the diagnoses can be used for individual family members, some relate specifically to the family, such as those pertaining to family coping, altered family processes, altered parenting, and parental role conflict.

The list of accepted nursing diagnoses from the NANDA national conferences still is being developed to reflect the range of health problems that require nursing interventions. This development and testing will take many years, and nurses in practice will continue to see the list of problems modified as diagnoses are validated or are unsupported through research.

The etiology (E) or related factors are the probable factors that are causing or contributing to the client's health problems. The etiological and contributing factors are connected to the diagnostic label with a "related to." For example,

- **P**: Constipation
- **E**: Related to immobility

The words *related to* imply a relationship between these two parts of the diagnostic statement. When the etiological factors are unknown, this wording may be included in the nursing diagnosis, for example, "altered family processes related to unknown etiology."

The defining characteristics are a cluster of signs and symptoms (S) that generally are observed with a particular nursing diagnosis. They represent the data used for making a diagnosis. Not all the defining characteristics need to be present to decide on a diagnosis. The nurse judges whether or not the signs and symptoms present in the patient represent a particular health problem. Defining characteristics are separated into major and minor designations (Carpenito, 1995, p. 13). Characteristics identified as "major" are usually present with the diagnosis; minor defining characteristics provide additional support for the diagnosis but may or may not be present to arrive at the diagnosis. These characteristics, then, allow the nurse to discriminate among diagnoses and determine a diagnostic label that represents the cluster of signs and symptoms. In the previous example, the defining characteristics may include, for instance, hard, formed stools and pain on defecation, among others.

Nursing diagnostic statements may be written with one, two, or three parts. In a one-part statement, only the diagnostic label is included (eg with wellness diagnoses such as potential for enhanced nutrition) (Carpenito, 1995, p. 22). Diagnostic statements that are two parts include: (1) the client's health problem (P) and (2) etiological (E) or related factors. When specific characteristics are present, the nurse is able to select a diagnostic category from an accepted list, such as the NANDA list. The "related to" phrase links the diagnostic label with the etiological or contributing factors. Thus, the diagnostic statement in the previous example would be:

$$P + E$$

or constipation related to immobility. The defining characteristics were present for the nurse to make this diagnosis.

TABLE 5–1. NANDA APPROVED NURSING DIAGNOSES

Pattern 1: Exchanging

Altered nutrition: More than body requirements
Altered nutrition: Less than body requirements
Altered nutrition: Potential for more than body requirements
Risk for infection
Risk for altered body temperature
Hypothermia
Hyperthermia
Ineffective thermoregulation
Dysreflexia
Constipation
Perceived constipation
Colonic constipation
Diarrhea
Bowel incontinence
Altered urinary elimination
Stress incontinence
Reflex incontinence
Urge incontinence
Functional incontinence
Total incontinence
Urinary retention
Altered (specify type) tissue perfusion (renal, cerebral, cardiopulmonary, gastrointestinal, peripheral)
Fluid volume excess
Fluid volume deficit
Risk for fluid volume deficit
Decreased cardiac output
Impaired gas exchange
Ineffective airway clearance
Ineffective breathing pattern
Inability to sustain spontaneous ventilation
Dysfunctional ventilatory weaning response (DVWR)
Risk for injury
Risk for suffocation
Risk for poisoning
Risk for trauma
Risk for aspiration
Risk for disuse syndrome
Altered protection
Impaired tissue integrity
Altered oral mucous membrane
Impaired skin integrity
Risk for impaired skin integrity
Decreased adaptive capacity: Intracranial
Field disturbance

Pattern 2: Communicating

Impaired verbal communication

Pattern 3: Relating

Impaired social interaction
Social isolation
Risk for loneliness
Altered role performance
Altered parenting
Risk for altered parenting
Risk for altered parent/infant/child attachment
Sexual dysfunction
Altered family processes
Caregiver role strain
Risk for caregiver role strain
Altered family process: Alcoholism
Parental role conflict
Altered sexuality patterns

Pattern 4: Valuing

Spiritual distress (distress of the human spirit)
Potential for enhanced spiritual well being

Pattern 5: Choosing

Ineffective individual coping
Impaired adjustment
Defensive coping
Ineffective denial
Ineffective family coping: Disabling
Ineffective family coping: Compromised
Family coping: Potential for growth
Potential for enhanced community coping
Ineffective community coping
Ineffective management of therapeutic regimen (individuals)
Noncompliance (specify)
Ineffective management of therapeutic regimen: Families
Ineffective management of therapeutic regimen: Community
Ineffective management of therapeutic regimen: Individual
Decisional conflict (specify)
Health-seeking behaviors (specify)

Pattern 6: Moving

Impaired physical mobility
Risk for peripheral neurovascular dysfunction
Risk for perioperative positioning injury

TABLE 5–1. NANDA APPROVED NURSING DIAGNOSES (*continued*)

Pattern 6: Moving (continued)
  Activity intolerance
  Fatigue
  Risk for activity intolerance
  Sleep pattern disturbance
  Diversional activity deficit
  Impaired home maintenance management
  Altered health maintenance
  Feeding self-care deficit
  Impaired swallowing
  Ineffective breastfeeding
  Interrupted breastfeeding
  Effective breastfeeding
  Ineffective infant feeding pattern
  Bathing/hygiene self-care deficit
  Dressing/grooming self-care deficit
  Toileting self-care deficit
  Altered growth and development
  Relocation stress syndrome
  Risk for disorganized infant behavior
  Disorganized infant behavior
  Potential for enhanced organized infant behavior

Pattern 7: Perceiving
  Body image disturbance
  Self-esteem disturbance
  Chronic low self-esteem
  Situational low self-esteem
  Personal identity disturbance

Sensory/perceptual alterations (specify; visual,
  auditory, kinesthetic, gustatory, tactile, olfactory)
Unilateral neglect
Hopelessness
Powerlessness

Pattern 8: Knowing
  Knowledge deficit (specify)
  Impaired environmental interpretation
    syndrome
  Acute confusion
  Chronic confusion
  Altered thought processes
  Impaired memory

Pattern 9: Feeling
  Pain
  Chronic pain
  Dysfunctional grieving
  Anticipatory grieving
  Risk for violence: Self-directed or directed at
    others
  Risk for self-mutilation
  Posttraumatic response
  Rape trauma syndrome
  Rape trauma syndrome: Compound reaction
  Rape trauma syndrome: Silent reaction
  Anxiety
  Fear

This list represents the NANDA approved nursing diagnoses for clinical use and testing (1994). (Reprinted from North American Nursing Diagnosis Association. (1994b). NANDA nursing diagnoses: Definitions and classifications, 1995–1996. Philadelphia: NANDA, with permission.)

Three-part statements include the diagnostic label reflecting the health problem (*P*), contributing factors (*E*), and signs and symptoms (*S*). For example,

- **P:** Constipation
- **E:** Related to mobility
- **S:** As manifested (or evidenced) by hard, formed stools and pain on defecation

A three-part diagnostic statement is possible only with an actual nursing diagnosis because the signs and symptoms are present. When potential nursing diagnoses are written, signs and symptoms are not present; thus, only a two-part statement is possible.

Historical Development of Nursing Diagnoses. Since the mid-1970s an effort has been made to identify nursing diagnoses. This work began formally in 1973 at the First National Conference for Classification of Nursing Diagnoses. At this time, NANDA was established as the formal group for identifying, reviewing, and endorsing nursing diagnoses. Conferences have been held since to consider additions and revisions to the list of accepted diagnoses. NANDA used retrospective recall for identifying nursing diagnoses by having nurses describe health conditions experienced in clinical practice. Nurses were asked to recall a particular patient problem from their practice, from which NANDA group members identified the nursing diagnosis. There is, of course, a bias to this method related to the nurse's recall of the patient problem.

The process used by NANDA has evolved from acceptance of the nursing diagnosis by small groups at the national conferences to a formal procedure for review. The review system includes a number of stages: comprehensive literature review, reanalysis of collected data, field studies, and collaboration with others for extensive field trials (NANDA, 1994a). Regardless of the review process used, some nurses have criticized the list in terms of clarity of the diagnoses and relevance to practice. No system of nursing diagnoses, however, will be accepted by all nurses, and nurses have the option of not using diagnoses they believe are questionable in their practice.

Planning

Nursing diagnosis provides the basis for the next phase of the nursing process, planning care, to address the client's health problems. Planning includes setting priorities, establishing goals, and selecting interventions.

Setting Priorities

Frequently, multiple nursing diagnoses are identified for a client, and priorities need to be set because not all diagnoses and goals can be or should be addressed at the same time. The first step in prioritizing problems is to identify the most important ones for the client. Some problems are life threatening and may have deleterious effects on the client; these must be taken care of immediately. The nature of the health problems, their immediate and potential effects on the client, and the client's overall health status also influence the priorities set by the nurse. Treatments received may have high priority if they adversely affect the patient. Factors such as availability of time, personnel, resources, cost, and coordination of care are important as well. Establishment of priorities results in a preferential order of goals that provides direction in planning care.

Establishing Goals of Care

Developing goals is an important step in the planning process because it identifies the desired outcomes of care. Doenges et al. (1995) define *goals* as the expected progress of the client in response to treatment (p. 76). Goals represent the desired level of wellness for the client. Goals set by nursing must be congruent with goals of other health professionals to ensure a coordinated approach to care.

The two types of goals are: (1) short-term goals, which are achieved quickly or as interim steps to meeting a goal that requires more time, and (2) long-term goals, which are met over a longer period. In some instances, long-term goals reflect the overall goal of care and may not be met before discharge.

Goals are stated in terms of patient *outcomes*, or what the patient will be able to accomplish rather than what the nurse plans to do. Goals should be specific to the client, reflecting the client's particular circumstances and should be both realistic and attainable. Goals may be written for each nursing diagnosis. For example, with the nursing diagnosis of constipation related to immobility, a goal might be stated as follows: "The client will demonstrate improved bowel elimination." With the nursing diagnosis of ineffective airway clearance related to postoperative immobility, a goal might be stated as follows: "The client will maintain a clear airway."

The literature reveals differences in the way in which goals should be stated. What is important, regardless of the model for stating goals, is that the goals represent the expected behaviors of the client and are derived from the nursing diagnoses.

Goals need to be stated in measurable terms because they provide criteria for determining the effectiveness of nursing interventions. Measurable verbs describe the exact behavior of the patient, family, or group. These behaviors may be cognitive (knowledge), psychomotor (skill), or affective (value). Table 5–2 provides a list of verbs in each of these three domains that are measurable and, therefore, appropriate for use in stating client goals.

Selecting Intervention Strategies

The planning process involves the selection of nursing interventions, nursing activities, and actions directed toward goal achievement. Bulechek and McCloskey (1992) define *nursing interventions* as direct care treatments that nurses perform on behalf of clients (p. 6). Nursing interventions include treatments for specific nursing diagnoses, physician-initiated treatments, and other nursing activities to assist the patient with "daily essential functions" (p. 7). Interventions directed toward nursing diagnoses reflect the etiology component of the nursing diagnostic statement. Nursing actions are planned to eliminate or at least reduce the effects of these contributing factors. With the nursing diagnosis of ineffective airway clearance related to postoperative immobility, interventions would be planned to reduce the effect of the immobility following surgery. With potential nursing diagnoses, interventions frequently focus on assessing client status to monitor the problem and avoid its becoming a reality.

Nursing practice requires multiple intervention strategies to meet client needs. Some patient problems are accompanied by prescribed nursing measures, actions typically performed for clients with a particular problem, such

TABLE 5–2. VERBS APPROPRIATE FOR WRITING OBJECTIVES IN THE COGNITIVE, AFFECTIVE, AND PSYCHOMOTOR DOMAINS

1. Cognitive		2. Affective	
Define	Apply	Acknowledge	Participate in
Identify	Use	Show awareness of	Respect
Name	Relate	Discuss willingly	Support
Recognize	Compare	Express satisfaction in	Assume responsibility
Give examples of	Contrast	Seek opportunities	Declare
State in own words	Detect	Accept	Defend
Demonstrate use of	Distinguish	Agree	Act consistently
Describe	Evaluate	Cooperate with	Is accountable
Explain	Classify		
Differentiate	Design	3. Psychomotor	
Discriminate	Develop	Follow example of	Demonstrate skill
Interpret	Modify	Imitate	Perform
Select	Organize	Follow procedure	Carry out
Conclude	Synthesize	Practice	
Determine	Assess		
Predict	Judge		

as interventions to reduce the effect of being immobilized—positioning, turning, coughing, and deep breathing. In other situations, however, the nurse needs to decide creatively on the best interventions for a particular patient and plan care because prescribed activities have not yet been established. In these situations, the nurse considers alternatives and consequences of different approaches to care if selected and determines the best action to take in terms of its benefits. Such decision making is important in choosing interventions that have an underlying scientific basis.

Bulechek and McCloskey (1992) suggest that nurses consider six areas when choosing an intervention:

1. Desired patient outcome
2. Characteristics of the nursing diagnosis
3. Research base of the intervention
4. Feasibility of successfully implementing the intervention
5. Acceptability of the intervention to the client
6. Capability of the nurse

It is important to consider what Bulechek and McCloskey refer to as the "research base of the intervention" because this base provides a scientific rationale for its use. Heater, Becker, and Olson (1988) reviewed 84 studies, both published and unpublished, that evaluated different interventions used in nursing practice and related patient outcomes. Findings suggest that research-based nursing interventions offer better outcomes for patients than routine procedural care.

In addition to activities specific to a nursing diagnosis, interventions such as counseling and teaching are necessary for many health problems. Therapeutic communication skills are critical to developing a relationship with the client and family and are important in planning and carrying out care. Teaching is a significant intervention strategy included in most plans of care, ranging from information sharing to assisting the client to develop new health behaviors.

The final step in the planning process is to document or write the plan of care. The plan of care includes important data about the client; the data are organized so that they communicate clearly the nursing diagnoses, goals, and intervention strategies. Although formats for care plans differ across institutions, each plan should provide a central source of information about the client essential in coordinating care and communicating with others involved in the care. Care plans may be computer-generated; standardized care plans that the nurse adapts, as needed, for the individual client; in the form of critical pathways, an abbreviated plan of care providing outcomes to be achieved within a specified time frame; and other formats, depending on the clinical agency.

Implementation

Implementation is the action phase of the nursing process in which the nurse carries out the plan of care. Although the plan provides a framework for intervening, the nurse continually makes judgments about modifying the planned actions or collecting additional data when client status changes and the client is not achieving the goals. The attitudes and values of the nurse are important because they influence the way in which the nurse interacts with the patient and family and carries out care. Respect for the dignity and worth of others is of particular importance in the implementation of care.

Because nursing textbooks contain detailed information on various interventions that nurses use in clinical practice, specific interventions are not presented in this chapter. In addition to these sources, Bulechek and McCloskey (1992) describe nursing interventions, their related research base, and protocols for using and evaluating the intervention. During implementation, the nurse continually assesses client responses and movement toward achieving the outcomes of care and obtains data for use in evaluating the effectiveness of nursing interventions and need for alternative actions. Implementation also includes documenting nursing care in the medical record. Documentation provides a means of communicating data about the patient's status and assists others in assessing client responses.

Evaluation

Evaluation, the final phase of the nursing process, provides a measure of the effectiveness of nursing care in promoting the achievement of client goals. Patient responses are evaluated to determine whether the desired outcomes of care have been achieved. Evaluation is concerned with the quality of care—whether or not goals were attained, the process used in care of the client, and the environment in which the care was delivered. Donabedian (1969) identified three components in the evaluation of the quality of health care: (1) outcomes of care, (2) process of care, and (3) structure in which the care is provided. Although evaluation of outcomes of care is generally the nurse's primary concern in terms of the nursing process, evaluation of process and structure also are important because they provide data for answering questions such as, What steps are taken in the care of the patient? and What are characteristics of the setting that may influence the outcomes and process of care?

Outcome evaluation focuses on changes in the client as a result of nursing interventions. In this type of evaluation, the nurse determines the degree to which client goals were achieved. These goals were established in the planning phase; now, through evaluation, the nurse judges whether they were met. The goals thus become the criteria for evaluation, which again highlights the importance of developing goals that are measurable and specific. Based on the results of the evaluation, modifications may be needed in the plan of care.

Process evaluation is another type of evaluation, but the focus is on the nurse rather than the client. Evaluation addresses the process of care for the client from assessment through implementation in terms of quality of nursing actions. The ANA (1991) standards of clinical nursing practice provide a framework for process evaluation because they specify characteristics of quality for each phase of the nursing process. Two types of standards are available. The first ones are generic standards that focus on nursing practice in all specialty areas:

1. *Assessment.* The nurse collects client health data.
2. *Diagnosis.* The nurse analyzes the assessment data in determining diagnoses.
3. *Outcome identification.* The nurse identifies expected outcomes individualized to the client.
4. *Planning.* The nurse develops a plan of care that prescribes interventions to attain expected outcomes.
5. *Implementation.* The nurse implements the interventions identified in the plan of care.
6. *Evaluation.* The nurse evaluates the client's progress toward attainment of outcomes.*

Standards are also available for specialized areas of nursing practice.

Structure evaluation focuses on the health care setting in which care is provided. This type of evaluation provides data on variables such as the agency's policies and procedures, quantity and characteristics of nursing and other staff, availability of resources needed for care, and the relation-

*Adapted from American Nurses Association. (1991). *Standards of clinical nursing practice.* Kansas City, MO: Author, with permission.

ship between financial resources of the institution and effect on the delivery of care (Reilly & Oermann, 1992).

Evaluation is an important phase of the nursing process because it is the phase in which the nurse ascertains the degree to which client goals have been met. It is a critical step that enables the nurse to judge the effectiveness of nursing interventions in promoting attainment of the outcomes of care and the overall quality of that care.

NURSING MODELS AS FRAMEWORK FOR NURSING PROCESS

Nursing models provide a framework for using the nursing process. The model suggests data to be collected from the client and others and how to organize the information. The model also provides a perspective of the meaning of the resulting nursing diagnoses and guidelines for planning, intervening, and evaluating care. Two examples are provided.

In an assessment based on Roy's adaptation model, the nurse collects data on four adaptive modes: (1) physiological, (2) self-concept, (3) role function, and (4) interdependence and on the related stimuli. Once data are gathered, the nurse judges whether the behaviors are adaptive or ineffective. Nursing diagnoses represent statements about the client's adaptive behavior and influencing factors. Appendix B provides an example of an assessment form based on Roy's model. Planning involves the establishment of goals with the intent of promoting adaptation. Interventions focus on the management of stimuli, and evaluation seeks to determine the effectiveness of these interventions in promoting adaptive behavior.

Using Orem's self-care model, the nurse collects data on universal, developmental, and health deviation self-care requisites and self-care agency. Appendices C and D provide assessment guides based on Orem's nursing conceptual model. Appendix C is for use in community health nursing and D for acute care. Nursing diagnoses represent actual or potential self-care deficits. Planning within Orem's model involves designing a system of nursing (wholly compensatory, partly compensatory, and supportive-educative) based on the client's self-care deficits. Nursing actions compensate for the client's self-care limitations and assist the client and family in developing self-care activities. Evaluation focuses on whether there is a decrease in self-care deficit and the patient can provide continuing self care.

THEORETICAL PERSPECTIVES OF CLINICAL JUDGMENT

In caring for clients, the nurse continually makes decisions about nursing diagnoses and interventions. Clinical judgment, the cognitive or intellectual process underlying these decisions, is known to be complex. It is viewed typically as a series of decisions made by the nurse: decisions about *which* data to observe and collect; inferential decisions for interpreting the data and arriving at the diagnosis; and decisions on nursing management (Tanner, 1983, p. 3). Alternate explanations for this critical thinking process have been proposed: information processing theory, decision theory, and phenomenology.

Information processing theory as applied to clinical judgment describes the actual thought process used by practitioners in deriving a nursing diagnosis or deciding on appropriate interventions. The process is similar across health care professions, although the types of decisions differ. Nurses decide on nursing diagnoses; physicians use a similar thinking process to derive medical diagnoses.

From early work by Elstein, Shulman, and Sprafka (1978) on the clinical judgment process used by physicians, a model of diagnostic reasoning, based on information processing theory, was developed. From this work and research in nursing, the diagnostic reasoning processes used by nurses have been described (Carnevali et al., 1984; Putzier, Padrick, Westfall, & Tanner, 1985; Tanner, 1983, 1987; Tanner, Padrick, Westfall, & Putzier, 1987; Westfall, Tanner, Putzier, & Padrick, 1986).

In diagnostic reasoning, the nurse engages in four major cognitive activities: (1) attending to available cues (signs, symptoms, and other data about the client and environment); (2) generating tentative hypotheses about the cues (possible explanations for clusters of cues); (3) gathering data about the tentative hypotheses to rule them in or out; and (4) evaluating each hypothesis based on the data to decide on the diagnoses (Putzier et al., 1985, p. 431). Research has indicated that these tentative diagnostic hypotheses are generated early in an assessment of a client (Elstein et al., 1972; Elstein et al., 1978; Putzier et al., 1985; Tanner, 1987). Arriving at early hypotheses is one strategy that helps practitioners manage the large amount of information to be processed. Early hypotheses about possible diagnoses guide subsequent data gathering in that information can be collected to rule in or out each hypothesis, thus providing a means of managing the data. As the nurse begins an assessment, clusters of cues suggest tentative hypotheses about the nursing diagnoses. Data then are gathered on these hypotheses until a diagnosis is made (Carnevali et al., 1984; Elstein et al., 1978; Putzier et al., 1985). This information assists the nurse in evaluating each hypothesis to decide which to keep or change and which to reject because the data no longer support that particular diagnosis for the client. The nurse then can select a diagnostic label to fit the data, the final stage in the process. After deciding on a nursing diagnosis, the nurse then can plan an appropriate course of action.

Decision theory provides another perspective to clinical judgment. Decision theory uses statistical models to make a diagnosis. Two models have been tested: (1) the Bayesian model, and (2) the lens model.

Research on clinical judgment based on *phenomenology* focuses on how decisions are made in real clinical practice and influences on those decisions. This perspective in nursing has been studied and advanced by Benner (1984). Through interviews and observations of nurses, Benner attempted to determine how nurses progressed from novices to experts in clinical nursing practice. Based on her research, Benner identified five stages of development:

Stage 1. *Novice.* Beginners or novices in nursing, lacking experience in clinical situations in which they need to perform, use context-free rules to guide their actions in the clinical setting. These general rules, or procedural lists of "things to do," unfortunately do not provide guidelines on the actions to take in the actual clinical situation.

Stage 2. *Advanced beginner.* Advanced beginners have had enough clinical experience to identify meaningful characteristics, or "aspects," of the clinical situation. These aspects are important to identify when making decisions about a client.

Stage 3. *Competence.* Competence, according to Benner, is typified by the nurse with 2 or 3 years of experience in similar clinical situations. This consistency of experience is needed to develop an ability to view nursing actions in terms of long-term goals and plans. Such planning requires consideration of what aspects of the present and future clinical situation are most important (p. 26). At this stage of development, the nurse is better able to cope with the demands of clinical nursing practice and is less dependent on rules to guide decision making.

Stage 4. *Proficient.* Because of prior experience with similar clinical situations, the proficient nurse has developed an ability to view the clinical situation as a whole, rather than focusing on specific aspects within it. The nurse has learned what to expect typically with a given client. Understanding the whole situation promotes decision making in that the nurse has a "perspective on which of the many existing attributes and aspects present are the important ones" (p. 29).

Stage 5. *Expert.* Extensive experience in the clinical field provides the expert with an "intuitive grasp" of the clinical situation and ability to focus quickly on the problem at hand. Decisions by experts are based on their perception of the clinical situation as a whole. Extensive experience in nursing has provided them with past concrete clinical situations that represent paradigm cases for making judgments about the client for whom they presently are caring. Past experience, therefore, "guides the expert's perceptions and actions and allows for a rapid perceptual grasp of the situation." (p. 8)

CRITICAL THINKING

There is much discussion in the literature about critical thinking and its use in nursing. The ability to think critically is essential to nursing practice and carrying out the nursing process. Nurses need to think critically to be "safe, competent, and skilled practitioners" (Miller & Malcolm, 1990, p. 67). Nurses who engage in critical thinking raise questions about care and interventions, search for answers, and consider multiple perspectives regarding care.

While accepted as an important cognitive skill used by nurses in clinical practice, varied definitions exist of critical thinking. Reilly and Oermann (1992) define critical thinking as rational thinking, an ability to evaluate statements and situations and base that evaluation on evidence. Paul (1993) describes critical thinking as purposeful and disciplined thinking based on intellectual standards. As a result, critical thinking yields well-reasoned answers. Nurses who engage in critical thinking do not accept statements outright but instead seek reasons for them.

Kataoka-Yahiro and Saylor (1994) define critical thinking as "reflective and reasonable thinking about nursing problems without a single solution and focused on deciding what to believe and do" (p. 352). In this conceptualization, the outcome of critical thinking is clinical judgment relevant to nursing problems (p. 352). These judgments may relate to decisions nurses make about clients as well as other nursing decisions such as ones pertaining to management and other dimensions of nursing practice.

While there are many views of critical thinking in nursing (Kataoka-Yahiro & Saylor, 1994), the perspective offered here is that critical thinking is the thought process underlying the nursing process and clinical judgment. Critical thinking is not the same as the nursing process. It is "much broader than nursing process alone" (Rane-Szostak & Robertson, 1996). In assessment, critical thinking enables the nurse to collect significant data, differentiate relevant from irrelevant information, identify cues in the data and cluster them, decide when additional data are needed to derive a nursing diagnosis, and make decisions about patient problems based on the data. Critical thinking enables the nurse to examine multiple problems and decide on nursing diagnoses. At this point in the nursing process, critical thought is needed to consider different problems which might be possible, to evaluate each one, and to decide on diagnoses. In the intervention phase, the nurse needs to generate all possible approaches and alternatives, evaluate strengths and weaknesses of each one, and decide on the best approach for the particular client. Alfaro-LeFevre (1995) suggests that in the evaluation phase, critical thinking enables the nurse to reassess, evaluate the accuracy of diagnoses, reexamine the appropriateness of goals, determine goal achievement, and evaluate factors promoting or impeding attainment of goals (p. 45).

SUMMARY

Nursing process is the methodology of nursing practice. It is the means through which the nurse delivers care to the individual client, family, groups, and community. The phases of the nursing process are interrelated and include assessment, diagnosis, planning, intervention, and evaluation. In assessment, the first phase, data are collected to make the nursing diagnoses. Studies in clinical judgment indicate that practitioners generate possible diagnoses about the client early in an assessment and gather data in relation to those diagnoses as a means of ruling them in or out. The data to be collected and ways in which they are organized vary with the conceptual model of nursing used and other frameworks such as functional health patterns.

The second phase of the nursing process, diagnosis, begins with an analysis of the data and concludes with an identification of the nursing diagnoses. Clinical judgment is the cognitive or intellectual process used by the nurse for analyzing data and deriving a nursing diagnosis, as well as deciding on nursing interventions. There are three components of a nursing diagnosis, referred to as the PES format: (1) health *p*roblem of the individual, family, group, or community; (2) *e*tiological or related factors; and (3) *s*igns and *s*ymptoms. The PES format provides a structure for writing diagnoses for clients and a means of communicating them to other practitioners. The NANDA list of accepted nursing diagnoses assists nurses in labeling the health problems of their clients. Research continues on the validation and testing of nursing diagnoses.

Nursing diagnoses provide the framework for planning care that addresses these health problems. Planning includes setting priorities of care, developing goals (outcomes of care), and choosing intervention strategies to achieve them. The implementation phase of the nursing process represents the action step in which the nurse carries out the plan of care. In the final phase, evaluation, the quality of the care delivered is judged, particularly as it relates to attainment of the outcomes of care.

Different theoretical perspectives have been offered to describe the clinical judgment process used by nurses and other health care practitioners. Theory and research indicate that the nurse attends initially to available cues. The nurse then generates tentative diagnostic hypotheses about possible explanations for clusters of cues and gathers data about the hypotheses to rule them in or out. Finally, the nurse evaluates each hypothesis based on the data collected to decide on the nursing diagnoses. Research also has suggested that these hypotheses about possible nursing diagnoses are generated early in an assessment and are used to direct subsequent data gathering. Critical thinking influences the nurse's judgments and decisions made in the practice setting.

REFERENCES

Alfaro-LeFevre, R. (1995). *Critical thinking in nursing.* Philadelphia: Saunders.

American Nurses Association. (1991). *Standards of clinical nursing practice.* Kansas City, MO: Author.

American Nurses Association. (1995). *Nursing's social policy statement.* Washington, DC: Author.

Benner, P. (1984). *From novice to expert: Excellence and power in clinical nursing practice.* Menlo Park, CA: Addison-Wesley.

Bulecheck, G. M., & McCloskey, J. C. (1992). *Nursing interventions: Essential nursing treatments* (2nd ed.). Philadelphia: Saunders.

Carnevali, D. L., Mitchell, P. H., Woods, N. F., & Tanner, C. A. (1984). *Diagnostic reasoning in nursing.* Philadelphia: Lippincott.

Carpenito, L. J. (1995). *Nursing diagnosis: Application to clinical practice* (6th ed.). Philadelphia: Lippincott.

Doenges, M. E., Moorhouse, M. F., & Burley, J. T. (1995). *Applications of nursing process and nursing diagnosis: An interactive text for diagnostic reasoning* (2nd ed.). Philadelphia: Davis.

Donabedian, A. (1969). *A guide to medical care administration. Vol. II: Medical care appraisal—Quality and utilization.* New York: American Public Health Association.

Elstein, A. S., Kagan, N., Shulman, L. S., Jason, H., & Loupe, M. J. (1972). Methods and theory in the study of medical inquiry. *Journal of Medical Education, 47,* 85–92.

Elstein, A. S., Shulman, L. S., & Sprafka, S. A. (1978). *Medical problem-solving.* Cambridge: Harvard University Press.

Gordon, M. (1987). *Nursing diagnosis: Process and application* (2nd ed.). New York: McGraw-Hill.

Gordon, M. (1995). *Manual of nursing diagnosis, 1995–1996* (7th ed.). St. Louis: Mosby.

Heater, B. S., Becker, A. M., & Olson, R. K. (1988). Nursing interventions and patient outcomes: A meta-analysis of studies. *Nursing Research, 37,* 303–307.

Kataoka-Yahiro, M., & Saylor, C. (1994). A critical thinking model for nursing judgment. *Journal of Nursing Education, 33,* 351–356.

Miller, M. A., & Malcolm, N. S. (1990). Critical thinking in the nursing curriculum. *Nursing & Health Care, 11,* 67–73.

NANDA. (1994a). NANDA News. *Nursing Diagnoses, 5*(2), 52–53.

NANDA. (1994b). *NANDA nursing diagnoses: Definitions and classifications 1995–1996.* Philadelphia: Author.

Paul, R. W. (1993). *Critical thinking: What every person needs to survive in a rapidly changing world.* Santa Rosa, CA: Foundation for Critical Thinking.

Putzier, D. J., Padrick, K., Westfall, U. E., & Tanner, C. A. (1985). Diagnostic reasoning in critical care nursing. *Heart & Lung, 14,* 430–437.

Rane-Szostak, D., & Robertson, J. F. (1996). Issues in measuring critical thinking: Meeting the challenge. *Journal of Nursing Education, 35,* 5–11.

Reilly, D. E., & Oermann, M. H. (1992). *Clinical teaching in nursing education* (2nd ed.). New York: National League for Nursing.

Tanner, C. A. (1983). Research on clinical judgment. In W. L. Holzemer (Ed.), *Review of research in nursing education* (pp. 2–32). Thorofare, NJ: Slack.

Tanner, C. A. (1987). Theoretical perspectives for research on clinical judgment. In K. J. Hannah, M. Reimer, W. C. Mills, & S. Letourneau (Eds.), *Clinical judgment and decision making: The future with nursing diagnosis* (pp. 21–28). New York: Wiley.

Tanner, C. A., Padrick, K. P., Westfall, U. E., & Putzier, D. J. (1987). Diagnostic reasoning strategies of nurses and nursing students. *Nursing Research, 36,* 358–363.

Westfall, U. E., Tanner, C. A., Putzier, D., & Padrick, K. P. (1986). Activating clinical inferences: A component of diagnostic reasoning in nursing. *Research in Nursing & Health, 9,* 269–277.

Yura, H., & Walsh, M. B. (1988). *The nursing process* (5th ed.). New York: Appleton-Century-Crofts.

Ziegler, S. M., Vaughan-Wrobel, B. C., & Erlen, J. A. (1986). *Nursing process, nursing diagnosis, nursing knowledge.* Norwalk, CT: Appleton-Century-Crofts.

BIBLIOGRAPHY

Ackley, B. J., & Ladwig, G. B. (1995). *Nursing diagnosis handbook: A guide to planning care* (2nd ed.). St. Louis: Mosby.

Andersen, J. E., & Briggs, L. L. (1988). Nursing diagnosis: A study of quality and supportive evidence. *Image: Journal of Nursing Scholarship, 20,* 141–144.

Bulechek, G. M., & McCloskey, J. C. (Eds.). (1992). *Nursing clinics of North America: Nursing interventions, 27*(2). Philadelphia: W.B. Saunders.

Carpenito, L. J. (1995). *Nursing care plans & documentation* (2nd ed.). Philadelphia: Lippincott.

Doenges, M. E. (1993). *Nurse's pocket guide: Nursing diagnoses with interventions* (4th ed.). Philadelphia: Davis.

Doenges, M. E., Moorhouse, M. F., & Geissler, A. C. (1993). *Nursing care plans* (3rd ed.). Philadelphia: Davis.

Facione, N. C., Facione, P. A., & Sanchez, C. A. (1994). Critical thinking disposition as a measure of competent clinical judgment: The development of the California Critical Thinking Disposition Inventory. *Journal of Nursing Education, 33,* 345–350.

Fernandez, R. (December 1994). Theory-based practice: A road to synthesis. *The International Orem Society Newsletter, 2*(5), 2–3.

Fernandez, R., Hebert, G., & Riggs, J. (1995). Transformational leadership: The partnership of theory-based practice and work redesign in a nursing care delivery system. In D. L. Flarey (Ed.), *Redesigning nursing care delivery systems: Transformation for the 90s.* Philadelphia: Lippincott.

Fernandez, R., & Wheeler, J. (1990). Organizing a nursing system through theory-based practice. In G. Gilbert, M. J. Madden, & E. Lawrenz (Eds.), *Patient care delivery models.* Rockville, MD: Aspen.

Gordon, M., Murphy, C. P., Candee, D., & Hiltunen, E. (1994). Clinical judgment: An integrated model. *Advances in Nursing Science, 16,* 55–70.

Griffiths, P. (1995). Progress in measuring nursing outcomes. *Journal of Advanced Nursing, 21,* 1092–1100.

Hammond, K. R., Kelly, K. J., Castellan, N. J., Jr., Schneider, R. J., & Vancini, M. (1966). Clinical inference in nursing: Use of information-seeking strategies by nurses. *Nursing Research, 15,* 330–336.

Hammond, K. R., Kelly, K. J., Schneider, R. J., & Vancini, M. (1966a). Clinical inference in nursing: Analyzing cognitive tasks representative of nursing problems. *Nursing Research, 15,* 134–138.

Hammond, K. R., Kelly, K. J., Schneider, R. J., & Vancini, M. (1966b). Clinical inference in nursing: Information units used. *Nursing Research, 15,* 236–243.

Harrington, P., & Kaniecki, N. (1988). Standards and QA—A common sense approach. *Nursing Management, 19*(1), 24–27.

Hartley, D., & Aukamp, V. (1994). Critical thinking ability of nurse educators and nursing students. *Journal of Nursing Education, 33,* 34–35.

Iowa Intervention Project. (1993). The NIC taxonomy structure. *Image: Journal of Nursing Scholarship, 25,* 187–192.

Iyer, P. W., & Camp, N. H. (1995). *Nursing documentation: A nursing process approach* (2nd ed.). St. Louis: Mosby.

Jenny, J. (1989). Classifying nursing diagnoses: A self-care approach. *Nursing & Health Care, 10,* 83–88.

Jones, J. A. (1988). Clinical reasoning in nursing. *Journal of Advanced Nursing, 13,* 185–192.

Kintgen-Andrews, J. (1991). Critical thinking and nursing education: Perplexities and insights. *Journal of Nursing Education, 30,* 152–157.

Lowe-Surge, R., Marvulli, C. M., & O'Brien, B. J. (1988). Staff nurses set standards for care. *Nursing Administration Quarterly, 12,* 63–67.

Lunney, M., & Paradiso, C. (1995). Accuracy of interpreting human responses. *Nursing Management, 26*(10), 48H–48K.

MacKenzie, S. J., & Laschinger, H. K. S. (1995). Correlates of nursing diagnosis quality in public health nursing. *Journal of Advanced Nursing, 21,* 800–808.

MacLeod, F., & MacTavish, M. (1988). Solving the nursing care plan dilemma: Nursing diagnosis makes the difference. *Journal of Nursing Staff Development, 4,* 70–73.

Maynard, C. A. (1996). Relationship of critical thinking ability to professional nursing competence. *Journal of Nursing Education, 35,* 12–18.

McCloskey, J. C., & Bulechek, G. M. (1996). *Nursing interventions classification (NIC)* (2nd ed.). St. Louis: Mosby.

McFarland, G. K., & McFarland, E. A. (1993). *Nursing diagnosis & intervention* (2nd ed.). St. Louis: Mosby.

Miller, G. A. (1956). The magical number seven, plus or minus two: Some limits on our capacity for processing information. *Psychological Review, 63,* 81–97.

Newell, A., & Simon, H. A. (1972). *Human problem-solving.* Englewood Cliffs, NJ: Prentice-Hall.

O'Connell, B. (1995). Diagnostic reliability: A study of the process. *Nursing Diagnosis, 6,* 99–107.

Radwin, L. E. (1995). Conceptualizations of decision making in nursing: Analytic models and "knowing the patient." *Nursing Diagnosis, 6,* 16–22.

Rasch, R. F. (1987). The nature of taxonomy. *Image: Journal of Nursing Scholarship, 19,* 147–149.

Roberts, S. L. (1987a). The future marriage between diagnosis related groups and nursing diagnosis related groups. *Critical Care Nursing Quarterly, 9*(4), 70–81.

Roberts, S. L. (1987b). The role of collaborative nursing diagnosis in critical care. *Critical Care Nurse, 7*(4), 81–86.

Rubenfeld, M. G., & Scheffer, B. K. (1995). *Critical thinking in nursing: An interactive approach.* Philadelphia: Lippincott.

Simon, H. A. (1978) Information-processing theory of human problem-solving. In W. K. Estes (Ed.), *Handbook of learning and cognitive processes: Human information processing* (Vol. 5, pp. 271–295). New York: Wiley.

Snyder, M. (1993). Critical thinking: A foundation for consumer-focused care. *Journal of Continuing Education in Nursing, 24*, 206–210.

Stark, J. (1995). Critical thinking: Taking the road less traveled. *Nursing 1995, 25*(11), 52–56.

Sternberg, R. J., & Lubart, T. I. (1995). *Defying the crowd*. New York: The Free Press.

Tanner, C. A. (1987). Teaching clinical judgment. In J. J. Fitzpatrick & R. L. Taunton (Eds.), *Annual review of nursing research* (Vol. 5, pp. 153–173). New York: Springer.

VanLeit, B. (1995). Using the case method to develop clinical reasoning skills in problem based learning. *American Journal of Occupational Therapy, 40*, 348–353.

Wells, D. L. (1995). The importance of critical theory to nursing: A description using research concerning discharge decision-making. *Canadian Journal of Nursing Research, 27*(2), 45–50.

White, J. E., Nativio, D. G., Kobert, S. N., & Engberg, S. J. (1992). Content and process in clinical decision-making by nurse practitioners. *Image: Journal of Nursing Scholarship, 24*, 153–158.

Woodtli, A. (1988). Identification of nursing diagnoses and defining characteristics: Two research models. *Research in Nursing & Health, 11*, 399–406.

Young, C. E. (1987). Intuition and nursing process. *Holistic Nursing Practice, 1*(3), 52–62.

Communication and Nursing Practice

Laurel L. Northouse

Effective communication is essential for nursing practice. Communication is the process that links nurses with clients and enables them to work together to achieve mutual, health-related goals. Communication also is necessary for satisfying relationships among health professionals. Through effective communication, nurses and other professionals develop collaborative relationships that enable them to provide well-coordinated, high-quality health care.

This chapter examines communication in nursing practice and provides guidelines to help nurses to improve their communication with clients and other health professionals. The first section of the chapter is a discussion of the importance of communication in health care. The second section provides a theoretical orientation for understanding communication in health care relationships. The developmental phases of the nurse–client relationship are discussed, as are specific factors that promote effective communication with clients and with other health professionals.

IMPORTANCE OF COMMUNICATION IN NURSING PRACTICE

Nursing has a long history of recognizing the importance of effective interpersonal relationships between nurses and clients. Peplau's (1952) seminal work, *Interpersonal Relations in Nursing*, underscores the critical role that interpersonal relationships play in client outcomes. Peplau (1965) argues that the interpersonal relationship between the nurse and client is the core of nursing.

Nurse investigators have continued to emphasize the importance of nurse–client communication. Studies have focused on areas such as empathy in nurse–client interactions (Olson, 1995; Reid-Ponte, 1992); the elements of a caring relationship (Larson, 1986); confirmation of communication behaviors (Drew, 1986; Heineken, 1982); and the role of nonverbal communication in nurse–client interactions (Bottorff, 1993). Furthermore, effective nurse–client communication is associated with increased coping ability (Drew, 1986) and greater compliance with health care regimens (Hanna, 1993; Street et al., 1993).

Although effective communication is associated with positive health outcomes, evidence suggests that nurse–client communication sometimes is limited or problematic (Fraser & Gallop, 1993). In a study of cancer patients, nearly half of the patients said that they did not discuss their problems with a nurse (Frank-Stromborg & Wright, 1984). Among the reasons given by patients for limited nurse–client communication were a general lack of contact with nurses and the perception that nurses were too busy. Many nurses recognize the importance of communication, but they have little time simply to interact and "be with" clients. Supportive interactions often have to occur while nurses are concurrently carrying out other physical tasks. In addition, nurses sometimes lack the communication skills necessary to deal with clients' complex psychosocial concerns. Perhaps it is not surprising that nurses often report a need for further education in communication.

Equally important to effective nurse–client communication is the quality of communication that exists between nurses and other health professionals. A number of studies report that the nature of the interpersonal relationships among professionals in health care settings has an impact on the kind and quality of health care provided to clients. Knaus, Draper, Wagner, and Zimmerman (1986) found that the quality of the relationships between physicians and nurses in intensive care units was a critical factor in lower patient mortality rates. Feiger and Schmitt (1979) reported that the degree of collegial interaction among health professionals was related to several positive health outcomes for clients. Effective professional–professional communication also is associated with higher job satisfaction and better job performance by nurses (Pincus, 1986). Taken together, these studies highlight the important role of effective communication in many areas of the health care delivery system.

THEORETICAL ORIENTATION TO INTERPERSONAL COMMUNICATION

A description of the theoretical assumptions that underlie the communication process is necessary to understand specific aspects of nurse–client communication and of professional–professional communication. Communication theory and King's nursing theory provide a basis for interpersonal communication.

Communication Theory

In studying how people communicate with one another, researchers delineate three basic assumptions about human communication (Berlo, 1960; Watzlawick, Beavin, & Jackson, 1967). These assumptions both guide and explain communication that occurs between individuals in health care settings.

Assumption 1: Interpersonal Communication Is a Process

The word *communication* often triggers the image of one person sending a message to another person. This image is based on a linear approach to communication. The linear approach, which also has been referred to as the *hypodermic approach*, assumes that one person instills or injects a message into another person (Burgoon, Heston, & McCroskey, 1974). From this perspective, communication is perceived as occurring in one direction with one person having a direct influence on a second person. A problem with the linear approach is that it is too restrictive. In real life, communication is more than a one-way linear event; it is an ongoing, ever-changing process (Berlo, 1960; Miller, 1972).

The assumption that human communication is a process is important because it underscores the complex nature of interpersonal communication in nursing practice. The assumption directs people to examine factors that affect both the nurse and the client and to determine how the continuous interchange between them will vary depending on the nature of the situation. Although an analysis of a single message created by one person and sent to another may be important, an analysis of communication as a process is even more important because it provides a richer understanding of how messages interact with and are influenced by other variables (Figure 6–1).

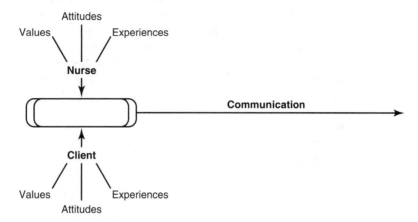

Figure 6–1. The Process Nature of Nurse–Client Communication

Assumption 2: Interpersonal Communication Is Transactional

The assumption that communication is transactional suggests that both individuals in an interaction affect and are affected by each other (Wilmot, 1979). Each individual is both a source and a receiver, and each has a reciprocal influence on the other. As a nurse constructs a message for a client, the nurse also is receiving cues from the client that influence the way in which the nurse formulates the message. A transactional approach forces individuals to consider the simultaneous interplay between the sender and the receiver of the message.

A transactional approach shifts the focus away from determining how one person affects the other; instead, the focus is on the relationship that has developed between two people and how it is maintained through their mutual influence on one another. For example, if a nurse chooses to be dominant with a client, it may be because the nurse desires to be dominant in general, or it may be because the nurse picks up clues from the client that seem to indicate that the client would prefer to be submissive. The interaction can be influenced by the preferences of the nurse or client, their perceptions of the other person's preferences, or by a combination of these factors working together. Forchuk (1995) found that a *combination* of nurse factors and client factors had a stronger effect on the quality of the therapeutic relationship that developed than either nurse or client factors alone. Forchuk's study underscores the importance of viewing relationships from a transactional perspective.

Assumption 3: Human Communication is Multidimensional

According to communication theorists, communication occurs on two levels: (1) the content dimension and (2) the relationship dimension (Watzlawick et al., 1967). The *content dimension* refers to the actual words or the information contained in a message, whereas the *relationship dimension* refers to the way in which the participants relate to one another.

To illustrate the two dimensions, consider the following hypothetical request made by a nurse to a new diabetic patient: "Please show me the procedure you follow for giving yourself insulin." The content dimension of this message refers to technique for insulin administration. The relationship dimension refers to how the nurse and client are associated with one another. It includes the nurse's attitude toward the client, the client's attitude toward the nurse, and their mutual feelings toward one another. The relationship dimension of a message implies how the content dimension should be interpreted, because the content alone can be interpreted in many ways. If, for example, a caring relationship exists between the nurse and the client, then the content ("Please show me the procedure you follow . . .") probably will be interpreted by the client as a helpful inquiry from a nurse who is concerned about the client's ability to administer his or her insulin. If, on the other hand, an impersonal or distant relationship exists between nurse and client, then the client may interpret the content of the message as an authoritative directive given by a nurse who wants to evaluate the client's competence. The two interpretations illustrate how the meaning of a message is not in words alone but in the interpretation given within the context of the participants' relationship.

The implication of this assumption for nursing practice is that nurses need to be aware of both *how* they communicate with clients and *what* they communicate. In a study of the communication between nurses and clients in an oncology setting, Thorne (1988) found that communication perceived as unhelpful by the client is associated with a lack of concern on the part of the nurse. Communication with clients is more effective if nurses pay attention to both the content and relationship dimensions of messages.

Moreover, a nonverbal dimension of interpersonal communication exists. Investigators estimate that 65% to 70% of the meaning in a message is nonverbal (Birdwhistell, 1970); others estimate that more than 90% of the meaning of a message can be accounted for by nonverbal communication (Mehrabian, 1971). Nonverbal communication is especially relevant in nursing practice because clients and family members attend closely to the nonverbal expressions of nurses and other health professionals. Clients often believe that important information is "leaked" through nonverbal behavior (Friedman, 1979); hence, clients often analyze the nonverbal behavior of health professionals to determine whether professionals are being completely honest with them.

A number of studies document the importance of nonverbal communication. Nonverbal communication is associated with increased verbal interaction between nurse and client in psychiatric settings (Aguilera, 1967); greater self-exploration by clients (Pattison, 1973); more positive evaluation of counseling sessions (Alagna, Whitehers, Fisher, & Wicas, 1979); lessened distress in hospitalized children (Triplett & Arneson, 1979); and decreased anxiety in institutionalized elderly clients (Simington & Laing, 1993). Nonverbal cues help both clients and professionals to validate verbal messages they receive from others.

Nursing Theory

King's (1971, 1981) conceptual framework provides another theoretical orientation for describing and understanding interpersonal communication in nursing practice. King uses a systems perspective to discuss the interrelationship among personal, interpersonal, and social systems in health care settings. King emphasizes the interpersonal system, especially the interpersonal relationships between nurses and client.

According to King, both nurses and clients make judgments about their situations and about one another. These judgments are based on their unique perceptions. King (1981) explains that interactions are influenced by the needs, goals, expectations, and past experiences of both the patient and the nurse. Transactions result from the reciprocal relationship established by nurse and client as they participate together to set mutual goals.

King's conceptual framework is useful for understanding communication that occurs between nurses and clients in nursing practice. The framework emphasizes the importance of looking at the perceptions that both nurse and client bring to an interaction, and it also underscores the need for mutual goal setting between nurse and client. Like the communication theory discussed previously, King's nursing theory views nurse–client communication as a transactional, ongoing process.

DEVELOPMENTAL PHASES OF NURSE–CLIENT RELATIONSHIPS

Effective nurse–client relationships do not just happen. Rather, they are influenced by the personal characteristics of the nurse and the client, the developmental stage of their relationship, and various contextual factors. This section of the chapter focuses on the developmental phases of the nurse–client relationship.

The nurse–client relationship develops through four sequential phases: (1) preparation, (2) initiation, (3) exploration, and (4) termination (Northouse & Northouse, 1992; Sundeen, Stuart, Rankin, & Cohen, 1994). For purposes of discussion, each phase is considered separately. In reality, however, these phases frequently overlap or blend.

Preparation Phase

The preparation phase occurs before the actual meeting between nurse and client. Often, the importance of this phase is minimized or even ignored. Planning for this phase, however, can have an impact on the development of subsequent phases.

For the nurse, the preparation phase entails planning for the first meeting with the client as well as assessing one's own strengths and limitations. Planning includes activities such as getting assessment forms ready, having educational materials available, and locating an appropriate place to meet. During an initial meeting, communication is more effective if the nurse has arranged for a private, comfortable setting where minimal interruptions will occur, although in the acute care setting this is often difficult to achieve.

For clients, the preparation phase entails actively seeking professional assistance by arranging for a home, office, or clinic visit. During this phase, clients also anticipate the kind of information or concerns that they will share with the professional. Some clients come to appointments with detailed lists of concerns; others mentally outline issues that need to be addressed. Clients form images and expectations about their initial meeting and work through anxieties about sharing information with someone new.

As nurses and clients anticipate their meeting, it is important that they are aware of any preconceptions they may have about the other person—

because these preconceptions can affect the development of a therapeutic relationship. Forchuk (1994) examined the preconceptions of both nurses and clients in 124 newly formed dyads in various psychiatric settings. She found that the preconceptions of the nurse and client developed very early in the course of their relationship and underwent almost no change over a 6-month period of assessment. Furthermore, she found that the more positive the preconceptions held by the nurse and the client, the faster they were able to develop an effective working alliance. Forchuk's findings suggest that nurses need to engage in self-assessment so that they can become aware of personal biases or preconceptions they may hold. Likewise, nurses need to determine whether clients have any negative preconceptions that may interfere with the client's ability to form an effective relationship with the nurse.

Initiation Phase

The initiation phase occurs when nurse and client have their first contact with one another. Sundeen and associates (1994) contend that the initiation phase is important because it sets the overall tone for the nurse–client relationship.

Specific tasks need to be accomplished during the initiation phase. First, the nurse needs to establish a therapeutic climate that will foster trust and understanding. Communication techniques such as reflection, restatement, and clarification help to create the therapeutic climate. Second, the nurse needs to clarify the purpose of the initial meeting. Benjamin (1981) points out that ambiguous statements such as "I think you know why we are meeting" lead to uncertainty between participants. Clear statements of purpose, on the other hand, structure the relationship and offer a sense of direction to the interaction. Third, nurses need to formulate a contract with the client. A contract is a mutual agreement or mutual expectation established between nurse and client. The fourth task is to establish mutual goals. Mutual goal setting fosters collaboration and provides a sense of direction for the relationship.

Exploration Phase

The exploration phase often is called the working phase because it is the phase of the relationship during which the nurse and client examine and work on the client's concerns. The overall goal of the exploration phase is to help clients to build skills for coping with problems and stress.

The first task of this phase is to explore clients' personal concerns. Typically, communication techniques are more direct in this phase. The nurse may seek clarification, question inconsistencies, or offer alternative explanations. The second task is to help clients to manage anxiety generated by the discussion of personal issues. A supportive atmosphere helps clients to express feelings without fear of rejection. The third task is to help clients to develop new coping skills. By exploring concerns, clients may question their previous behavior and consider new options for dealing with personal concerns or health problems.

The exploration phase does not always proceed smoothly. Sayre (1978) reports some of the common mistakes made by nurses during this phase, such as changing topics prematurely, giving insufficient feedback, giving inappropriate advice, and responding in stereotypical ways. The direction and flow in the exploration phase vary according to characteristics of the nurse and client and the nature of the concerns being discussed. As exploration occurs, however, goals are addressed, plans are formulated, and the termination phase emerges.

Termination Phase

During this phase, the nurse assists the client to find closure to problems and concerns. The first task for this phase is to plan for closure. If the nurse and client are meeting for only one session, they may use termination time to finish covering a particular topic or to discuss plans for referral. If they have two or three sessions remaining before they terminate, they may want to discuss how they will use the time they have left. A second task for the nurse in the termination phase is to summarize issues that were raised or accomplishments that occurred. Summaries are most useful if they are brief and specify progress that has been made during the relationship.

Communication problems that have been observed more frequently during the termination phase are: (1) ending an interaction prematurely, (2) leaving insufficient time to deal with termination issues, (3) avoiding termination, and (4) bringing up new issues just as closure is about to occur (Sayre, 1978). These problems can be eliminated for the most part by attending to the tasks of termination.

Developing the nurse–client relationship takes time. Nurses in psychiatric and rehabilitation settings have more time to nurture the development of interpersonal relationships than of nurses in screening clinics, short-stay ambulatory settings, and hospitals. Nevertheless, by attending to the tasks of each phase, nurses can facilitate the development of effective therapeutic relationships.

FACTORS THAT ENHANCE NURSE–CLIENT RELATIONSHIPS

Although many factors can influence the effectiveness of nurse–client relationships, the discussion in this section focuses on three key factors: (1) responding with empathy, (2) providing confirmation, and (3) sharing information. These factors have received the greatest attention in the area of health communication and appear to have an impact on the overall effectiveness of the nurse–client relationship.

Responding with Empathy

Empathy is considered one of the most essential and at the same time one of the most complex factors affecting the communication between nurses and clients. Over the years, empathy has been defined in many ways. However, in most nursing research studies, *empathy* is defined as the ability of the nurse to perceive the meanings and feelings of the client and to communicate that understanding to the client (Gagan, 1983).

Empathy is not the same as sympathy. *Sympathy* is the concern or compassion shown by one person toward another person. Empathy, on the other hand, is an attempt by one person to *feel with* another person and to understand that person's point of view. According to Kalisch (1973), there are two reasons why sympathy is less helpful than empathy. First, when the nurse views the client in terms of how the nurse would feel if in a similar situation (sympathy), the nurse is not necessarily accurate in his or her perception. The client's reaction may be different from the nurse's reaction. Second, in sympathy, the nurse becomes preoccupied with her or his similarity to the client, which interferes with the nurse's ability to concentrate on the client and the client's point of view.

Several attempts have been made to measure the amount of empathy that nurses demonstrate toward clients. One approach is to ask a panel of experts to judge tape-recorded interactions between nurses and clients and to determine the degree to which the nurse is responding to the client in an empathetic manner (Williams, 1979). Another approach is to ask nurses to read several case studies of counseling situations and to choose, from a list of several responses, the response that would be the most empathetic (Forsyth, 1979). Another way of measuring empathy and one of the more widely used approaches is to ask clients to rate the amount of empathy that they perceive from nurses (Forsyth, 1979). Most investigators using this approach use the Barrett-Lennard Relationship Inventory, a 16-item questionnaire that asks one person (for example, the client) to rate another person (the nurse) on such items as "She/He tries to see things through my eyes" and "She/He understands me" (Barrett-Lennard, 1962).

Forsyth (1979) explored the amount of empathy between nurses and clients in a variety of clinical settings using two of the aforementioned approaches. Using the case study method, Forsyth found that only 50% of the nurses demonstrated high empathic ability based on the types of responses they would make to clients in the case studies. When clients were asked to actually rate their nurses' empathic abilities, however, 98% rated their nurses as highly empathetic. The study reveals that different methods for measuring empathy may produce different results.

Olson (1995) examined the relationship between nurse-expressed empathy and two outcomes: patient-perceived empathy and patient distress in an acute care setting. The results of the study indicated that as nurses expressed more empathy, patients felt more understood and reported less anxiety, depression, and anger. Olson's research highlights the important role that empathic communication plays in patients' response to illness and also lends support for continued efforts to teach empathy skills to nurses.

Some investigators believe that empathy is communicated along the nonverbal dimensions of an interaction. Hardin and Halaris (1983) studied the nonverbal behavior of nurses who were rated as highly empathetic or not empathetic by patients. The investigators found a general pattern of differences: high-empathy nurses smiled but laughed less than low-empathy nurses; they engaged in moderate versus frequent gesturing; and they kept their legs still versus moving their legs frequently. These investigators contend that nonverbal communication and specific nonverbal behaviors may be associated with empathy.

For the most part, studies on empathy indicate that empathy has a positive effect on client outcomes (Olson, 1995; Williams, 1979). Empathy reduces clients' feelings of alienation and helps them to feel understood (Rogers, 1983). As clients feel understood in a nonjudgmental way, they feel more positive about their own value and worth. Although several communication techniques can be used to communicate empathy, such as reflection, restatement, and clarification, these techniques cannot be used in a mechanical or "rote" manner. Rather, they need to be used in the context of a caring relationship in which the nurse tries actively to understand the world of the client and then communicates this understanding to the client.

Providing Confirmation

In recent years, there has been a growing interest in the concept of confirmation and its relevance to nursing practice (Drew, 1986; Fraser & Gallop, 1993; Heineken, 1983). *Confirmation* refers to the verbal or nonverbal messages that one person sends to another that acknowledge, accept, or endorse the receiver of the message (Heineken, 1983). Although confirmation overlaps in many ways with the concept of empathy, it also is a distinct concept that requires further consideration.

According to communication research done by Sieburg (1969), interpersonal messages can be grouped into either confirming responses or disconfirming responses. *Confirming responses* acknowledge and validate the other person's perspective. They are responses that communicate to others that their opinions are of value even if they are different from one's own opinion. Examples of confirming responses include:

- Responding directly to a person's statements
- Nodding one's head
- Asking questions related to the same topic
- Showing verbal and nonverbal interest and awareness of what is being said
- Expressing agreement, disagreement, or neutrality

- Expanding or elaborating on content, expressing feelings about the content, or requesting clarification of what the other said (Heineken & Roberts, 1983, p. 78)

Disconfirming responses, on the other hand, exhibit indifference to and deny the experiences of others. Hence, they are responses that make the recipient feel discounted and negated. Examples of disconfirming responses include:

- Making irrelevant comments
- Responding ambiguously
- Interrupting
- Keeping silent when a response is indicated or failing to acknowledge an individual's communication
- Using impersonal language
- Introducing a different, unrelated topic
- Shifting the focus to a tangential subject
- Avoiding or shifting eye contact
- Turning away from the speaker
- Tapping one's feet or fingers
- Making demeaning or disparaging remarks
- Talking to another instead of deferring to the person speaking (Heineken & Roberts, 1983, pp. 78–79)

Heineken (1982) was one of the first nurses to study confirmation in a nursing practice setting. She compared the interpersonal responses of four groups of psychiatric clients with the responses of a group of people without psychiatric problems. She found that psychiatric clients engaged in significantly more disconfirming communication than did the people in the control group. An important implication of the study is that when psychiatric clients use primarily disconfirming communication, they are likely to receive disconfirming responses from others (Heineken, 1983). Over time, an ongoing pattern of dysfunctional communication can occur. Based on her research, Heineken encourages nurses to observe clients' interactions and, if necessary, to teach clients ways to use more confirming communication with others.

How does disconfirming behavior from a nurse affect a client? Drew (1986) studied confirming and excluding (disconfirming) responses between hospitalized patients and their caregivers. Drew found that patients who felt excluded by a caregiver experienced fear and anger and perceived themselves as a bother to the caregiver. In addition, these patients hesitated to ask the caregiver questions and found disconfirming interactions energy depleting, leaving them with less energy to cope with their health problems. Conversely, patients who experienced confirming responses from caregivers said that the caregiver's warm, nurturing responses gave them feelings of strength and relaxation. Patients also experienced more confidence in their own ability to cope with their situations, and they felt that they had more energy to direct toward their own recovery.

Based on patients' comments, Drew (1986) developed a composite of behaviors characteristic of caregivers who confirm rather than exclude clients. Caregivers who engage in excluding behaviors lack warmth, seem hurried, avoid eye contact with the patient, use a flat tone of voice or an abrupt manner of speaking, use jargon as a distancing maneuver, and avoid closeness to the patient. Conversely, caregivers who engage in confirming behaviors have a wider range of affective responses; have a relaxed, yet energetic manner; maintain eye contact during interactions; use a more expressive voice tone; avoid jargon; and maintain a closer position to the patient while speaking.

There is some indication that confirming and disconfirming responses are reciprocal in nature (Sundell, 1972). That is, when one person is confirming, the other person's response will be confirming; or when one person is disconfirming, the other person's response will be disconfirming. In some situations, a cycle of either confirming or disconfirming communication can occur (Northouse & Northouse, 1992). For example, a nurse who is physically exhausted by the events of the day may react in a disconfirming manner to a client's concern. In response, the client may disconfirm the nurse. The nurse again reacts negatively to the client's response and further disconfirms the client. This pattern can continue until the interaction terminates or until one of the participants in the interaction interrupts the cycle of disconfirming responses. Effective communication in nursing practice depends on nurses who continually assess their interactions with clients. Conscious attempts to use confirming communication responses will enhance the effectiveness of the nurse–client relationship and will assist clients to cope more effectively with their circumstances.

Sharing Information

Sharing information is another important component of nurse–client relationships. Information is important to clients because it helps to reduce their sense of uncertainty and gives them a framework for understanding events around them. Some investigators go so far as to say that communicating information to clients can improve their psychological responses to treatment (Waitzkin & Stoeckle, 1972). Given that information is important for clients, nurses frequently are confronted with questions such as how much information patients want, what kind of information patients need, and what is the best way to communicate information to clients.

Several factors make sharing information a more complex process for nurses than it initially appears. First, clients differ in their levels of comprehension (Greenwald & Nevitt, 1982), levels of competence (Schoene-Seifert & Childress, 1986), and preferences for information (Cassileth, Rupkis, Sutton-Smith, & March, 1980). Nurses need to consider these individual differences as they share information with clients. Second, information-giving sessions in many health care settings typically occur within a short period (Morse et al., 1992). Thus, there is little opportunity for questions, clarification, or even nursing assessment of the extent to which clients or family members understand the information. Third, the perceptions of nurses and clients about the kind of information that clients need can differ. To illustrate, Lauer, Murphy, and Powers (1982) studied how nurses and cancer patients ranked patients' educational needs. They found that patients ranked getting information about side effects as their major need, whereas nurses ranked dealing with feelings as patients' most important need. This example of different perceptions underscores the complexity of providing information. Nurses need to be sure that they are addressing the information needs of clients and not projecting their own perceptions of those needs onto clients.

Nurses also confront another problem in sharing information: they often are not viewed as a legitimate source of information for clients. Historically, when clients and family members asked a nurse for information about their blood pressure or temperature, the nurse told them to ask the physician. This practice of evading clients' questions or referring them to others distorted clients' perceptions of nurses as legitimate sources of information. Although nurses' attitudes have changed and nurses now recognize that it is within the scope of nursing practice to provide information, some research indicates that clients' and family members' perceptions of the nurse have not changed. For example, in a study of family members of cancer patients, Dyck and Wright (1986) reported that the majority of the family members did not view the nurse as having a major information-giving role. Approximately one third of the family members thought that releasing information was contrary to the nurse's code of ethics and beyond the nurse's scope of practice. Some family members said they were hesitant to ask a nurse for information because they thought that it would put the nurse in an awkward position. Other investigators report that patients perceive that physicians rather than nurses are the primary source of information about disease and treatment questions (Dodd, 1982; Frank-Stromborg & Wright, 1984).

What strategies can nurses use to facilitate sharing information with clients? First, nurses need to recognize and accept that they have a legitimate role to provide clients and family members with information. The social policy statement developed by the American Nurses Association (1995) mandates that nurses have the responsibility to assist clients with actual and potential problems and to help them find ways to alleviate health problems. Second, nurses must teach clients that they are available to provide them with information as well as with comfort and support. Third, nurses need to assume a more active role in *initiating* information-giving sessions with clients. Bond (1982) studied the relationships between nurses and family members and found that in all but one of the nurse–family interactions that occurred, the responsibility for initiating the interaction fell on family members. Given that other investigators report that clients and family members are hesitant to approach nurses because they think nurses are "too busy" or are not legitimate sources of information, it is essential that nurses assume a greater role in seeking out clients' concerns and questions. Fourth, nurses need to assess the amount and type of information clients want as well as the degree to which clients understand information they are given.

Empathy and confirmation focus primarily on the relationship dimension of the communication process, whereas sharing information centers primarily on the content dimension of the communication process. Because the content and relationship dimensions of interpersonal communication are interwoven, more effective communication will occur when nurses share information in an empathetic, confirming relationship.

FACTORS THAT PROMOTE EFFECTIVE INTERPERSONAL RELATIONSHIPS

A spirit of collegiality among nurses and other health professionals is essential to deliver high-quality health care. Health professionals need to collaborate to solve complex health care problems. Too often, however, conflicts and misunderstandings occur between professionals that interfere with effective working relationships. This section of the chapter focuses on three factors that promote effective relationships among health professionals: (1) clarifying roles, (2) sharing control, and (3) maintaining contact.

Clarifying Roles

Although health professionals work in close proximity, there is often little understanding of one another's roles. Leininger (1971) notes that health professionals spend anywhere from 2 to 8 years in professional education programs, yet have minimal exposure to the roles or expertise of other health professionals. Milne (1980) finds that students in various health disciplines have only a rough idea of each other's professional roles. This lack of understanding is a major factor in role confusion and territorial disputes between various health professionals (Fagin, 1992; Williams & Williams, 1982).

How can lack of knowledge of other people's roles create problems in interpersonal relationships? First, it can cause health professionals to make demands on one another that are inconsistent with their view of their own professional role (Northouse & Northouse, 1992). Nurses, for example, become frustrated when they are expected to do non-nursing tasks such as retrieve patients' charts, transport patients, or transcribe medical orders. These tasks are inconsistent with nurses' views of themselves as competent providers of complex patient care. Second, misunderstandings can lead to underutilization of one another's unique expertise. Nurses who spend their time carrying out the work of ward clerks have less time to perform expert nursing roles. Third, misunderstandings of one another's roles can increase territorial disputes. For example, social workers and clinical nurse specialists who do not understand the unique contribution of each other to the health care team can get caught in role struggles.

Although it seems obvious that nurses and other professionals need to clarify their roles with one another, it is not a simple task. One of the problems professionals encounter is that there is considerable overlap among roles. Weiss (1983) asked a sample of nurses, physicians, and consumers to identify whether 417 behaviors were appropriate to the nurse's role, the physician's role, or both. Of the 417 behaviors, 82% were rated by all three groups as being equally within the role of physician and nurse. Further adding to the role overlap is the fact that many tasks formerly considered solely the physician's tasks now are commonly carried out by nurses or shared with nurses (Mechanic & Aiken, 1982). Tasks such as monitoring electrocardiogram readings, administering intravenous medications, or assessing lung sounds are only a few of the tasks that have shifted to nurses. This shift has created confusion about the role of nursing in relation to medicine (Mechanic & Aiken, 1982).

Although all health professionals need to clarify their roles, it is especially important for nurses. Nurses' work often is invisible to others (Fagin, 1992). Nurses spend a great deal of time observing and assessing the health status of clients, but these activities often go unnoticed by other professionals and consumers. In many situations, other professionals and consumers often are unaware of the unique expertise of nurses. In Weiss's (1983) study with a group of physicians, nurses, and consumers, none of the professional behaviors was rated as solely in the domain of nursing, whereas a number of behaviors were rated solely in the domain of medicine. Furthermore, Weiss reported that nurse participants in the study could not agree on the behaviors that belonged solely to their professional domain. Weiss's study points out that nurses need to delineate their unique contribution to health care and then articulate their roles to others. Health professionals who understand and respect one another's areas of expertise will be in a better position to combine their collective resources and provide the comprehensive services that are needed in current health care settings.

Sharing Control

Equally important to clarifying roles is sharing control. *Sharing control* is the process in which health professionals attempt to have a mutual influence but no one particular group tries to dominate another. According to communication theory, control is manifested through "relational control" in interpersonal relationships (Watzlawick et al., 1967). *Relational control* is a transactional process that occurs as individuals decide how they are going to relate to one another and as they determine who has greater control in the relationship.

Three kinds of relationships emerge, depending on how relational control is negotiated among individuals (Figure 6–2). In the first kind of relationship, a *complementary relationship*, one person is dominant and the other is submissive. Control is not divided equally between the two participants. Historically, physicians and nurses have functioned in a complementary relationship. Physicians assumed the head position on the health care team, and nurses functioned in a dependent role carrying out physicians' orders (Kalisch & Kalisch, 1977). Although complementary relationships often are stable and predictable because individuals know where they stand with one another, they also can be repressive because they inhibit creativity and independent thinking in the subordinate person.

In the second kind of relationship, a *symmetrical relationship*, control is more evenly distributed between the two participants. Participants exchange ideas and are free to express their opinions. Although this kind of relationship initially appears ideal, power struggles can occur in symmetrical relationships when participants compete to acquire or give up control. For example, in a symmetrical nurse–physician relationship, if both assume dominant positions, conflict can occur as they struggle to determine who will have the final say in a treatment decision.

In the third kind of relationship, a *parallel relationship*, control moves back and forth between the two participants. Participants take turns holding and giving control, depending on the circumstances, rather than competing for control. For example, in a parallel nurse–physician relationship, the nurse may assume greater control than the physician in patient education areas, whereas the physician may assume greater control in pharmacological decisions. For the most part, parallel relationships are characterized by more effective and flexible communication among participants (Wilmot, 1979).

Relational control often is manifested in the degree of collaboration that occurs among health professionals. *Collaboration* is the ongoing inter-

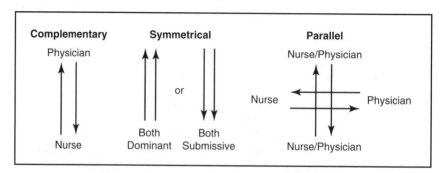

Figure 6–2. Types of Relationships Among Health Professionals

action that occurs between professionals in which each person contributes to the problem-solving effort that results in a new assessment, problem definition, or plan (Lamb & Napodano, 1984). It implies trust and respect of one another and of each person's work and perspective. Collaboration also incorporates the notion that a synergistic alliance forms among the participants that maximizes each person's contribution to the health care team (Pike, 1991). Collaboration also implies a distribution of control or a give-and-take of control rather than a fixed dominance of one professional over another. More and more professionals are realizing that to solve the complex health care problems confronting clients, they need expertise and input from a variety of health professionals.

Although collaboration seems essential, there are indications that professional collaboration is lacking in many health care settings. Lamb and Napodano (1984) studied the interactions between nurse practitioners and physicians and found minimal collaboration. Rather, they more often observed independent practice by each professional with only occasional consultations with one another. Feiger and Schmitt (1979) also report little collegiality among doctors, nurses, and nutritionists on health care teams. Among the health care teams they studied, a hierarchical pattern of interaction tended to persist, with the physician demonstrating the most active, influencing form of interaction.

What factors promote greater collaboration among professionals? According to Alt-White, Charns, and Strayer (1983), certain managerial and organizational factors enhance collaboration. These investigators found greater collaboration among physicians and nurses on primary care nursing and critical care units. Units characterized by more open communication and the ability to deal with conflict constructively also show greater nurse–physician collaboration. However, on units where nurses perceive considerable organizational stress, for example, difficulty getting supplies and frustrating work, there is less nurse–physician collaboration. Furthermore, units with more effective nursing coordination, such as discussions with nurse managers and use of nursing rounds, have greater nurse–physician collaboration.

In addition to these organizational factors, individual characteristics of physicians and nurses can affect collaborative efforts. Feiger and Schmitt (1979) find that the degree of nurse–physician collaboration differs according to the interactional style of the physician. Whereas some physicians in their study encouraged a high degree of participation from nurses, other physicians were indifferent to nurses' comments and discouraged team collaboration. Weiss and Remen (1983) report that nurses who minimize their professional expertise hinder the development of collaborative relationships with physicians. According to Pike (1991), nurses need to gain a sense of empowerment that enables them to overcome feelings of timidity, self-doubt, and subservience and allows them to function as full participants in the health care team. From a transactional perspective, both nurses and physicians influence the nature of their relationship and the degree of collaboration they can attain.

Collaboration is essential in community settings as well as in acute care settings. The increasing shift of health care services from hospital-based to community-based settings necessitates that health professionals engage in more collaborative efforts with consumers, community leaders, and professionals from a variety of community agencies. Chrislip and Larson (1994) identified several keys to developing successful collaboration in community settings (Table 6–1). These components highlight the importance of broad-based involvement by a variety of individuals, effective communication, skilled leadership, and the ability to move away from individual interests to the broader concerns of the community.

The dramatic changes in health care demand even greater interdisciplinary collaboration than has been seen in the past. Single discipline-centered approaches will not be able to address the complex biopsychosocial needs of clients and their family caregivers in either hospital or community-based settings (Fagin, 1992). Collaboration and the synergy that it creates give professionals a more comprehensive understanding of clients' situations than an individual clinician or discipline can achieve alone (Pike, 1991). Furthermore, because collaborative efforts have been associated with better patient outcomes (Feiger & Schmidt, 1979; Rubenstein et al., 1984) and with decreased health care costs (Fagin, 1992), it is imperative that health care professionals learn to share control and work together to improve patient care.

TABLE 6–1. KEYS TO SUCCESSFUL COLLABORATION IN COMMUNITY SETTINGS

Keys to Successful Collaboration	Rationale
Good timing and clear need	Provides momentum for collaborative effort
Broad-based involvement	Ensures that a variety of key participants are included
Credibility and openness of process	Helps process to be viewed as fair
Involvement by high-level, visible leaders	Brings credibility to process
Support of "established" authorities	Prevents undermining powers that be
Strong leadership of the process	Helps to enforce positive group norms
Interim successes	Maintains momentum
Shift to broader concerns	Enables participants to move from individual interests to community interests

Adapted from Chrislip, D., & Larson, C. (1994). Collaborative leadership. San Francisco: Jossey-Bass, pp. 52–54, with permission.

Maintaining Contact

A third factor that affects professional communication is the amount of time that health professionals spend interacting with one another. According to some investigators, there is surprisingly little interaction between health professionals on a day-to-day basis. Katzman and Roberts (1988) studied nurse–physician communication in a hospital setting and found that no built-in mechanism existed for regular communication between nurses and physicians. Over a 3-month period, the investigators observed that the majority of physicians came to the unit and left without ever interacting with a nurse. The investigators also report that it was common for a nurse to literally run after a physician as the physician was leaving the unit to obtain specific information about a client. Lamb and Napodano (1984) also report minimal interaction between nurse practitioners and physicians in a primary care setting. In the few instances in which interactions did occur, these investigators found that they were almost always initiated by a nurse. Morse and Piland (1981) studied the communication in nurse–patient, nurse–nurse, and nurse–physician dyads. The investigators report that nurse–patient and nurse–nurse communication was fairly open but that nurse–physician communication typically was closed, with little two-way exchange.

Although the responsibility for initiating interactions frequently rests with the nurse, studies indicate that nurses are hesitant at times to approach physicians, even though safe nursing care requires such interaction. Katzman and Roberts (1988) report several instances in which staff nurses hesitated to call physicians. Nurses in these situations expressed fears about asking "dumb" questions of physicians and also said they were hesitant to speak up frequently, saying, "I don't know enough," "I'm afraid to speak up," and "It's the physician's show" (p. 587). Other investigators report that nurses behave in deferent ways toward physicians, making tentative suggestions rather than direct statements about ways to improve or alter patient care (Kalisch & Kalisch, 1977; Mauksch, 1983). Katzman and Roberts (1988) attribute the communication problems between nurses and physicians to nurses' feelings of inferiority, physicians' lack of recognition of nurses' roles, and nurses' inability to articulate the importance of nursing interventions.

Clearly, effective communication is necessary among all members of the health care team, because quality patient care depends on it. Nurses can facilitate effective interactions by using more direct, informed, and confident patterns of communication with physicians. This more assertive, collegial approach needs to emerge from nurses' greater awareness, acceptance, and articulation of their unique contribution to the care of patients and family members. Physicians, on the other hand, can facilitate more effective interactions with nurses by communicating in more egalitarian ways, recognizing nurses' unique expertise, and seeking input from nurses on an ongoing basis.

Organizations also need to take a more active role in developing organizational structures that facilitate better working relationships between nurses and physicians. Knaus and associates (1986) compared 13 intensive care units on various organizational components and patient care outcomes. The investigators found that the hospital with the best performance in terms of patient outcomes had more comprehensive nursing education support systems, better nurse–physician communication, and an atmosphere of mutual respect among the health professionals. The hospital receiving the lowest ranking in terms of patient care outcomes lacked a comprehensive support system for nurses, had no established routine for discussing patient care plans, exhibited poor nurse–physician communication, and displayed an atmosphere of distrust. This study highlights the need for a multifaceted approach to facilitate effective relationships among health professionals and ensure optimal patient care outcomes.

The three communication factors—(1) clarifying roles, (2) sharing control, and (3) maintaining contact—promote effective interprofessional relationships. These factors do not operate in isolation from one another; they are interdependent. As professionals clarify their roles through more frequent interactions, they will be more willing to share control with others in important health care decisions.

SUMMARY

Communication is essential in nursing practice. Because of the rapid changes and increased complexity in health care, nurses need to communicate more effectively with clients and with other health professionals.

Communication theory and King's (1981) nursing theory provide a theoretical basis for understanding interpersonal relationships in health care settings. According to communication theory, three basic assumptions regarding human communication exist: (1) interpersonal communication is a process; (2) it is transactional; and (3) it is multidimensional because it has both a content and relationship component. According to King's nursing theory, interpersonal communication is affected by the perceptions that both nurse and client bring to their interaction. King's theory also emphasizes the importance of mutual goal setting between nurse and client.

There are four developmental phases in the nurse–client relationship: (1) the preparation phase, (2) the initiation phase, (3) the exploratory phase, and (4) the termination phase. Various tasks need to occur within each phase to ensure the development of a productive, therapeutic relationship.

The three factors that can enhance the effectiveness of nurse–client relationships are: (1) responding with empathy; (2) providing confirmation; and (3) sharing information. These three factors are interrelated and collectively address both the content and relationship dimension of interpersonal communication.

Other factors also can promote better relationships between health professions: clarifying roles, sharing control, and maintaining contact. These factors will assist professionals not only in developing better working relationships but also ultimately in improving the quality of patient care.

REFERENCES

Aguilera, A. D. (1967). Relationship between physical contact and verbal interaction between nurses and patients. *Journal of Psychiatric Nursing, 5*(1), 5–21.

Alagna, F., Whitehers, S., Fisher, J., & Wicas, E. (1979). Evaluative reaction to interpersonal touch in a counseling interview. *Journal of Counseling Psychology, 26,* 465–472.

Alt-White, A. C., Charns, M., & Strayer, R. (1983). Personal, organizational and managerial factors related to nurse–physician collaboration. *Nursing Administration Quarterly, 8*(1), 8–18.

American Nurses Association. (1995). *Nursing's social policy statement.* Washington, DC: Author.

Barrett-Lennard, G. T. (1962). Dimensions of therapist response as causal factors in therapeutic change. *Psychological Monographs, 76*(43), 1–36.

Benjamin, A. (1981). *The helping interview* (3rd ed.). Boston: Houghton Mifflin.

Berlo, D. K. (1960). *The process of communication.* New York: Holt, Rinehart, & Winston.

Birdwhistell, R. L. (1970). *Kinesics and context.* Philadelphia: University of Pennsylvania Press.

Bond, S. (1982). Communicating with families of cancer patients. 2. The nurses. *Nursing Times, 78,* 1027–1029.

Bottorff, J. L. (1993). The use and meaning of touch in caring for patients with cancer. *Oncology Nursing Forum, 20,* 1531–1538.

Burgoon, M., Heston, J. K., & McCroskey, J. (1974). *Small group communication: A functional approach.* New York: Holt, Rinehart, & Winston.

Cassileth, B. R., Rupkis, R. V., Sutton-Smith, K., & March, V. (1980). Information and participation preferences among cancer patients. *Annals of Internal Medicine, 92,* 832–836.

Chrislip, D. D., & Larson, C. E. (1994). *Collaborative leadership.* San Francisco: Jossey-Bass.

Dodd, M. (1982). Assessing patient self-care for side effects of cancer chemotherapy—Part I. *Cancer Nursing, 5,* 447–451.

Drew, N. (1986). Exclusion and confirmation: A phenomenology of patients' experiences with caregivers. *Image: Journal of Nursing Scholarship, 18*(2), 39–43.

Dyck, S., & Wright, K. (1986). Family perceptions: The role of the nurse throughout an adult's cancer experience. *Oncology Nursing Forum, 12*(5), 53–56.

Fagin, C. M. (1992). Collaboration between nurses and physicians: No longer a choice. *Academic Medicine, 67,* 295–303.

Feiger, S. M., & Schmitt, M. (1979). Collegiality in interdisciplinary health teams: Its measurement and its effects. *Social Science and Medicine, 13A,* 217–229.

Forchuk, C. (1994). The orientation phase of the nurse–client relationship: Testing Peplau's theory. *Journal of Advanced Nursing, 20,* 532–537.

Forchuk, C. (1995). Uniqueness within the nurse–client relationship. *Archives of Psychiatric Nursing, 9*, 34–39.

Forsyth, G. L. (1979). Exploration of empathy in nurse–client interaction. *Advances in Nursing Science, 1*(2), 53–61.

Frank-Stromborg, M., & Wright, P. (1984). Ambulatory cancer patients' perceptions of the physical and psychological changes in their lives since the diagnosis of cancer. *Cancer Nursing, 7*, 117–130.

Fraser, K., & Gallop, R. (1993). Nurses' confirming/disconfirming responses to patients diagnosed with borderline personality disorder. *Archives of Psychiatric Nursing, 7*, 336–341.

Friedman, H. S. (1979). Nonverbal communication between patients and medical practitioners. *Journal of Social Issues, 35*(1), 82–100.

Gagan, J. (1983). Methodological notes on empathy. *Advances in Nursing Science, 5*(2), 65–72.

Greenwald, H. P., & Nevitt, M. C. (1982). Physicians' attitudes toward communication with cancer patients. *Social Science and Medicine, 16*, 591–594.

Hanna, K. M. (1993). Effect of nurse–client transaction on female adolescents' oral contraceptive adherence. *Image: Journal of Nursing Scholarship, 25*, 285–290.

Hardin, S., & Halaris, A. (1983). Nonverbal communication of patients and high and low empathy nurses. *Journal of Psychiatric and Mental Health Services, 21*(1), 14–20.

Heineken, J. (1982). Disconfirmation in dysfunctional communication. *Nursing Research, 31*(4), 211–213.

Heineken, J. (1983). Treating the disconfirmed psychiatric client. *Journal of Psychiatric Nursing and Mental Health Sciences, 21*(1), 21–25.

Heineken, J., & Roberts, F. B. (1983). Confirming, not disconfirming: Communicating in a more positive manner. *American Journal of Maternal Child Nursing, 8*(1), 78–80.

Kalisch, B. (1973). What is empathy? *American Journal of Nursing, 73*, 1548–1552.

Kalisch, B. J., & Kalisch, P. A. (1977). An analysis of the sources of physician–nurse conflict. *Journal of Nursing Administration, 7*(1), 51–57.

Katzman, E. M., & Roberts, J. I. (1988). Nurse-physician conflicts as barriers to the enactment of nursing roles. *Western Journal of Nursing Research, 10*, 576–590.

King, I. M. (1971). *A theory for nursing: General concepts of human behavior.* New York: Wiley.

King, I. M. (1981). *Toward a theory for nursing: Systems, concepts, process.* New York: Wiley.

Knaus, W. A., Draper, E. A., Wagner, D. P., & Zimmerman, J. E. (1986). An evaluation of outcomes from intensive care in major medical centers. *Annals of Internal Medicine, 104*, 410–418.

Lamb, G. S., & Napodano, R. J. (1984). Physician–nurse practitioner interaction patterns in primary care practices. *American Journal of Public Health, 74*(1), 26–29.

Larson, P. (1986). Cancer nurses' perceptions of caring. *Cancer Nursing, 9*(2), 86–91.

Lauer, P., Murphy, S., & Powers, M. (1982). Learning needs of cancer patients: A comparison of nurse and practitioner perceptions. *Nursing Research, 31*(1), 11–16.

Leininger, M. (1971). This I believe . . . about interdisciplinary health education for the future. *Nursing Outlook, 19*, 787–791.

Mauksch, I. (1983). An analysis of some critical contemporary issues in nursing. *Journal of Continuing Education in Nursing, 14*(1), 4–14.

Mechanic, D., & Aiken, L. H. (1982). A cooperative agenda for medicine and nursing. *New England Journal of Medicine, 307*(12), 747–750.

Mehrabian, A. (1971). *Silent messages.* Belmont, CA: Wadsworth.

Miller, G. R. (1972). *An introduction to speech communication* (2nd ed.). New York: Bobbs-Merrill.

Milne, M. A. (1980). Training for the team. *Journal of Advanced Nursing, 5,* 579–589.

Morse, B. W., & Piland, R. N. (1981). An assessment of communication competencies needed by intermediate-level health care providers: A study of nurse–patient, nurse–doctor, nurse–nurse communication relationships. *Journal of Applied Communications Research, 9*(1), 30–41.

Morse, J. M., Anderson, G., Bottorff, J. L., Yonge, O., O'Brien, B., Solberg, S. M., & McIlveen, K. H. (1992). Exploring empathy: A conceptual fit for nursing practice. *Image: Journal of Nursing Scholarship, 24,* 273–280.

Northouse, P. G., & Northouse, L. L. (1992). *Health communication: Strategies for health professionals.* Norwalk, CT: Appleton & Lange.

Olson, J. K. (1995). Relationships between nurse-expressed empathy, patient perceived empathy, and patient distress. *Image: Journal of Nursing Scholarship, 27,* 317–322.

Pattison, J. (1973). Effects of touch on self-exploration and the therapeutic relationship. *Journal of Consulting and Clinical Psychology, 40,* 170–175.

Peplau, H. E. (1952). *Interpersonal relations in nursing: A conceptual frame of reference for psychodynamic nursing.* New York: Putnam.

Peplau, H. E. (1965). The heart of nursing: Interpersonal relations. *Canadian Nurse, 61,* 273–275.

Pike, A. W. (1991). Moral outrage and moral discourse in nurse–physician collaboration. *Journal of Professional Nursing, 7,* 351–363.

Pincus, J. D. (1986). Communication: Key contributor to effectiveness—The research. *Journal of Nursing Administration, 16*(9), 19–28.

Reid-Ponte, P. (1992). Distress in cancer patients and primary nurses' empathy skills. *Cancer Nursing, 15,* 283–292.

Rogers, C. R. (1983). *Freedom to learn for the 80's.* Columbus, OH: Merrill.

Rubinstein, L. Z., Josephson, K. R., Wieland, G. D., English, D. A., Sayre, J. A., & Kane, R. L. (1984). Effectiveness of geriatric evaluation unit. *New England Journal of Medicine, 311,* 1664–1670.

Sayre, J. (1978). Common errors in communication made by students in psychiatric nursing. *Perspectives in Psychiatric Care, 16,* 175–183.

Schoene-Seifert, B., & Childress, J. F. (1986). How much should the cancer patient know and decide? *Ca—A Cancer Journal for Clinicians, 36*(2), 85–94.

Sieburg, E. (1969). *Dysfunctional communication and interpersonal responsiveness in small groups.* Unpublished doctoral dissertation, University of Denver.

Simington, J. A., & Laing, G. P. (1993). Effects of therapeutic touch on anxiety in the institutional elderly. *Clinical Nursing Research, 2,* 438–450.

Street, R. L., Piziak, V. K., Carpenter, W. S., Herzog, J., Hejl, J., Skinner, G., & McLellan, L. (1993). Provider–patient communication and metabolic control. *Diabetes Care, 16,* 714–721.

Sundeen, S., Stuart, G. W., Rankin, E. D., & Cohen, S. A. (1994). *Nurse–client interaction: Implementing the nursing process.* St. Louis: Mosby.

Sundell, W. (1972). *The operation of confirming and disconfirming verbal behavior in selected teacher–student interactions.* Unpublished doctoral dissertation, University of Denver.

Thorne, S. (1988). Helpful and unhelpful communications in cancer care: The patient perspective. *Oncology Nursing Forum, 15*(2), 167–172.

Triplett, J., & Arneson, S. (1979). The use of verbal and tactile comfort to alleviate distress in young hospitalized children. *Research in Nursing & Health, 2,* 17–23.

Waitzkin, H., & Stoeckle, J. D. (1972). The communication of information about illness: Clinical, sociological and methodological consideration. *Advances in Psychosomatic Medicine, 8,* 180–215.

Watzlawick, P., Beavin, J., & Jackson, D. D. (1967). *Pragmatics of human communication.* New York: Norton.

Weiss, S. J. (1983). Role differentiation between nurse and physician: Implications for nursing. *Nursing Research, 32,* 133–139.

Weiss, S. J., & Remen, N. (1983). Self-limiting patterns of nursing behavior within a tripartite context involving consumers and physicians. *Western Journal of Nursing Research, 5,* 77–89.

Williams, C. (1979). Empathic communication and its effect on client outcome. *Issues in Mental Health Nursing, 2*(1), 16–26.

Williams, R., & Williams, C. (1982). Hospital social workers and nurses: Interprofessional perceptions and experiences. *Journal of Nursing Education, 21*(5), 16–21.

Wilmot, W. W. (1979). *Dyadic communication: A transactional perspective* (2nd ed.). Reading, MA: Addison-Wesley.

BIBLIOGRAPHY

Baggs, J. G., & Schmitt, M. H. (1988). Collaboration between nurses and physicians. *Image: Journal of Nursing Scholarship, 20,* 145–149.

Bates, B. (1970). Doctor and nurse: Changing roles and relations. *New England Journal of Medicine, 283*(3), 129–134.

Christensen, C., & Larson, J. R. (1993). Collaborative medical decision making. *Medical Decision Making, 13,* 339–346.

Daniels, T. G., Denny, A., & Andrews, D. (1988). Using microcounseling to teach RN nursing students skills of therapeutic communication. *Journal of Nursing Education, 27,* 246–252.

Disalvo, V. S., Larsen, J. K., & Backus, D. K. (1986). *Communication Education, 35,* 231–242.

Donovan, C. (1992). Nurse participation in decisions regarding limitation of treatment. *The Yale Journal of Biology and Medicine, 65,* 131–136.

Farley, R. C., & Baher, A. J. (1987). Training on selected self-management techniques and the generalization and maintenance of interpersonal skills for registered nurse students. *Journal of Nursing Education, 26,* 99–103.

Garvin, B. J., & Kennedy, C. W. (1986). Confirmation and disconfirmation in nurse/physician communications. *Journal of Applied Communication Research, 14*(1), 1–19.

Glenn, J. K., Williamson, H. A., Hector, M. G., Dally, J., & Reid, J. (1987). Communications among nurse practitioners and physicians in team-delivered ambulatory care. *Medical Care, 25,* 570–576.

Harrison, T. M., Pistolessi, T. V., & Stephen, T. D. (1989). Assessing nurses' communication: A cross-sectional study. *Western Journal of Nursing Research, 11,* 75–91.

Inui, T. S., & Carter, W. B. (1985). Problems and prospects for health services research on provider–patient communication. *Medical Care, 23*(5), 521–538.

Kasch, C. (1986). Establishing a collaborative nurse–patient relationship: A distinct focus of nursing action in primary care. *Image: Journal of Nursing Scholarship, 18*(2), 44–47.

Kasch, C., & Dine, J. (1988). Person-centered communication and social perspective taking. *Western Journal of Nursing Research, 10,* 317–326.

Kennedy, C. W., & Garvin, B. J. (1986). Confirmation–disconfirmation: A framework for the study of interpersonal relationships. In P. Chinn (Ed.), *Nursing research and methodology* (pp. 221–235). Rockville, MD: Aspen.

Loveridge, C. E., & Heineken, J. (1988). Confirming interactions. *Journal of Gerontological Nursing, 14*(5), 27–30.

Prescott, P. A., & Bowen, S. A. (1985). Physician-nurse relationships. *Annals of Internal Medicine, 103,* 127–133.

Rosse, J. G., & Rosse, D. H. (1981). Role conflict and ambiguity: An empirical investigation of nursing personnel. *Evaluation and the Health Professions, 4,* 385–405.

Topf, M. (1988). Verbal interpersonal responsiveness. *Journal of Psychosocial Nursing, 26*(7), 8–16.

Weiss, S. (1985). The influence of discourse on collaboration among nurses, physicians, and consumers. *Research in Nursing & Health, 8,* 49–59.

Health Teaching in Nursing Practice

Marlyn D. Boyd

The role of the nurse as a health teacher started in America with colonization. Over the next 200 years, nurses' health teaching continued and became an expected component of nursing practice. Today, nurses enjoy the right and responsibility to instruct, counsel, and educate patients and consumers as an independent nursing function. This chapter provides an overview of the legal and ethical responsibility of nurses to provide health teaching and of key constructs necessary for successful teaching and learning: readiness to learn, assessment, planning, choosing appropriate teaching strategies and methods, evaluation, and documentation of health teaching.

Because of the limitations of the amount of information that can be presented, this chapter provides a skeletal framework for health teaching. Health teaching is founded on ongoing research from a multitude of areas such as education, educational psychology, health psychology, health education, and nursing. The reader is encouraged to consult health teaching texts and professional periodicals to expand his or her understanding of the theories and research that serve as the foundation for the process of health teaching.

MANDATES FOR HEALTH TEACHING

Health teaching has long been an expected component of competent and comprehensive nursing care. Health teaching is increasingly becoming more important as the landscape of health care changes to focus on cost containment. Shorter hospital stays, increasing numbers of procedures performed on an outpatient basis, home health care, and hospice all necessitate an emphasis on health teaching.

Another factor that has propelled health teaching into the forefront of nursing practice is the realization that many of the health problems in the United States are related to lifestyle choices. Heart disease and many cancers, including skin, lung, colorectal, liver, prostate, and cervical cancers, have a heavy lifestyle component. Smoking and the resultant cardiovascular disease and lung cancer; obesity and the resultant cardiovascular, autoimmune, and cancer risks; alcohol intake and cirrhosis of the liver; sexually transmitted disease; and AIDS all have contributing factors that stem from lifestyle choices.

Primary prevention of diseases such as these begins with health teaching in the schools, in the community, within families, and with individuals to change lifestyle behaviors to reduce risks. To diminish the potential morbidity and mortality from such diseases, secondary prevention aims at educating and encouraging persons at risk to participate in regular screenings. Finally, tertiary prevention involves health teaching as persons undergo treatment for the resultant complications of diseases or conditions.

From an ethical perspective, nurses provide health teaching because of their belief that individuals have the right of self-determination and autonomy over their bodies. Nurses also believe that individuals are responsible for their own health promotion and maintenance.

If nurses' ethical persuasions are not enough to encourage them to provide quality health teaching, then legal mandates require them to make health teaching a part of their practice. Nurses' legal obligations to provide quality health teaching are provided on national, state, and local levels.

On the national level, the American Nurses Association (ANA) delineates health teaching as one of the six basic functions of nursing practice. National organizations that guide nursing education, national specialty groups such as the Critical Care Nurses' Association, Enterostomal Nurses' Association, Public Health Nurses' Association, Joint Commission on Accreditation of Health Care Organizations (JCAHO), and others all include health teaching as a primary role responsibility of the registered nurse (RN). Statements from groups such as these establish on a national level that health teaching is an expected part of nursing practice (Boyd, 1992a).

On a state level, the primary legal mandate that nurses have to provide health teaching is provided through each state's nurse practice act. All 50 state boards of nursing have formal statements that outline the expectations of nursing practice within each state and that refer to health teaching, guidance, or counseling as part of the expected practice of nursing.

On a local level, expectations for nurses' involvement in health teaching can be found in health care agencies' mission statements, RNs' job descriptions, procedure and policy manuals that direct care, and in the Patient Bill of Rights adopted in some form by virtually every provider group (Boyd, 1992a).

It is clear from the multitude of supportive statements from groups such as those mentioned, that registered nurses are expected to teach and that their patients and consumers have a right to expect such a professional service. What if there is no formal program in place, such as a diabetes education or a cardiac rehabilitation program? What if there is no designated person, such as a diabetes educator, to do the teaching? Should the patient expect health teaching from his or her assigned nurse? What if health teaching is omitted or done incorrectly? What if a patient comes to harm because of the lack of teaching or learning? Is the nurse legally responsible? The answers to these questions from both the ethical and legal perspective is yes. Individuals should expect adequate instruction so they can understand and sufficiently take care of themselves to improve their health status, maintain functioning, and avoid injury or poor outcomes. Can the RN be held legally liable for omission of health teaching or inadequate health teaching and insufficient learning? Yes, health teaching is an independent nursing function, and the nurse can be held accountable for the omission of teaching or inadequate, incomplete, or inappropriate teaching (malpractice). Even when nurses share teaching responsibilities with other health care professionals, the nurse is still held solely accountable for his or her teaching (Boyd, 1992b).

Health teaching is legally held to the same standards as any other component of nursing practice. Registered nurses have been sued for lack of teaching, inadequate instruction, and poor patient outcomes related to the patient's inability to be able to take proper action. Some of these suits were settled against the nurse; in others, the nurse had carried out his or her teaching responsibility and the suit was settled in the nurse's favor. Health teaching is not an option for the registered nurse, it is a legal mandate (Boyd, 1992a).

LEARNING AND MOTIVATION

Learning is a complex process, and how it is accomplished and what initiates the process vary somewhat from person to person. Learning first involves an individual's paying attention to a stimulus. Second, learning involves the individual's incorporating the information or psychomotor skill into short-term memory storage. Next, learning involves an individual's transferring what was learned into long-term memory. Finally, learning involves the individual being able to retrieve what was learned and use it as needed. Before doing this, however, the learner must want to learn the information or task and be ready mentally, physically, and psychologically to undergo the "learning." These two factors are referred to as readiness to learn and motivation for learning.

Readiness to learn involves the individual's ability and energy to learn. In contrast, motivation stems from the individual's desire to learn. Before successful teaching and learning can take place, these two factors must be assessed. Readiness to learn is covered in the following section on assessing learning ability.

Motivation

Motivation for learning often is misunderstood. Nurses cannot motivate individuals to learn. Motivation is an internal process and is innate to an individual. Motivation is based on basic physiological drives such as the need for food, water, air, and shelter, and on desires, such as socialization and acceptance. In addition, much of what motivates individuals to learn comes from a complex mix of their heredity and sociocultural and spiritual backgrounds (Whitman, 1992b, d; Rankin & Duffy, 1993).

In health teaching, motivation answers the questions: Why does someone want to gain new information or change their behavior? Why does someone have the desire to learn or change behavior? Answers to these questions will vary from individual to individual. What serves as a motivator for learning and changing behaviors for one individual may not serve as a motivator for another individual. For example, one woman maintains her weight and exercises regularly to stay physically attractive; another woman engages in the same behaviors but does so because of a strong family history of heart disease and fear of an early death. Moreover, motivators may change for an individual over time and as circumstances change.

Motivation often is associated with the individual's developmental tasks or needs. Nurses can use their knowledge of individuals' developmental tasks to help learners to understand how health teaching and the consequences of changes in health behaviors can help them to accomplish their developmental tasks. This is often referred to as making the material relevant to the learner.

How can nurses determine an individual's developmental task? By asking the learner. What is the most important thing to you right now? What bothers you the most about having _____ or knowing that you need to _____? Nurses will often find that individuals' primary concern is not about their health or the sequela of some health diagnosis or procedure, but about losing their job, for example, and the resulting financial difficulty. For others, motivation for change may be lack of peer acceptance, not being sexually attractive, not being able to have children, not being able to care for their children long-term, or impending death. How can health teaching help these individuals to prevent, cope with, or resolve these concerns? How can learning and changing behavior help them do what is important for them? These issues are their motivators for learning and changing behavior.

Some examples of using motivators and developmental tasks might include showing a teenager, whose desire for physical attractiveness and peer acceptance is a primary motivator for her behavior, that a well-balanced diet can help her hair to be healthier and shinier, her nails to be stronger, or her skin to be healthier. A 35-year-old auto mechanic keeps missing work because he is not keeping his diabetes under control. He is concerned about losing his job and the financial consequences of that on his family. He needs to make the connection between his diabetes self-care and keeping the job that provides financial security for him and his family. If he is conscientious with his care regimen, he will miss less work and his financial security is less threatened.

What many people refer to as motivators are actually *reinforcers.* Both positive or negative consequences can serve as reinforcers to increase or decrease the likelihood of a behavior being repeated. Reinforcers, however, do not instill motivation; they are consequences to behaviors based on a motivation.

Reinforcers are an important part of teaching and learning. Positive reinforcement lets individuals know that they are headed in the right direction, that they are competent, and that they have mastered a skill. Positive reinforcement also can help to bolster self-esteem and to foster independence and self-responsibility. Individuals are more likely to repeat a behavior when it has positive consequences for them. Negative reinforcement also can be effective in that individuals will experience the undesired consequences of behavior choices.

ASSESSMENT OF LEARNING ABILITY

An individual's ability to learn can be assessed by gathering data in four broad categories: health status; health values; cognitive, psychological, and psychomotor abilities and previous learning experiences; and developmental characteristics (Whitman, 1992b, c).

Health Status

Health status assessment involves the nurse gathering data about the individual's energy level for learning, comfort status, sensory status, and adjustment to health status. Before successful teaching can begin and learning occur, the individual must have adequate physical and mental energy to learn. If the person is spending the majority of his or her physical energy on recuperating from an illness, surgical procedure, or treatment, the individual will not be able to focus attention on the learning.

Assessment of energy level can be included in a physical assessment, noting the amount of time that has passed since a particular treatment or procedure and the person's general activity level. Does the person pay attention to what is being said? Does he or she give eye contact? The nurse can also ask the learner if he or she feels up to talking about a particular issue.

If an individual is coping with a recent unfavorable diagnosis, he or she will not have the psychological energy to focus on learning. An assessment of the individual's psychological energy would include noting the amount of time since receiving a procedure, diagnosis, or unfavorable prognosis; physical energy level; eye contact; change in the amount and style of oral communication; and withdrawal. Emotions such as fear, anxiety, anger, and grief will diminish an individual's ability to concentrate and learn (Potter & Perry, 1991). Again, the nurse can simply ask the learner if he or she wants to begin learning about some issue or whether another time would be better.

As anyone who has sat through a long lecture on a hard seat or tried to concentrate on learning when hungry can attest, comfort status does affect learning. Pain, hunger, fatigue, thirst, lack of sleep, and other physical discomforts can all decrease an individual's ability to concentrate on learning. Before beginning teaching sessions, the nurse should assess the comfort status of the learner or learners and increase their comfort level as much as possible. If the learner is in pain, pain medication can be given and teaching timed to coincide with its peak effect. If discomfort cannot be diminished, then short, to-the-point teaching sessions may be necessary.

Sensory status assessment involves the nurse's determining the extent of functioning of the learner's five senses: vision, hearing, taste, touch, and smell. Before teaching begins, glasses should be cleaned and in place and hearing aids cleaned and batteries checked. Depending on the degree of impairment of vision or hearing, teaching strategies may need to be adapted (Whitman, 1992a).

Adjustment to health state entails determining whether the individual is ready to learn both psychologically and physically. If the learner is still in the grieving stages of denial, anger, or depression, he or she may have difficulty learning. For example, if a person with a new colostomy refuses to look at it or touch the appliance, then he or she is not ready for self-care teaching. The learner is not emotionally or psychologically ready to learn. Likewise, if an individual with a new prosthesis has not completely healed, prothesis use cannot be taught. The individual is not physically ready to learn.

Health Values

As with motivation, how health is valued and how it is ranked within an individual's value system vary depending on a variety of factors, including heredity, sociocultural factors, and personal experiences. Nurses cannot assume that individuals hold optimal health as their highest value, which is to say that their health is the number-one driving force behind their behaviors. Improving, maintaining, or optimizing health are low priorities or not priorities at all for some people. Therefore, if the nurse just "tells them what they need to do," it is unlikely that health behaviors will change.

Health values assessment is crucial before teaching begins. If an individual does not believe that changing his diet will have any effect on his potential for a myocardial infarction, he will probably not modify his diet. If a mother does not believe that immunizations are that important for her child's health, she may not make the effort to have the child immunized.

Likewise, if a woman does not believe that smoking during pregnancy is harmful to her unborn child, she will continue to smoke. What individuals believe has a strong impact on their health behavior. Their beliefs may be based on factual information, past experiences, vicarious experiences, or cultural myth.

Health values can be assessed by using different theoretical models. Perhaps one of the best known and researched theories of health behavior is the Health Belief Model constructs of seriousness, susceptibility, benefits, barriers, and cue to action (Becker, 1974; Rosenstock, 1990). For example, a nurse has a 47-year-old, obese, hypertensive, and sedentary male client. She is assessing his perception of risk for heart disease and a possible myocardial infarction. Questions she would ask might include: "How serious do you believe that heart disease is?" "How serious do you believe it would be if you had a heart attack?" "Do you believe you are more likely to have a heart attack if you do not lose weight and get your high blood pressure down to a safe level?" "What would make it hard for you to lose weight?" "What good things would come from you losing weight?" The patient is more likely to change his health behaviors if he believes that heart disease is serious, that he is likely to have a heart attack if he does not lose weight, and that there are barriers to his weight loss but that the benefits outweigh the barriers. If the patient does not hold these beliefs, he is less likely to change his diet and exercise behavior.

Finally, cues to action or triggers for the change in health behavior need to be identified. Triggers for the inception of behavioral change may be a personal event such as a myocardial infarction or an accident while driving intoxicated; a social expectation (stop smoking); or a legal mandate (wearing seatbelts). Individuals may be able to identify what event would precipitate a change in health behavior. The nurse can ask, for example, what it would take the patient to stay on a diet and exercise regularly or to stop smoking. Questions such as these help learners to identify possible sequelae to their behaviors and provide the nurse with an indication of the magnitude of impact the trigger must have to initiate behavioral change.

Another factor to assess is whether individuals believe that they can successfully make changes and that there will be positive consequences to those changes. The degree to which individuals believe that they have control over the outcomes of their actions is termed *locus of control*. Individuals' perceptions of their ability to have control or power over their health is a *health* locus of control (Wallston, Wallston, Kaplan, & Maides, 1976). If individuals believe that chance, luck, fate, or powerful others have control over their health, then they may believe that they are powerless to make changes. This is called having an *external* locus of control. In contrast, if individuals believe that they can influence their health by taking action and changing behaviors, they are considered to have an *internal* locus of control. Locus of control can be assessed by asking the learner questions such as, Why do you think you have/got_____? Is there anything that you could have done to avoid _____? If you made up your mind to do it, do you think you could _____?

If the learner has an internal locus of control, the nurse may find that he or she only needs to help the learner to acquire the knowledge and skills necessary to change the selected behavior. The nurse/teacher will serve as a resource and facilitator for learning. If the learner has an external locus of control, the nurse will need to structure learning to provide greater direction and emphasize the learner's ability to influence his or her health.

Closely related to health locus of control, although it has a different impact on health behavior, is *self-efficacy*. Locus of control tends to be consistent over time, whereas self-efficacy often is situation specific. Self-efficacy refers to individuals' beliefs about their ability to perform a certain behavior in the future (Bandura, 1986). An individual may feel confident that he or she can reduce dietary fat, yet believe that it will be impossible to stop smoking. Another person will believe that he or she can stop smoking but not exercise on a regular basis. The exciting part of this concept is that individuals' perceptions of self-efficacy can change. Nurses are in an ideal position to help to raise individuals' sense of self-efficacy. A successful method of helping individuals to increase their sense of self-efficacy is to help them to master a physical activity. Breaking down the task into smaller units of behavior helps the individual to master the activity. This success will make the learner more confident that he can repeat the skill at a later time (Bandura, 1986; O'Leary, 1985).

Cognitive, Psychological, and Psychomotor Abilities

To successfully plan teaching sessions, the nurse must assess individuals' cognitive, psychological, and physical abilities available to learn and use new information or skills. These abilities will vary from person to person and across the life span. Children's abilities in these areas change as they grow, whereas adults' abilities change as they age. Cognitive assessment is done to determine what cognitive skills individuals have and how extensive their abilities are. For example, if a person has a below-average IQ, the nurse's approach with teaching would be very different than if the person has a college degree. If the individual cannot read or write, then the nurse would need to use supporting materials other than written materials to reinforce the teaching and could not depend on a written test to evaluate learning.

Baseline data for cognitive assessment include determining the individual's orientation to space, time, and person. Once it has been established that the person is oriented, then the nurse can assess his or her basic level of cognitive abilities to communicate orally, use written information, and understand and remember new information. These assessments can be made by answering questions such as: At what level can the person communicate? Is the learner in concrete thought and having difficulty with abstract ideas such as what is happening inside his or her body? If the individual is having difficulty with abstract concepts, then teaching needs to include concrete examples, analogies, demonstrations, pictures, and others to help the individual to understand the concept. Is the learner able to grasp abstract concepts such as physiology? If so, then teaching can involve more explanations and information.

How extensive is his or her vocabulary? Does he or she have difficulty articulating questions or responses? Does he or she use medical terminology correctly? Can the learner use nuances of terms such as hot versus burning or stabbing versus sharp? Answers to questions such as these help the nurse to use an appropriate level of vocabulary to communicate health information.

What type of work does/did the person do? If the person was involved in information exchange (reading, writing, and using new information), he or she will be more likely to feel comfortable and confident learning something new. However, if the person did not use new information and repeated the same manual tasks repetitively over years, he or she may be less comfortable and less confident about learning, for example, how to manage newly diagnosed diabetes.

How far did the learner go in school? How long ago did he or she leave school? Does the learner read? If so, what and how often? These questions can help the nurse to assess an individual's ability to use written communications and ability to use abstract concepts. The less formal education a person has had and the longer it has been since he or she completed formal education, the more limited an individual's abilities will be in these areas (Boyd, 1992c; Doak, Doak, & Root, 1985). Likewise, typically people who can successfully gain information or pleasure from reading will read frequently. Most public information such as newspapers, Reader's Digest, tabloid papers, and the like are written on about an eighth-grade reading level. Unfortunately, it is not uncommon for health teaching materials to be written on a twelfth-grade reading level or above. In general, people tend to read three to five grade levels below their grade completion (Boyd, 1992b). In choosing written health teaching materials, the nurse needs to keep in mind that the average reading level for adults in the United States is eighth grade and that approximately one in four adults cannot read well enough to use written materials to gain information (Department of Health and Human Services, 1991; Doak et al., 1985; Weiss et al., 1994).

Finally, does the learner pay attention to what you say or does his or her attention wander? Is the person uncomfortable or experiencing pain? Is the learner emotionally distracted? Tired? Does he or she have the necessary energy to learn? Is he or she grieving and in denial? If the individual is not physically and psychologically ready to learn, the nurse must help to move the learner to a stage of readiness.

Assessing a learner's psychomotor abilities is necessary to plan teaching skills such as self-injection of insulin, self-care of wounds, ostomies, and other self-care activities. Does the learner have any deficits in physical mobility? Are fine motor skills diminished? For example, self-care behaviors for learners with arthritis may need to be adapted because of diminished fine motor control and range of motion. Learners who have neurological or musculoskeletal diseases and conditions may need to have teaching adapted to accommodate their limited psychomotor functions.

The learner's general understanding of health topics such as anatomy and physiology, nutrition, exercise, and risk reduction behaviors will influence the nurse's planning for health teaching. Nurses must not assume that just because someone is well educated or communicates in sophisticated language that he or she has a general knowledge of health-related information. Likewise, just because an individual has not had the opportunity to receive a formal education does not mean that he or she has below-average intelligence or that he or she cannot learn. If the individual is health oriented and engages in diet management, exercise, or other health promotive behaviors, the nurse can discuss these activities to determine the extent of the learner's general health knowledge and identify any misconceptions or inaccurate information that the learner may have. Learners may undertake changes in health behaviors without accurate information. Individuals practice health behaviors for many reasons. Their understanding of the underlying principles for their behaviors may or may not be based on sound scientific principles. Moreover, an individual may have a great deal of knowledge in one area of health self-care management and little in another area. For example, a learner may have in-depth knowledge of nutrition as it relates to weight loss but have only a cursory knowledge of how to start and maintain an exercise regimen.

Previous Learning Experiences

Past behaviors and experiences are brought with the learner to a new learning situation and strongly influence new learning. An assessment of a learner's past health behaviors can provide the nurse with a wealth of information about the individual's health practices and the importance that the person places on health. Likewise, such an assessment can help the nurse to identify areas where the individual has had a bad experience in the past, has had poor outcomes, or was not successful in changing behavior. Such information helps the nurse to plan teaching strategies. For example, if an individual is overweight and is being instructed in diet management and exercise, it is important for the nurse to know whether the individual has tried to manage his or her weight in the past and has been unsuccessful. Another example would be discussing contraceptive choices with a woman whose partner refuses to use a condom or with a woman who has become pregnant because she does not like to put in a diaphragm or cannot remember to take her oral contraceptive. If an individual has not been successful in adopting a health behavior in the past, the nurse will plan more time to help the learner to identify barriers to successful behavioral change. Once these barriers are identified, the nurse can help the learner to plan to minimize barriers and, therefore, be successful in changing health behaviors.

Developmental Characteristics

Individuals' developmental stages influence cognitive, psychological, and psychomotor abilities for learning (Whitman, 1992c). Children's abilities in these areas change as they grow and mature. Children's mental, psychological, and psychomotor abilities for learning increase as they move from infancy through adolescence. Their abilities to learn primarily depend on their physical and mental maturation. In contrast, adult learning is primarily influenced by developmental tasks. Teaching adults focuses on collaboration and involvement in the teaching/learning process (Knowles, 1984). Successful teaching takes these developmental changes into consideration. Table 7–1 provides a comparison of learner characteristics between children and adults, and Table 7–2 lists considerations for teaching adults who are aging and experiencing a decline in their physical abilities.

Learner assessments can be part of physical and mental assessments. They can be conducted at the time of admission, while providing treatments or procedures, or during social interactions to establish rapport. It is important for the nurse to give assessment of learning abilities and past experi-

TABLE 7–1. COMPARISON OF HEALTH TEACHING FOR CHILDREN AND ADULTS

Characteristics	Children	Adults
Readiness to learn	Based primarily on biological development	Determined by life tasks, roles and immediate problems
Application of learning	Postponed application; subject centered	Immediate application related relevant problems
Orientation to learning	Dependent	Independent
Value of experience	Experiences seen as external events	Experiences are internalized; provide foundation for further learning; and may contribute to resistance to change
Rate of learning	Quickly masters isolated facts	Resistant to learning nonrelevant materials; aging process increases time needed to complete some learning tasks
Barriers to learning	Few competing responsibilities for learning time; accustomed to formal learning through school experiences	Family, work, and community may compete for learning time and energy

Reproduced with permission from Whitman, N. (1992). Developmental characteristics. In N. Whitman, C. Gliet, B. Graham, & M. D. Boyd. Teaching in nursing practice: A professional model (2nd ed.), (p. 125). East Norwalk, CT: Appleton & Lange.

TABLE 7–2. COMMON AGING CHANGES THAT AFFECT LEARNING

Changes with Aging	Adaptation for Teaching
Hearing	
Loss of ability to discriminate sounds	Speak clearly, sit close to "good ear"
Decreased conduction of sound	Do not shout. Speak in a normal tone or lower pitch slightly
Loss of ability to hear high frequency	
Decreased ability to distinguish words with S, Z, T, F, and G	Face learner to aid lip reading
	Use audiovisual aids to reinforce teaching
	Write key words in large black letters to reinforce oral communication
	Decrease extraneous noise
Vision	
Decreased visual acuity	Make sure glasses are clean and in place
Decreased ability to discriminate between blue, violet, and green. Colors tend to fade.	Use print materials with large 14-point type
Lens become thicker and more yellow with decreased accommodation	Use distinct large configurations, high contrast to help discrimination (black on white)
Pupil smaller, leading to less light reaching retina	Avoid or limit the use of blue, green, and violet
Decreased depth perception	Use soft white light to decrease glare
Decreased peripheral vision	Have light behind learner
	Avoid making room completely dark for audiovisual presentations
	Accommodate changes by taking more time for learner to explore depths
Smell, Touch, Taste, Vibration, and Temperature	
Decreased abilities in each of these	Teach alternate ways of assessing odors
	Offer fluids at periodic intervals during teaching
	Increase teaching time for psychomotor skills and allow time for repetitions
	Teach about using thermometers to check temperatures
Neurological	
Slowed cognitive functioning	Slow pace of presentation
Decreased short-term memory	Give smaller amounts of information at a time
Decreased ability to think abstractly	Repeat information frequently
Decreased ability to concentrate on material	Reinforce information frequently
Increased reaction time (slower to respond)	Reinforce oral teaching with written and audiovisual aids
	Use analogies and examples to illustrate abstract concepts
	Decrease outside stimuli
	Allow more time for learners to express themselves
Musculoskeletal	
Decreased muscle tone	Fatigues more easily; take frequent breaks
Osteoporosis	Have chairs with arm rests

TABLE 7–2. COMMON AGING CHANGES THAT AFFECT LEARNING (*continued*)

Changes with Aging	Adaptation for Teaching
Musculoskeletal (continued)	
Osteoarthritic changes	Teach low-impact exercises; provide mats for exercise; slow speed of exercise; increase warm-up and cool-down time
Thigh muscles flaccid	
Decreased rate and magnitude of reflex	
Decreased sense of balance	Increase safety precautions
Gait shorter and slower	Have nearby supports
Decreased fine motor coordination	
Psychological/Emotional	
Ego integrity versus despair (Erickson)	Establish reachable short-term goals
Well-developed lifestyle habits	Encourage participation in decision making and planning
Changes in roles due to retirement, etc.	
Changes in body image due to effects of aging	Integrate new behaviors with previously established ones
Decreased independence	Involve family members
	Focus on problem solving
	Apply teaching to the present
	Show relevance of teaching to everyday life
	Bolster self-esteem for learning
Respiratory	
Decreased blood flow to pulmonary circulation	Shorten length of teaching session
Tires more easily	Take frequent breaks
Cardiovascular	
Decreased oxygen to the cardiac muscle	Rise slowly
Decreased circulatory force may result in orthostatic hypotension	Change positions slowly
Genitourinary	
Prostate enlargement	More frequent bathroom breaks
Difficulty starting to urinate	
Loss of muscle tone in perineal floor leading to urgency and stress incontinence in females	
Endocrine	
Decreased heat regulation results in increased sense of being cold	Comfort may be an issue
	Have rooms warm
	Have learners bring sweaters or lap robes

Adapted from Weinrich, S. P., Boyd, M. D., & Nussbaum, J. (1989). Journal of Gerontological Nursing, 15 (11), 17–20, 33–34, with permission.

ences the same importance as other types of nursing assessments. For example, a nurse would not begin a nursing intervention for a patient in respiratory distress without first doing a physical assessment. To do so would anchor the nurse's intervention on a lack of necessary information, a hunch, or a guess and would not conform to standards of nursing practice. The outcomes of the nurse's actions may or may not bring about the desired result. Likewise, teaching without an accurate assessment may or may not result in successful teaching and learning. Moreover, teaching without assessing the learner is outside the standards for nursing practice.

PLANNING TEACHING

The teaching/learning process is a planned and sequential educational activity that nurses undertake to identify individual, family, and community learning needs and use to promote learning and the successful adoption of health behaviors. As discussed, the first step is to assess the learner. Once the assessment is completed, the nurse can identify learning needs, make nursing diagnoses, identify teaching and learning objectives, and plan teaching strategies. Evaluation of the success of the teaching and learning flow from the behavioral objectives.

Because health teaching can influence health behaviors and health outcomes, nurses must prioritize teaching content. Some content is essential to the individual's health, whereas other content may be desired but not necessary to promote health, maintain functioning, or prevent illness or disease. Another factor in planning teaching is the reality that the amount of time that realistically can be devoted to health teaching often is limited. Therefore, nurses must identify immediate learning needs (urgent), specific learning needs (necessary for that particular learner), and survival learning needs (life-sustaining). These must be put ahead of long-term learning needs (those that can be met at a later time), general learning needs (generic health information), and well-being learning needs (nice but not necessary) (George, 1982).

In addition, the nurse must incorporate those needs identified by the learner into planning teaching. Incorporating learner needs serves several purposes. It involves the learner in setting the teaching agenda and helps to invest the learner in the outcomes. It helps to remove the sense of paternalism that the nurse knows what is best and the learner should be a good learner and do it. Learner involvement also helps to place the responsibility of learning and behavioral change with the learner, not the nurse. It also provides an opportunity for the nurse to meet learning needs that may or may not be related to the immediate need. Collaboration between the learner and nurse in planning teaching content is essential to maximize learning.

After assessing which learning need must be met, nursing diagnoses related to teaching/learning are made. For example, if an individual is overweight because he or she does not know how to plan and prepare low-fat, nutritious meals, the nursing diagnosis would be "knowledge deficit related to nutrition and food preparation." If the learner does not know how to take a newly prescribed medication, the nursing diagnosis would be "knowledge deficit related to new medication." If the learner does not know how to perform a new psychomotor skill, then the nursing diagnosis would be "skills deficit related to ostomy self-care or skills deficit related to self-injection of insulin." Examples of nursing diagnoses related to health teaching are:

- Knowledge deficit related to preparation of low-fat meals
- Knowledge deficit related to new medication
- Psychomotor skills deficit related to self-injection of insulin
- Lack of exercise due to sedentary lifestyle
- Noncompliance of medication regimen due to belief of fatalism regarding health

Once learning needs are identified and nursing diagnoses made, goals and objectives for teaching must be delineated. Goals are broad general statements that describe what is expected to occur as a result of the teaching/learning. Planning teaching/learning can be analogous to planning a trip. The nurse has to know where he or she is going before planning on how to get there. Examples of goal statements are:

- Understands how to prepare low-fat, nutritious meals
- Understands how to take new medication
- Decreases blood cholesterol level
- Plans an exercise program
- Displays affection for new infant
  /of taking care of colostomy

Once this statement of learning destination is made, then the specific directions (behavioral objectives) can be formulated (Boyd, 1992d). Examples of behavioral objectives are found in Table 7–3.

TABLE 7–3. BEHAVIORAL OBJECTIVES

Who	What	Conditions	How Well	By When
Mrs. Smith	Will identify foods high in saturated fats	From a list of 20 foods	15 or more	Before discharge
Mr. Brown	Will demonstrate crutch walking	Without assistance	Using proper technique	By 4/23/97
Mrs. Jones	Will hold her infant close to her body	During feedings	Each time she feeds the infant	Before discharge
Mr. Long	Will change his wound dressing	With use of a checklist	Using sterile technique	Before discharge

Unlike goal statements, which are not measurable, behavioral objectives are specific about who will do what and under what circumstances, as defined by a given unit of measurement. If teachers have behavioral objectives, they can plan teaching content and methods to help the learner to meet the objectives (Reilly & Oermann, 1990). Learners can use behavioral objectives to know what is expected of them and as yardsticks of success. Moreover, behavioral objectives are the cornerstones of teaching/learning evaluations (Boyd, 1992d).

TEACHING STRATEGIES

Teaching strategies encompass instructional methods, educational methods, behavioral strategies, and teaching aids. Choosing the best methods and materials to facilitate learning is based on the nurse's assessment. Selected strategies that are commonly used in the clinical setting are presented here from each of these categories.

Instructional Methods

Instructional methods refer to how the nurse will structure the teaching session. Instructional methods include one-to-one instruction, lecture, lecture-discussion, demonstration, return demonstration, role playing, games, case presentations, simulations, and field trips. In most instances the nurse/teacher will use more than one of these methods to facilitate learning.

Instructional methods are chosen to facilitate a particular type of learning. For example, if information delivery is the primary objective, then a lecture format would be suitable. If, however, the learner is expected to master a skill, then demonstration and return demonstration would be the methods of choice. With objectives that focus on attitudinal change, discussion, role playing, and simulations would be the instructional methods of choice.

Educational Methods

Educational methods refer to strategies that have been shown to facilitate learning. The effectiveness of educational strategies increase if they are age specific. Educational strategies that are commonly used in health teaching include using a hierarchy of learning, advanced organizers, specificity, brevity, repetition, primacy, relevancy, and reinforcement.

Hierarchy of Learning

Learning must progress from simple to complex and from concrete to abstract in content. Moreover, learners need to have an understandable foundation on which to build more complex information or skills. This educational premise is evident in virtually every formal educational program. Individuals begin with the easiest information and necessary background information before moving on to higher-level material. An example of this principle is found in nursing education. Nursing students do not begin their nursing education by taking care of patients in an intensive care unit; rather, they learn about a host of interrelated materials and skills one course at a time, building gradually on their knowledge and abilities to eventually reach the point of competency to care for the critically ill. This is not to say that learners cannot successfully carry out health care recommendations without fully understanding them. The goal of health teaching is not to produce experts in a particular area but to assist individuals to acquire adequate knowledge and skills to effectively maintain or promote their health and well being and avoid a decrease in their health status.

One way to determine what information a learner needs is to organize it into *nice to know* and *need to know* information and skills. Once this has been determined, then using a hierarchical approach will help the learner to master the content or skill.

Advanced Organizers

Advanced organizers involve telling the learner what is to be learned, then cuing the learner to each point, and when the teaching session is finished, summarizing what was covered. For example, the nurse would say, "Mr. Smith, today I'm going to go over your heart medicine. I'll be talking about four things. It's important that you remember each of these so you can take your medicine correctly at home. I'll be sharing with you: (1) The name of your heart medicine; (2) Why you need to take it; (3) How to take it; and (4) What side effects you will need to tell your doctor about. Now, let's start with (1). The name of your heart medicine is _____" Once the nurse has covered each of these areas, she or he can summarize each of the four key points and have the learner review them to check for comprehension and accuracy of the information retained.

Specificity

Specificity, or making the information clear and to the point, increases the learner's ability to remember it. The learner can cue in easily on the expected behavior. For example, a learner will have a much clearer idea of what is expected of him or her when the nurse instructs the learner to walk 15 minutes each day, 5 days a week until the return appointment rather than telling the learner to "get some exercise." Long, detailed discussions may not get the point across as effectively.

Brevity

Brevity has many advantages for teaching and learning. People can remember small amounts of information better than large amounts, and fortunately, short teaching sessions are more realistic for nurses to incorporate into their clinical practice. Again, it is important to prioritize the content, focus on necessary information, and leave the *nice to know* information to be covered once crucial content has been mastered.

Repetition

Repetition strengthens learning. Using a variety of methods to present information also strengthens learning by having the learner use more than one way of experiencing the information. Repeating the information by oral, written, and audiovisual methods and through physical involvement increases retention of the information or skill and reinforces learning.

Primacy

Regardless of what information is presented, people remember the first one-third and the last one-fourth of the information best (Ley, 1972). Therefore, it behooves the nurse/teacher to structure health teaching in such a manner that the most important content is presented first and a summary of the key points is made in closing.

Relevancy

Making the material relevant to the learner and his or her needs and interest is necessary to ensure that the learner will see the need to apply the learning to his or her life. For example, why would an individual exert time and energy to learning information about diabetes unless there was a need or particular interest involved? The nurse should ask how the information can be presented so the learner sees its utility to his or her health and daily functioning.

Reinforcement

Reinforcement of learning provides the learner with feedback, increases retention, and increases the learner's ability to master the content or skill. Positive reinforcement can help an individual to feel confident for self-care and increase his or her self-efficacy.

Behavioral Strategies

Behavioral strategies encompass those methods that have been shown to increase the likelihood of behavioral change. These strategies include contracting, graduated behavioral change, tailoring, and self-monitoring.

Contracting

Contracting has been shown to be an effective method of promoting behavioral change. In contracting, the teacher and learner mutually develop a contract of behavior and rewards. The reward must be something that the learner chooses. The contract should be fair; the terms should be clear; and the reward should be positive. The contracts and procedures should be consistent, and at least one other person should participate in the behavior change (Mahoney & Thoresen, 1974).

Graduated Behavioral Change

Graduated behavioral change is accomplished through the learner's making small increments of change over time. This strategy services several purposes. It makes the task seem manageable; it does not overwhelm the learner with new behavior; it increases the possibility for success; and it increases odds of the behavior continuing as an ingrained habit. For example, it would be easier for an individual to decrease gradually the fat in his or her diet starting with those items that he or she perceives as the easiest to change or give up than to suddenly and totally change the diet. Another example would be a smoker who does not believe that he or she can quit "cold turkey" but is willing to decrease the nicotine content of the cigarettes and gradually decrease the number smoked each day.

Tailoring

Tailoring is a successful behavioral strategy for increasing adherence to behavioral change. Tailoring involves "fitting" a prescribed regimen into a learner's lifestyle. The objective of tailoring is to try and disrupt the individual's daily routine as little as possible when incorporating a new health behavior. For example, a once-a-day medication such as a diuretic may be prescribed. Typically it is taken in the morning. If the nurse does not assess the patient's lifestyle, she or he may not learn that the patient works nights and sleeps during the day. The patient may stop taking the diuretic because it interrupts his sleep. For patients who do not have easy access to a bathroom, such as truck drivers and high-rise construction workers, tailoring a diuretic medication to their lifestyle may greatly increase their medication compliance.

Self-Monitoring

Self-monitoring works well with literate and highly motivated learners. Having learners keep a diary of their health behaviors, such as eating patterns, can help them to determine what, how much, where, and when they eat. They can use this information to analyze their eating behaviors and plan for change. Other behaviors such as monitoring stress and anger also can be changed through self-monitoring.

Teaching Aids

Teaching aids are those materials that the nurse uses to help to get the information across to the learner. Teaching aids include pictures, props, audiovisuals (overhead transparencies, slides, and television), print materials, three-dimensional objects such as models, and computer-assisted instruction. Teaching aids are helpful because they allow the concepts to be presented in a variety of formats and require the learner to use multiple senses in learning. Teaching aids should be chosen with care to ensure that they are accurate, up to date, culturally sensitive, literacy appropriate, and relevant to the learning.

Throughout the teaching/learning process, the nurse needs to make sure that the teaching style and content are culturally sensitive and literacy appropriate. If the teaching process and materials are not culturally sensitive, the learner may not believe that they are relevant to him or her or may find the teaching materials offensive. If literacy abilities are not taken into account before teaching, the learner may not understand what is being taught and may exhibit poor compliance because he or she does not understand what is expected of him or her.

EVALUATION OF TEACHING AND LEARNING

Evaluation of teaching and learning involves assessing both the process and the outcomes of learning. Evaluation is an ongoing aspect of teaching that allows the nurse to adjust the teaching process as he or she gains more information. Continual evaluation helps the nurse to tailor the teaching process to the learner. Evaluation also serves as the basis for documenting learning.

Formative Evaluation

The process of formative evaluation focuses on the nurse and the teaching process and involves the nurse's assessing the effectiveness of the stages of assessment, planning, and implementation (Boyd, 1992d). Were pertinent data collected to identify learning needs and to form accurate nursing diagnoses? Was the choice of teaching methods and materials appropriate to the learner and the information or skill to be learned? What problems or difficulties occurred during the process? The nurse will use this information to improve the quality of teaching. Formative evaluation also enables the nurse to identify patients with difficulty learning; early in the teaching in some situations, the teaching may need to focus on the caregiver or family member rather than the patient.

Outcome Evaluation

Outcome evaluation, or impact evaluation, focuses on the learner. Behavioral objectives are used to measure the success of learning. Did the learner meet the behavioral objectives? Was the teaching process successful in promoting learning?

Evaluation methods can include written tests, checklists, interviews, observation of behavior, and physiological outcomes such as blood pressure and cholesterol levels. The nurse must use a method that is appropriate to the learning being evaluated and that is reasonable given the clinical setting. Common evaluation methods include having learners review what they have learned and return the demonstration. Another method that helps the nurse to assess the learner's ability to use the information is to have the learner solve hypothetical situations based on the desired information and skills that he or she has learned. The nurse must be careful in choosing evaluation methods to make sure that they evaluate what the learner needs to know. For example, one cardiac rehabilitation program's evaluation of class content focused on the prevalence of cardiovascular disease and national mortality statistics. The test did not address the information that individuals in the program needed to know to identify symptoms of angina, what to do with the onset of angina, and so forth. The test was evaluating *nice to know* information, not the learners' retention of *need to know* information.

Another consideration in choosing evaluation methods is the learner's abilities and comfort level with using that particular method. Many learners may feel threatened by formal evaluation such as written tests. A more relaxed and informal method of discussion or return demonstration may be more suitable.

Methods appropriate for evaluating cognitive learning would include written tests, checklists, oral summaries, and discussions. Methods suitable for evaluating psychomotor skills include checklists, simulations, observation, and return demonstrations. Evaluation of attitudinal change might include discussions, role playing, observation, and attitudinal-oriented written tests.

DOCUMENTATION OF HEALTH TEACHING

Documentation of health teaching is just as important and necessary as documentation of any other nursing activity. Documentation serves several purposes. It provides a permanent record of teaching and learning (documentation materials must remain in the permanent record). It serves as a communication medium among various health professionals. It is required for accreditation of many agencies, and it is required for third-party reimbursement such as Medicare (Boyd, 1992a; Joint Commission on Accreditation of Health Care Organizations, 1994). Most important, documentation serves to record the nurse's planned and purposeful approach to teaching and the learner's ability to learn and use the information or skills. This documentation would prove invaluable in a court of law.

Documentation of health teaching does not need to be lengthy or time consuming. Flowcharts, checklists, and standardized teaching care plans can be used to streamline documentation. If anecdotal notes are used, the nurse can note content, learner response, and the learner's ability to use the information or skill appropriately. What is most important is that the nurse documents that teaching occurred, the extent of learning in objective terms, and the learner's ability to use the knowledge or skills learned with sufficient mastery to avoid coming to harm.

SUMMARY

Health teaching is a challenging, yet immensely rewarding, part of nursing practice. The nurse has the ethical and legal responsibility to provide quality health teaching to each patient and consumer under his or her care. The process of health teaching is based on data gleaned from a vast array of professions and is constantly changing and growing. Health teaching is a planned and purposeful activity that moves through the phases of assessment, planning, and evaluation. The nurse chooses appropriate instructional methods, educational and behavioral strategies, and teaching aids based on the assessment. Evaluating both the teaching process and the learner's ability to use information and skills is necessary to determine the success of the process. The outcomes of health teaching must be documented to communicate that teaching and learning have occurred and to serve as a legal record.

REFERENCES

Bandura, A. (1986). *Foundation of thought and action: A social cognitive theory.* Englewood Cliffs, NJ: Prentice-Hall.

Becker, M. (1974). *The health belief model and personal health behavior.* Thorofare, NJ: Slack.

Boyd, M. D. (1992a). Policies, guidelines and legal mandates for health teaching. In N. Whitman, C. Gliet, B. Graham, & M. D. Boyd (Eds.), *Teaching in nursing practice: A professional model* (pp. 17–30). East Norwalk, CT: Appleton & Lange.

Boyd, M. D. (1992b). Strategies for effective health teaching. In N. Whitman, C. Gliet, B. Graham, & M. D. Boyd, *Teaching in nursing practice: A professional model* (pp. 171–194). East Norwalk, CT: Appleton & Lange.

Boyd, M. D. (1992c). Teaching populations with special needs. In N. Whitman, C. Gliet, B. Graham, & M. D. Boyd, *Teaching in nursing practice: A professional model* (pp. 235–259). East Norwalk, CT: Appleton & Lange.

Boyd, M. D. (1992d). The teaching process. In N. Whitman, C. Gliet, B. Graham, & M. D. Boyd, *Teaching in nursing practice: A professional model* (pp. 155–170). East Norwalk, CT: Appleton & Lange.

Department of Health and Human Services. (1991). *Literacy and health in the United States: Selected annotations.* Atlanta: Center for Disease Control, Department of Health and Human Services, Public Health Service.

Doak, C. C., Doak, L. G., & Root, J. H. (1985). *Teaching patients with low literacy skills.* Philadelphia: Lippincott.

George, G. (1982, May). If patient teaching tries your patience, try this plan. *Nursing '82, 12,* 50–55.

Joint Commission on Accreditation of Health Care Organizations. (1994). *The Joint Commission standards for nursing care* (2nd ed.). Oakbrook Terrace, IL: Author.

Knowles, M. S. (1984). *Andragogy in action.* San Francisco: Jossey-Bass.

Ley, P. (1972). Primary rated importance and recall of medical statements. *Journal of Health and Social Behavior, 13,* 311–317.

Mahoney, M. J., & Thoresen, C. E. (1974). *Self-control: Power to person*. Monterey, CA: Brooks-Cole.

O'Leary, A. (1985). Self-efficacy and health. *Behavioral research and therapy, 23*, 437–451.

Potter, P. A., & Perry, A. G. (1991). *Basic nursing: Theory and practice*. St. Louis: Mosby.

Rankin, S. H., & Duffy, K. L. (1993). *Patient education: Issues, principles, and guidelines*. Philadelphia: Lippincott.

Reilly, D. E., & Oermann, M. H. (1990). *Behavioral objectives: Evaluation in nursing* (3rd ed.). New York: National League for Nursing.

Rosenstock, I. M. (1990). The health belief model: Explaining health behavior through expectancies. In R. Glanz, B. Rimer, & F. Lewis (Eds.), *Health behavior and health education: Theory, research and practice*. San Francisco: Jossey-Bass.

Wallston, B. S., Wallston, K. A., Kaplan, G. D., & Maides, S. A. (1976). Development and validation of the health locus of control scales. *Journal of Consulting and Clinical Psychology, 44*, 580–585.

Weiss, B. D., Blanchard, J. S., McGee, D. L., Hart, G., Warren, B., Burgoon, M., et al. (1994). Illiteracy among Medicaid recipients and its relationship to health care costs. *Journal of Health Care for the Poor and Underserved, 5*, 99–111.

Whitman, N. (1992a). Age related factors influencing selection of teaching strategies. In N. Whitman, C. Gliet, B. Graham, & M. D. Boyd (Eds.), *Teaching in nursing practice: A professional model* (pp. 195–216). East Norwalk, CT: Appleton & Lange.

Whitman, N. (1992b). Assessment of the learner. In N. Whitman, C. Gliet, B. Graham, & M. D. Boyd (Eds.), *Teaching in nursing practice: A professional model* (pp. 133–152). East Norwalk, CT: Appleton & Lange.

Whitman, N. (1992c). Developmental characteristics. In N. Whitman, C. Gliet, B. Graham, & M. D. Boyd (Eds.), *Teaching in nursing practice: A professional model* (pp. 115–131). East Norwalk, CT: Appleton & Lange.

Whitman, N. (1992d). Learner readiness: Factors affecting the client as a learner. In N. Whitman, C. Gliet, B. Graham, & M. D. Boyd (Eds.), *Teaching in nursing practice: A professional model* (pp. 89–90). East Norwalk, CT: Appleton & Lange.

BIBLIOGRAPHY

Cordell, B., & Smith-Blair, N. (1994). Streamlined charting for patient education. *Nursing '94, 1*, 57–59.

Dellasega, C., Clark, D., McCreary, D., Helmuth, A., & Schan, P. (1994). Nursing process: Teaching elderly clients. *Journal of Gerontological Nursing, 1*, 31–38.

Griffiths, M., & Leek, C. (1995). Patient education needs: Opinions of oncology nurses and their patients. *Oncology Nursing Forum, 22*, 139–144.

Lorig, K. (1992). *Patient education: A practical approach*. St. Louis: Mosby.

Miller, B., & Bodie, M. (1995). Determination of reading comprehension level for effective patient health-education materials. *Nursing Research, 43*, 118–119.

Miller, M. (1995). Culture, spirituality, and women's health. *Journal of Obstetrics, Gynecology and Neonatal Nursing, 24*, 257–263.

Office of Education and Improvement. (1993). *Adult literacy in America: A first look at the results of the National Adult Literacy Survey* (2nd ed.). Washington, DC: Department of Education.

Redman, B. L. (1988). *The process of patient education* (6th ed.). St. Louis: Mosby.

Theis, S. L., & Johnson, J. H. (1995). Strategies for teaching patients: A meta-analysis. *Clinical Nurse Specialist, 9*, 100–105, 120.

Tolsma, D. D. (1993). Patient education objectives in Healthy People 2000: Policy and research issues. *Patient Education and Counseling, 22*, 7–14.

Weinrich, S. P., Weinrich, M. C., Boyd, M. D., Atwood, J., & Cervanka, B. (1994). Teaching older adults by adapting for aging changes. *Cancer Nursing, 17*, 494–500.

Whitman, N., Gliet, C., Graham, B., & Boyd, M. D. (Eds.) (1992). *Teaching in nursing practice: A professional model* (2nd ed.). East Norwalk, CT: Appleton & Lange.

Computers in Nursing Practice

Patricia A. Brown and Sally S. Kellum

The integration of computer applications into health care has proven to be one of the most exciting technological advances in the field. The impact of computers on nursing, in particular, has been dramatic. Computers are helping to improve the quality and efficiency of nursing care delivery through the use of information systems that facilitate the input, processing, and retrieval of patient information. Electronic access to discussion groups, journals, books, and databases via electronic networking provides practitioners with current resources for improving the quality of care. Nursing care planning programs are assisting nurses with decision making. Computer-based instruction programs are adding a new dimension to professional and patient education. Word processing, spreadsheet, and database programs are facilitating administrative tasks and increasing productivity. As these uses become more sophisticated and widespread, computers will be integrated in nursing practice in ways that have yet to be imagined.

The nurse of today and tomorrow must have a sound knowledge base in computer technology and its nursing practice applications in order to function competently in settings in which these applications are integral to nursing care delivery. This chapter provides a foundation in the basics of computer technology and its applications.

COMPUTER TECHNOLOGY

One need not be an engineer or mathematician to understand what a computer is or how it works. A computer, or more appropriately, a computer system, is a combination of devices interconnected and working together in a synchronized fashion to perform tasks for people (users) by processing information that is stored in the computer or entered into it. Some computer systems are more powerful than others; that is, they can store more information and execute sophisticated jobs more quickly, thus increasing their capacity for task performance.

The three major categories or types of computers are: (1) mainframe computers, (2) minicomputers, and (3) microcomputers. Mainframes are the largest, most expensive, and most powerful computers. They are used typically by large organizations, such as hospitals or corporations, and can serve multiple users simultaneously. Minicomputers are somewhat smaller than mainframes, less expensive, and less powerful. They are generally used by large organizations as well and also can serve multiple users simultaneously. Microcomputers, or personal computers (PCs), are the smallest and least powerful of the computer systems and also the least expensive. The technology of personal computers, however, has progressed rapidly. Currently, PCs match or exceed the capabilities of the minicomputers of only a few years ago. Today's PCs can serve multiple users simultaneously via PC networks. Because PCs are now able to perform tasks previously limited to mainframes and minicomputers, PCs have been displacing these more expensive and more specialized machines.

The devices or equipment that are integral to any computer system are called hardware; software refers to the special instructions, or programs, written for and executed by computer hardware. Computer hardware enables computer software to perform its designated task.

Computer Hardware

A computer system consists of various hardware components, the primary being the *central processing unit (CPU)*. The CPU of a computer system executes instructions from programs that are loaded into the system, retrieving and processing information from memory (part of the computer where programs and data are stored) as necessary. Computer memory also is built into the hardware of a computer system, and in many computer systems additional memory capacity may be added at a later time, if needed. The CPU and computer memory usually are housed in the same box or chassis and constitute what is commonly referred to as "the computer."

All interactions with computers are accomplished using hardware called *peripherals*. All commands, or instructions, to the computer CPU are sent through peripherals, and all output from the computer CPU is presented through peripherals. Peripherals include such devices as computer keyboards and monitors.

Information (data) can be entered into a computer system through a variety of peripherals called *input devices*. These input devices are connected to the CPU of a computer system by cables.

- *Keyboard*. A keyboard that resembles a typewriter keyboard is the most common input device. Information is entered into the computer by pressing the keys.
- *Light pen*. A light pen resembles a writing pen attached to a thin wire. When held up to and moved against the surface of a computer display screen, the light pen allows the user to control the software application. Light pens require software that is specifically designed to be used with them.
- *Mouse*. A mouse is a small rectangular device, about the size and shape of a note pad, with one to three buttons on it. By moving the mouse, users can control the movement of an on-screen pointer or cursor. Depending on the application in use, clicking the mouse enables specific tasks to be completed.
- *Optical scanner*. Optical scanners vary in size, shape, and capabilities. They can transfer printed material (text) and pictures (graphics) into a computer system by scanning materials that are inserted into the scanner or moved across the surface of the scanner.
- *Voice recognition*. Some computers are equipped to understand speech, although in a limited way. Speech that is understood is entered into the CPU and causes the computer to execute certain tasks.

A variety of peripherals are used to transfer information from the computer to the user. These are commonly known as output devices. As with input devices, they are connected to the CPU of a computer system by cables:

- *Computer monitor*. A computer monitor displays information, text, and graphics from a computer on a screen for the user to read. Monitors can be either monochrome (black and white) or color. Most desktop PCs use cathode ray tube (CRT) monitors, identical to those used in televisions. Portable PCs, known as laptop or notebook PCs, use various types of liquid crystal display (LCD) monitors. When a monitor functions as a "touch screen," or a light pen is used with a monitor, the user touches the monitor to make selections or enter information into the computer. In this way, a computer monitor can also serve as an input device.
- *Printer*. A printer provides printed pages, or hard copy, of information from the computer to the user. The output is identical to the information that can be displayed to users on a computer monitor. There are different types of printers, varying in size, speed, cost, capabilities, and quality of print. Dot-matrix, ink jet, and laser printers are commonly used with PCs. Laser printers are the fastest and provide the highest quality of print, although they are more expensive.

A *computer terminal* serves as both an input and output device. The term *computer terminal* refers to a monitor and keyboard, usually when these are linked to a more powerful computer. In a mainframe or minicomputer environment, computer terminals usually have limited processing power of their own, whereas in a PC network, the individual terminals are PCs that have their own processing power.

An additional piece of hardware that serves as both an input and output device is the *modem*. A modem, which stands for modulator/demodulator, is connected to the CPU of a computer system either within the same chassis or through an external cable connection. It is a small device that, when functioning, enables a computer system to communicate with other computer systems via ordinary telephone lines. Information can be transferred from system to system. It is through a modem that users can connect to various on-line services. As with other types of hardware, modems vary in cost and capability, and the most expensive modems usually provide the quickest transfer of information from computer system to computer system.

Computer Software

A computer program, or software, is a group or set of instructions that have been developed by computer programmers for the purpose of carrying out a specific task or tasks. Computer programs are written in various languages, such as BASIC, C, and PASCAL; the type of language utilized depends on the task to be accomplished, expertise of the programmer, and type of hardware with which the software will be used. Each computer program has specific hardware requirements; software designed for one type of hardware will not "run" (work) on other hardware, unless the hardware has been designated as compatible. One need not be a computer programmer to run software; well-designed software should be "user-friendly," that is, easy to use.

Computer programs or data are stored on floppy disks, also called diskettes; fixed hard disks; or CD-ROMs (compact disk read-only-memory). Floppy disks are portable and compact but have a limited capacity. A hard disk is a device, housed in the chassis with the CPU, that has the capacity to store vast amounts of data or programs. The largest floppy disks hold the equivalent of 500 typewritten pages, whereas the largest hard disks can hold the equivalent of millions of typewritten pages. CD-ROMs are portable and compact, like floppy disks, and can store the equivalent of hundreds of thousands of typewritten pages. Unlike floppy disks and hard disks, however, CD-ROMs are read-only, that is, the data or programs on them cannot be altered.

As mentioned, computer hardware enables computer software to perform its designated task. However, the user is an indispensable part of this whole process, for it is the user who must enter specific commands into the CPU through an input device instructing it to run a specified program, access specific data, or perform another function.

Most computer programs are copyrighted; that is, they belong to the copyright holder and can be used only as specified by the agreement that accompanies the program. Many agreements specify that the software can be used only on one machine at a time. Although many programs are copy-protected, difficult, if not impossible, to physically copy on to another disk, the user still may be able to copy them to other diskettes and thus have more than one copy available for use. Unless a licensing agreement specifically states that this is permissible, however, doing so would be illegal and unethical. Unfortunately, "pirating" of computer software is a major problem, one that must be discouraged as unlawful and unethical. Programs designated as public domain can be freely used without violating any copyright. On-line computer networks enable access to many public domain programs that legally can be *downloaded*, that is, transmitted from a remote site to a local computer system, for later use.

Computer programs perform many different kinds of tasks with the greatest accuracy and efficiency. Some general-purpose software includes word processing, spreadsheet, database, communications, graphics, desktop publishing, and presentation software:

- *Word processing software.* A word processor allows users to create a document as it would be done on a typewriter. However, the words and paragraphs can be edited, saved, and retrieved as necessary, making it unnecessary to totally recreate the document to make corrections. The editing capabilities of a word processor vary. A good word processor, however, will permit users easily to delete letters, words, and paragraphs; move blocks of text from one part of a document to another; locate specific words or phrases; change margins; paginate; and highlight specific parts of a document with underlining, boldface, italics, and so forth. Many word processors also include a spelling checker that can detect and correct misspelled words. A document created with a word processor can even be used in conjunction with a grammar checker program so that basic grammatical errors can be detected and corrected. Documents created with a word processor are given a file name and can be saved on a floppy or hard disk and/or printed (hard copy) and retrieved as necessary.
- *Spreadsheet software.* A spreadsheet program provides the user with an array or matrix of "cells" into which numbers, formulas, or text can be entered. The spreadsheet program enables the user to link the cells as desired.
- *Database software.* With the use of database software, users can store, sort, and retrieve information from databases. Databases are comprised of records, where each record can include a variety of information. Software is available that allows the user to create databases from scratch, that is, the user defines the record structure and enters data into the records. Data stored in databases can be sorted, searched, and extracted depending on various criteria.

- *Communications software.* Communications software, used in conjunction with a telephone line and modem, allows users to access other computer systems. General-purpose communications software allows users to connect to various on-line services, computer bulletin boards, or computer networks such as the Internet. More specialized communications software provides access to specific networks.
- *Graphics software.* Graphics software allows users to create images on a computer monitor, modify them as necessary, and save and/or print them. With the use of graphics software, illustrations can be created for printed documents as well as audiovisuals, such as slides and overhead transparencies. Collections of graphics images, sometimes referred to as clip-art libraries, can also be purchased and used with other computer applications.
- *Desktop publishing.* Desktop publishing software includes word processing and graphics capabilities in the same software program. With the use of desktop publishing software, manuscripts that include both text and illustrations can be created and, in combination with high-quality printers, made ready for publication. Desktop publishing programs also can be used to create high-quality educational materials.
- *Presentation software.* Presentation software allows users to create presentations that integrate graphics, clips from videos or software programs, and even sound with text. These presentations are referred to as *multimedia*. The more traditional style of presentation, which involved using overhead transparencies or slides that were activated at specific times during a presentation, is fast being replaced by multimedia presentations developed and managed by presentation software. The presentation requires the use of a monitor large enough to be seen by the audience or a transparent LCD panel placed on an overhead projector. The presentation is controlled by a keyboard or mouse.

COMPUTERS IN HEALTH CARE DELIVERY AND NURSING

Computer technology, still evolving in health care delivery, has had a tremendous impact on patient care. Computers have helped to make medical diagnosis quicker and more accurate and medical treatment more efficient. They also have enabled health care providers and consumers to access health information more readily. Likewise, computers have helped to make the delivery of nursing care more efficient.

Nursing informatics, broadly defined early on as "the use of computers in nursing clinical practice, administration, research, and education" (Ball, Hannah, Jelger, & Peterson, 1988, p. xv), has emerged as a nursing specialty. Nursing informatics uses "computer science, information science, and nursing science . . . to assist in the management and processing of nursing data, information, and knowledge to support the practice of nursing and the delivery of nursing care" (Graves & Corcoran, 1989, p. 227). Informatics nurses "analyze, design, develop, modify, implement, evaluate, or maintain information handling technologies that collect patient and client data to support the practice of nursing" (ANA, 1995, p. iii) and, in doing so, assume varied roles in a wide range of settings (Carty, 1994). Certification as an Informatics Nurse is now offered through the American Nurses Credentialing Center.

The overview of computer applications described encompasses the possibilities currently offered by computers, although they may not yet be apparent in all settings. Integrating computer technology in professional practice and health care delivery systems requires thoughtful planning, financial commitment, and user education. Nurses' experiences with computers will vary.

Computers in Clinical Practice

The clinical practice applications of computer technology are some of the most exciting and widespread of all computer health care applications.

Medical Diagnosis and Treatment

Although this area of application is not directly related to nursing practice, each nurse should be familiar with the ways in which computers are used to facilitate medical diagnosis and treatment. Often, the nurse is required to educate patients about diagnostic procedures and treatments. In order to do so effectively, he or she should be well informed about the procedures or treatments and the underlying technology.

Before the computer era, medical diagnosis was commonly a long and tedious process that was often unsuccessful until it was too late. Today, with the help of computer technology, diagnosis is quicker and more accurate. Computer systems that are used in medical diagnosis are usually *dedicated systems*, that is, they are designed to perform specialized tasks and are not used for other purposes.

Computers are frequently used today for medical imaging, such as computed tomography (CT) scans, magnetic resonance imaging (MRI), and ultrasound. Precise images of tissue can be generated with a CT scan of tissue. The procedure involves the noninvasive scanning of tissue with a radiographic beam and subsequent computerized analysis to produce a three-dimensional image of the scanned tissue or organ, showing its position and shape. Pictures produced by CT scan are far superior to those produced by non-CT scans and can eliminate the need for further diagnostic testing to distinguish among types of soft-tissue pathologies, such as blood, clot, cyst, and tumor (Bronzino, 1982). An MRI machine uses magnetic fields that cause energy to be absorbed and emitted from tissue, depending on the chemical and physical environment present. A computer analyzes differences in energy and generates even more explicit images that provide information about the chemical composition of the tissue, its structure, and function (Green, Modic, & Steinmetz, 1987). In addition to CT scan and MRI, images produced from ultrasound techniques, which use sound waves to differentiate tissues, that were originally generated without computer intervention are now more accurate because of the introduction of computers to medical imaging (Friedman & Street, 1986–87). More recently, computed radiography has emerged. This technology promises to convert all general radiological films to an electronic form. Radiology may someday be a filmless process that will allow multiple users to view X-ray results on monitors in different areas of a hospital and even at remote sites, such as a physician's office. "The 'filmless' hospital has been demonstrated as a model for the future" (Shannon, 1985, p. 295).

Computers also have made laboratory analysis of specimens more accurate, efficient, and objective. Analysis of blood and tissue specimens has been computerized. Subjective, tedious, microscopic analysis of cells has been replaced by flow cytometry (which collects data from each cell) and computerized cell analysis (which compiles the data from cells). These computer analyses produce quantitative and objective information about cells and tissues (Friedman & Street, 1986–87). In today's environment of managed care and cost consciousness, many laboratories are negotiating outreach programs. As a by-product of these affiliations, facilities will be networked with these outreach sites to enhance ordering tests and receiving results.

In addition to the use of computers for medical imaging and laboratory analysis, computer systems also have been developed to serve interpretive functions. As described by Bronzino (1982), these systems enhance care by facilitating the accuracy of results and diagnosis and by returning the results quickly. For example, ECG (electrocardiogram) and pulmonary function test interpretation are accomplished with systems dedicated to these specific functions. A typical ECG interpretative system functions via telephone lines that transmit ECG signals to the computer system; the system analyzes the signals based on predetermined criteria entered into the system and interprets the ECG, generating a diagnosis, for example, a specific dysrhythmia. Computerized ECG interpretation also is used to assess patient response to physical exercise, such as during a stress test and for ambulatory (Holter) monitoring (VanBemmel, 1987). A computerized pulmonary function lab analyzes and processes data from measurement devices that determine the partial pressures of gases, lung volume, and gas and fluid flow. Utilizing predetermined criteria and calculations, the computer system interprets these results for the user (Bronzino, 1982).

Health Care Information Systems

In a variety of clinical practice settings, computer technology is making the delivery of care more efficient and cost effective through the development and implementation of information systems that increase productivity. Information systems can be designed to manage the data and functions inherent in any setting, such as an entire hospital, one department in a hospital, an ambulatory care practice, or a statewide health department. An information system can run on a mainframe, minicomputer, or PC, depending on the capacity of the system. Using an information system, data are processed and organized. The content and design of the system are determined by eventual users who access the system via PCs or terminals. Information systems require significant financial and time commitment for research and development and for implementation. Systems are developed in-house or purchased from vendors, who tailor generic systems to individual users. Integration of computer-driven information systems is needed for medical practice (Shannon, 1985, p. 295) and health care in general.

The most common categories of information systems include hospital information systems (HIS), nursing information systems (NIS), and patient data management systems (PDMS).

Hospital Information Systems. An HIS is a network of computer terminals linked to a central mainframe or minicomputer housed in a specific location in a hospital. The main computer system is programmed at varying levels of complexity to facilitate the tasks that must be accomplished throughout the hospital. Inherent in the system is a design to maintain patients' records in a consistent fashion. Patient information can be stored in the system and retrieved as necessary. Information systems can improve discharge planning and patient follow-up and monitor quality of care by automatically comparing actual care to predetermined standards (Gross, 1988). Allocation of nursing resources can be accomplished using patient acuity classification systems that predict the staffing of nursing personnel (Saba, 1988).

Users in various departments throughout the hospital access an HIS via terminals located in their respective departments. At these terminals, data can be entered, processed, or retrieved, and tasks specific to the department can be accomplished. From terminals located in the admissions office, admissions information can be entered and a patient's file started. From terminals in the laboratory, results of lab tests can be entered into a patient's file. In an operating room setting, scheduling, staff records, inventory control, infection control, room use, equipment use and needs, and costs can be managed (Robinson, 1985; Warnock-Matheron & Hannah, 1988). From central supply areas and the pharmacy, information regarding supplies and drugs used by individual patients can be entered. In fully integrated systems, information from one department links to information in other departments, for example, with the department responsible for compiling a patient's bill. This enables billing to be accomplished automatically by the system. Medical orders and physicians' notes can be entered into the system and instantaneously printed in the appropriate departments. Fully integrated hospital information systems allow all departments to communicate with each other. Some HISs include a variety of individual information systems for different areas, such as billing, some of which may have been purchased from different vendors. These systems should interface easily with each other; data should not be duplicated but integrated. Specific nursing applications are often integral to an HIS. Nurses use a computerized hospital information system more than any other group of heath care professionals (Hannah, Ball, & Edwards, 1994).

Nursing Information Systems. Nursing information systems have been described as systems that use computer technology to support the administration of nursing services and the delivery of patient care (Saba, 1988). An NIS should be integral to an HIS or easily interfaced. With the use of an NIS, nursing functions that involve recording patient information or accessing relevant patient information are accomplished via a computer terminal, strategically placed on the nursing unit either in the nurses' station or, more recently, point-of-care terminals at a patient's bedside. In critical care areas, the bedside terminal can be mounted on a rolling device that can be raised for standing or lowered for use in a chair. A long cord allows the device to be moved outside the patient's room, if necessary, for privacy or isolation cases. The current trend is for the point-of-care terminal to be portable. Many facilities are implementing wireless systems that connect via airwaves to the NIS or HIS. These resemble laptop computers and are being used on rounds for implementing orders while observing the patient (Figure 8–1). The computer moves with the practitioner, eliminating the need for notes and later transcription. A speech-input interface for computerized charting, intended to be more convenient and easier to use than keyboard or keypad entry, also has been introduced. "The addition of a speech-input interface that frees the nurse's hands and eyes may fill the current void for a well-accepted, productivity-enhancing, and nursing specific computer interface" (Dillon, McDowell, Norcio, & DeHaemer, 1994).

With an NIS, documentation of nursing care is accomplished on the computer rather than handwritten in a patient's chart. Progress notes and clinical observations, for example, vital signs and intake and output, can be edited as they are entered; after they are entered, however, they cannot be modified or deleted.

The majority of the literature has supported the success of nursing information systems and computerized charting. With an information system in place, personnel can be used more effectively, duplication of effort can be avoided, and time previously spent on clerical activities can be reduced (Hannah et al., 1994). With computerized documentation, time spent on charting can be reduced (Minda & Brundage, 1994; Pabst, Scherubel, & Minnick, 1996) and time spent in patient care increased (Pabst et al.). As de-

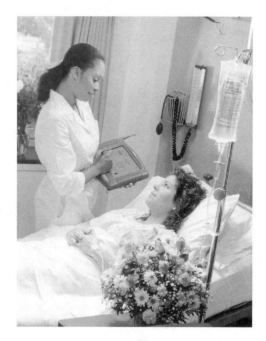

Figure 8–1. A nurse uses a hand-held wireless device to chart at a patient's bedside. *(Telxon Corporation, Akron, Ohio, with permission.)*

scribed by McKinney (1988), nurses report that they are more organized and efficient when fully functioning computer terminals are located at each patient's bedside. Nurses have responded positively to computerized bedside nursing systems particularly with regard to comprehensiveness and timeliness of documentation. In particular, nurses found on-screen prompts that reminded them about tasks to be done or when to document especially helpful (Hendrickson, Kovner, Knickman, & Finkler, 1995). Using a hand-held computer for home care visits, nursing productivity and cost savings increased dramatically (Gogola, 1995).

Nursing care planning programs also can be integrated into an NIS. Many systems include a directory of standardized care plans based on medical and/or nursing diagnoses that can be generated from the system and modified as necessary to individualize them. Care plans can be stored in the computer and retrieved and updated as necessary. A printed copy of a care plan can be generated for easy insertion into a kardex if needed.

Decision support systems (DSSs) may some day be an integral part of or complementary to an NIS. Decision support systems are designed using artificial intelligence techniques, a branch of computer science based on logic, in which the knowledge and logical thinking of a domain expert is encoded into a computer program (Brennan, 1988). This process also is referred to as *knowledge engineering*. The result, an expert system, acts as a computerized consultant for making decisions. Expert systems have the potential for improving the quality of nursing care through dissemination of knowledge that may not otherwise be readily available to assist with decision making (McFarland, 1995).

Most expert systems in nursing are being developed to assist nurses with generating nursing diagnoses, care planning, and patient assessment (McFarland, 1995). The Creighton On-line Multiple Modular Expert System (COMMES), the first expert system in nursing and the only one that has moved beyond the prototype stage, is a large database of nursing knowledge that helps nurses to develop nursing diagnoses and determine protocols for patient care (Expert Systems for Nursing, 1988; McFarland, 1995). The Computer-Aided Nursing Diagnosis and Intervention system (CANDI) compares assessment data entered by the nurse with its database of information about nursing problems and diagnoses. Possible nursing diagnoses are suggested and refined (Chang, Roth, Gonzales, Caswell, & DiStefano, 1988). The Urological Nursing Information System (UNIS) assists in the assessment of elderly patients with urinary incontinence (Petrucci & Petrucci, 1991).

Expert system development in nursing poses many challenges for nurse informaticists who choose to specialize in this area (McFarland, 1995). Careful thought must be given to identifying areas of practice that would benefit from expert systems. When an area of practice has been selected, experts must be identified. After experts are identified, knowledge must be obtained from the experts and subsequently arranged and translated so that it can be processed by a computer. The use of experts in this process has been problematic. Recently, Henry (1995) has suggested using an inductive algorithm approach for acquiring knowledge from an existing research database as an alternative to the use of experts.

Patient Data Management Systems. The management of high-volume clinical information, such as that commonly obtained on patients in critical care units, emergency rooms, step-down units, postanesthesia care units, and the operating room, also can be facilitated with the use of information systems dedicated solely to this function. The earliest systems were simply computer-based monitoring systems that automatically collected data on selected physiological parameters (Milholland, 1988). Sensing devices attached to a patient relayed data such as heart rate, ECG, pulse rate, temperature, venous and arterial blood pressure, cardiac output, pulmonary artery pressure, pulmonary wedge pressure, intracranial pressure, and respiratory values to the computerized monitoring system. Once the data were entered into the computer, the computer displayed the readings on the screen or printer.

More recently, Patient Data Management Systems (PDMS) have emerged in critical care settings (Milholland, 1988). These more advanced systems rely on computerized patient monitoring but also allow for the storage and integration of data from these systems. For example, data displayed on a bedside monitor are automatically entered into a computerized patient chart (Figure 8–2). Prior to storage, the accuracy of the data is determined by appropriate care providers. Data also can be manually entered, such as patient assessments, care plans, and treatment records, or made available to the sys-

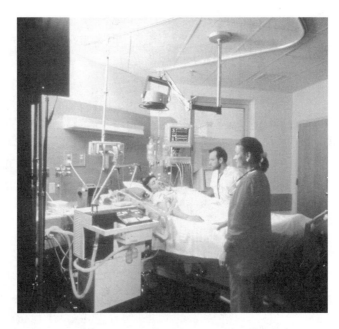

Figure 8–2. Computerized monitoring at a patient's bedside.
(Hewlett-Packard Company, Andover, Massachusetts, with permission.)

tem through linkage with other parts of the hospital, such as the laboratory (Figure 8–3). More advanced systems are designed to identify life-threatening emergencies by comparing data entering the system with predetermined parameters that represent dangerous deviations from the norm (Fairless, 1986). Some systems trend minute-to-minute data capture of ECG and pressure waveforms for critical review. This feature is useful in evaluating a patient for trends in cardiac rhythm patterns or reviewing events after cardiac arrest. Inherent in many of the advanced systems are a variety of calculations, including those used to determine optimal drug dosages and administration intervals in selected situations. PDMSs are available from a variety of vendors, and in many cases, they cannot be linked with the institutional NIS or HIS. Interfaces need to be developed to link these "stand-alone" systems with established HISs, so that the potential offered by fully integrated HISs, access to information from any terminal within a facility, can be realized.

A number of ethical and legal issues have emerged with the use of information systems. Ensuring the confidentiality of computerized patient information has been and continues to be a major concern (Albarado, McCall, & Thrane, 1990; Frawley, 1995; Romano, 1987). Individual patient records should be inaccessible to "unauthorized" personnel, that is, anyone not directly responsible for that person's care. Generally, this can be accomplished by assigning authorized user-specific access codes or passwords. In

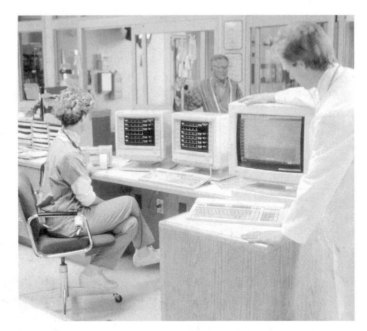

Figure 8–3. From the nurses' station, a patient's clinical information is viewed at a terminal. *(Hewlett-Packard Company, Andover, Massachusetts, with permission.)*

many cases, these codes can be used only to access certain kinds of data from terminals at specific locations. Nursing involvement in the initial design and ongoing development of information systems helps to ensure that systems are useful to nursing and that patients' rights to privacy and confidentiality continue to be met.

Computer-based patient records (CPRs) can provide comprehensive, accessible, accurate, and legible patient information for a variety of purposes, including close monitoring of patient progress for case management purposes and instant availability of the patient record for review (Bliss-Holtz, 1995). Uniform computerized databases enabled by information systems and computer-based patient records can also be used for quality control purposes (Denwood, 1996).

The most current trend is to generate a comprehensive interdisciplinary plan of care that is updated throughout all encounters with a health care system, both inpatient and outpatient. An integrated health care delivery system must be capable of allowing a patient to enter the system at any point of service and have all necessary and appropriate information available to the caregiver (Keever, 1995). The fully developed longitudinal computer-based patient record of the future "will consist of all of the clinical information concerning a single patient throughout his or her life" (Andrew & Dick, 1995).

Large hospitals are merging with smaller hospitals, clinics, and physicians' offices. With managed care, the HIS of tomorrow will need to link a variety of sites across a single state, the nation, and in some cases, across the world. The term *telemedicine* is currently being used to describe this type of communication (Flaherty, 1995).

Computers for Professional Growth and Networking

Using a PC, modem, telephone, and communications software, nurses can contact remote sites (on-line services or networks) for immediate access to discussion groups and forums, meetings, bulletin boards, databases, expert advice, books, journals, newsletters, practice guidelines, research reports, and continuing education offerings. Via E-mail, available on many networks, nurses can communicate with each other electronically. The Internet, also known as the "information superhighway," is a worldwide network of computer networks (Introduction to the Internet, 1995). Like other on-line services, the Internet allows nurses in clinical practice to collaborate and share ideas for patient care, access recent research findings and related databases and literature, and post questions for experts. Because of its sheer size, the large number of academic institutions represented, and the vast amount of data available, the Internet is probably the best single on-line resource available to nurses.

Computers in Nursing Administration

Many NISs include programs that assist with the allocation of nursing resources, especially staffing. In addition, personnel information, such as continuing education information data and licensing information, can be maintained on an automated record and easily accessed. Budget preparation also can be facilitated with the use of computer technology. Database and spreadsheet programs form the basis of many administrative applications. Programs that perform these tasks can be integral to an NIS or can be purchased or developed as separate applications that can function on independent PCs.

The administrative tasks of nurses and other professionals in private practice also can be facilitated by using computers. Database, spreadsheet, and financial management applications maintain accurate corporate records, client lists, and billing information. Some applications easily identify patients who need follow-up care.

Computers in Nursing Research

Computers have revolutionized the management of research data (Fawcett & Buhle, 1995, p. 273). With the use of computer technology, research is easier to accomplish than ever before. Literature reviews, for both research and clinical purposes, are facilitated with the assistance of computerized database searching. "These databases offer speed, flexibility, currency, and convenience in retrieving health information" (Fried, Killion, & Schick, 1988, p. 244). As mentioned, large databases of medical and/or nursing resources can be quickly accessed. Traditionally, libraries have provided database searching services. More recently, individuals have been given the opportunity to perform database searching with their own PCs from their home or office. With PCs supporting CD-ROM bibliographic and full-text databases, nurses can perform literature searches efficiently in clinical settings as well. In one hospital setting, nurses successfully used a PC-based literature search and retrieval system to answer questions about patient care and general health issues (Boyle, Blythe, Potvin, Oolup, & Chan, 1995).

When doing research, contact with other researchers is important. With electronic networking via E-mail, nurses and other health care professionals can easily identify and communicate with peers who have similar interests.

The writing of research proposals and reports also is greatly facilitated by using computers, word processing, and desktop publishing applications. Data can be entered directly into laptop PCs at data collections sites. Database programs can help organize data obtained from subjects, questionnaires, and other measurement instruments. The Internet can even be used for data collection (Fawcett & Buhle, 1995). Statistical programs, available to run on PCs, perform complex data analyses that would be extremely time-consuming to compute by hand.

"Through computerized information systems, nurses can collect, manipulate, and retrieve nursing data in systematic ways to advance nursing knowledge" (Werley, 1985, p. 2). The research possibilities offered by the vast amount of nursing data captured through computers is endless. Potentially, nursing data can be collected and compared at local, regional, national, and international levels (Werley, Devine, & Zorn, 1988). For this to be accomplished, however, nursing databases must be standardized so that grouping and comparison of data collected from different sites is possible (Werley, 1985). Currently, efforts continue to determine a Nursing Minimum Data Set, that is, uniform standards for the collection of minimum, essential nursing data (Werley et al., 1988).

Computers in Professional and Patient Education

The introduction of computer technology has had a tremendous impact on the teaching/learning process. Word processing programs have made it easier for students at any level to write, edit, and print papers to fulfill course requirements. Spreadsheet programs have facilitated grading processes and record keeping. Distance education, enabled by computer technology, has made the "electronic classroom" a reality: "Through the 'electronic classroom' . . . students, teachers, and preceptors, through synchronous or asynchronous communication, discuss topics, report on learning activities, solicit input, and receive feedback from the teacher or peers as they would in face-to-face situations" (Johnston & Lewis, 1995, p. 238).

In both nursing programs and clinical settings, nursing students and clinicians are using computer-based instructional materials for learning, reinforcement, remediation, and continuing education purposes. Currently, these programs are available primarily as computer-assisted instruction (CAI) and interactive videodisc. *Computer-assisted instruction* refers generally to media located on a floppy disk and requires a computer to run the program. Text can be combined with sound, color, and graphics to add interest or help to make a point. Interactive videodisc (IVD) refers to media located on optical discs and requires an analog videodisc player and a computer to run the program. Interactive videodisc systems integrate the use of full-screen full-motion video with computer-assisted learning in an automatic, interactive fashion. The combination of video and CAI makes learning even more stimulating and realistic. For example, certification and recertification in cardiopulmonary resuscitation and advanced cardiac life support can be accomplished using the Actronics Learning System, which simulates medical emergencies and utilizes sensorized manikins to determine if compression and inflation techniques performed by the user are correct (Figure 8–4). CD-ROM interactive systems also have been developed, although they are not yet widely available.

Computer-assisted instruction programs include games, tutorials, drill and practice programs, and simulations; most interactive videodisc programs are primarily simulations. CAI games provide users with a "fun" way of learning about some content area. For example, crossword puzzles are commonly used. A tutorial assumes the role of teacher and can stand alone, instructing the user in some content area. Drill and practice programs provide repetitive practice in applying previously learned content. Drill and practice CAI is useful particularly when continued practice is needed to master specific skills. Many nursing education programs use drill and practice programs to assist nursing students in achieving competence in performing drug calculations. Simulations allow users to apply knowledge of some content area in a simulated, "real-life" situation described on a computer screen; decision-making abilities can be tested with this type of program. In a well-developed simulation, users are given the opportunity to see the results of different choices made throughout the situation presented. Many programs integrate the tutorial, drill and practice, and simulation components in one software program; users identify their own learning needs and progress at their own pace in learning and applying the content of the program.

Computer-based education provides a self-directed and cost-effective means of learning that is a viable alternative to traditional teaching meth-

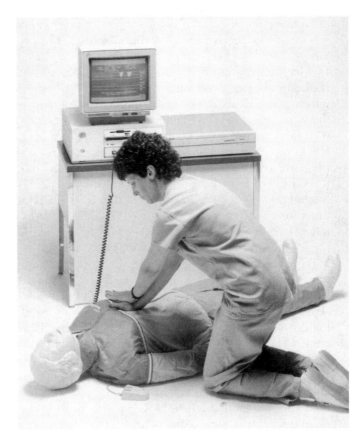

Figure 8–4. A nurse performs chest compressions that are monitored by the Actronics Learning System. *(Actronics, Inc., Pittsburgh, Pennsylvania, with permission.)*

ods. In addition, many programs maintain records of each user's performance, providing documentation of teaching/learning activities for legal, continuing education, and/or accreditation purposes. Well-developed programs are personalized; use colorful, entertaining designs and pictures or video; provide feedback about the learning that has taken place; summarize a user's overall progress in learning the content; and are easy to use.

The use of computer-based learning materials has progressed rapidly in health care. The waiting rooms of many health care providers now contain PCs and a library of programs on various health topics. Patients use programs that are applicable to their specific health care needs, as identified by the nurse and other health care providers. Computer-based instruction materials can be purchased from vendors or developed using multimedia authoring software.

Computers and the Role of the Nurse

Nurses should make every attempt to update their knowledge of new applications for computers in health care settings. Information about computer applications can be obtained through attending conferences and continuing education programs. Professional journals and books also provide sources of information regarding computer applications. The journal *Computers in Nursing* is devoted entirely to the topic of computer use in nursing; the journal *Computers in Health Care* focuses on the use of computers in a variety of health care settings. Professional organizations encompass subgroups of individuals with specific interests in computer applications, such as the National League for Nursing Council on Nursing Informatics. All these avenues are open to nurses who want to stay informed about computer use in nursing and health care.

If computers are to be incorporated into a health care setting, nurses *must* be involved in the planning phase so the computer applications that are devised and developed are appropriate and useful to nursing. Nurses should be continually involved in the evaluation of computer systems that include nursing applications to ensure that the systems meet nursing and patient care needs. Many large medical centers with hospital information systems have developed specific roles for nurses whose primary responsibility is to provide or augment nursing care through the use of computers.

SUMMARY

Every nurse should have some working knowledge of computers. It is likely that all nurses will be using computers in their practice in some capacity in the future. In addition, it is imperative that nurses be creative with regard to the potential uses of computers in practice settings so that the impact on improving the quality of care can be fully realized.

REFERENCES

Albarado, R. S., McCall, V., & Thrane, J. M. (1990). Computerized nursing documentation. *Nursing Management, 21* (7), 64–65.

American Nurses Association. (1995). *Standards of practice for nursing informatics.* Washington, DC: Author.

Andrew, W., & Dick, R. (1995). Applied information technology: A clinical perspective (Feature focus: The computer-based patient record, Part 2). *Computers in Nursing, 13*, 118–122.

Ball, M. J., Hannah, K. J., Jelger, U. G., & Peterson, H. (Eds.). (1988). *Nursing informatics: Where caring and technology meet.* New York: Springer-Verlag.

Bliss-Holtz, J. (1995). Computerized support for case management. *Computers in Nursing, 13*, 289–294.

Boyle, J., Blythe, J., Potvin, C., Oolup, P., & Chan, I. (1995). Literature search and retrieval in the workplace. *Computers in Nursing, 13*, 25–31.

Brennan, P. (1988). DSS, ES, AI: The lexicon of decision support. *Nursing & Health Care, 9*, 501–503.

Bronzino, J. D. (1982). *Computer applications for patient care.* Menlo Park, CA: Addison-Wesley.

Carty, B. (1994). The protean nature of the nurse informaticist. *Nursing & Health Care, 15*, 174–177.

Chang, B. L., Roth, K., Gonzales, E. Caswell, D., & DiStefano, J. (1988). CANDI: A knowledge-based system for nursing diagnosis. *Computers in Nursing, 6*(1), 13–21.

Denwood, R. (1996). Data capture for quality management nursing opportunity. *Computers in Nursing, 14*, 39–44.

Dillon, T., McDowell, D., Norcio, A., & DeHaemer, M. (1994). Nursing acceptance of a speech-input interface: A preliminary investigation. *Computers in Nursing, 12*, 264–271.

Expert Systems for Nursing. (1988, December/January). *Nursing Educators Microworld*, p. 2.

Fairless, P. R. (1986). 9 ways a computer can make your work easier. *Nursing 86, 16*(9), 55–56.

Fawcett, J., & Buhle, Jr., E. (1995). Using the Internet for data collection: An innovative electronic strategy. *Computers in Nursing, 13*, 273–279.

Flaherty, R. (1995). Electronic bulletin board systems extend the advantages of telemedicine. *Computers in Nursing, 13*, 8–10.

Frawley, K. (1995). Achieving the CPR while keeping an ancient oath. *healthcare Informatics, 12*(4), pp. 28–30.

Fried, A. K., Killion, V. J., & Schick, L. C. (1988). Computerized databases in nursing. *Computers in Nursing, 6*, 244–252.

Friedman, J., & Street, G. (1986–87, Winter). Computers advance treatment and learning at medical centers. *The Magazine*, pp. 17–23.

Gogola, M. (1995). A joint hospital/vendor project brings CQI and point-of-care technology to home care. *Computers in Nursing, 13*, 143–150.

Graves, J., & Corcoran, S. (1989). The study of nursing informatics. *Image: Journal of Nursing Scholarship, 21*, 227–230.

Green, A. M., Modic, M. T., & Steinmetz, N. D. (1987). Should you be using MR imaging? *Patient Care, 21*(2), 26–37.

Gross, M. S. (1988). The potential of information systems in nursing. *Nursing & Health Care, 9*, 477–479.

Hannah, K. J., Ball, M. J., & Edwards, M. J. (1994). *Introduction to nursing informatics.* New York: Springer-Verlag.

Hendrickson, G., Kovner, C., Knickman, J., & Finkler, S. (1995). Implementation of computerized bedside monitoring systems in 17 New Jersey hospitals. *Computers in Nursing, 13*, 96–102.

Henry, S. (1995). An inductive algorithm approach to knowledge acquisition for expert system development. *Computers in Nursing, 13*, 226–232.

Introduction to the Internet. (1995). *Interactive Healthcare Newsletter, 11*(9/10), 2–8.

Johnston, M., & Lewis, J. (1995). Reaching RNs through the electronic classroom. *Nursing & Health Care, 16*, 237–238.

Keever, G. W. (1995). Integrated delivery systems: Virtuality becomes reality. *healthcare Informatics, 12*(10), 47–50.

McFarland, M. (1995). Knowledge engineering of expert systems for nursing. *Computers in Nursing, 13*, 32–37.

McKinney, P. (1988). Can point of care terminals ease the threat? *Computers in Healthcare, 9*(4), 62.

Milholland, J. (1988). Patient data management systems. *Computers in Nursing, 6*, 237–241.

Minda, S., & Brundage, D. (1994). Time differences in handwritten and computer documentation of nursing assessment. *Computers in Nursing, 12*, 277–279.

Pabst, M., Scherubel, J., & Minnick, A. (1996). The impact of computerized documentation on nurses' use of time. *Computers in Nursing, 14*, 25–30.

Petrucci, K., & Petrucci, P. (1991). Expert systems and nursing. *Nursing Economics, 9*, 188–190.

Robinson, L. W. (1985). Computers to the OR STAT! *Today's OR Nurse, 7*(10), 10–15.

Romano, C. A. (1987). Privacy, confidentiality, and security of computerized systems: The nursing responsibility. *Computers in Nursing, 5*, 99–104.

Saba, V. K. (1988). Taming the computer jungle of NISs. *Nursing & Health Care, 9*, 487–491.

Shannon, R. H. (1985). Computer-enhanced radiology: A transformation to imaging. In M. J. Ball, D. W. Simborg, J. W. Albright, & J. V. Douglas (Eds.), *Healthcare information management systems: A practical guide* (pp. 283–296). New York: Springer-Verlag.

VanBemmel, J. H. (1987). Computer-assisted care in nursing. *Computers in Nursing, 5*, 132–139.

Warnock-Matheron, A. G., & Hannah, K. J. (1988). Comparative analysis of computer-based operating room information systems. *Computers in Nursing, 6*, 147–156.

Werley, H. H. (1985). School hosts invitational conference to develop nursing minimum data sets. *Input/Output, 1*(3), 1–4.

Werley, H. H., Devine, E. C., & Zorn, C. R. (1988). Nursing needs its own minimum data set. *American Journal of Nursing, 88*, 1651–1653.

BIBLIOGRAPHY

Ahijevych, K., Boyle, K. K., & Burger, K. (1985). Microcomputers enhance student health fairs. *Journal of Nursing Education, 24*, 16–20.

Andreoli, K., & Mussner, L. A. (1985). Computers in nursing care: The state of the art. *Nursing Outlook, 33*(1), 16–21.

Andrew, W. (1995). Applied information technology: A clinical perspective (Feature focus: The continuum of interoperability). *Computers in Nursing, 13*, 38–40.

Andrew, W., & Dick, R. (1995a). Applied information technology: A clinical perspective (Feature focus: The computer-based patient record [Part 1]). *Computers in Nursing, 13*, 80–84.

Andrew, W., & Dick, R. (1995b). Applied information technology: A clinical perspective (Feature focus: The computer-based patient record [Part 3]). *Computers in Nursing, 13*, 176–181.

Andris, J., & Sykes, R. (1995). Faculty authoring of course-specific software for disadvantaged nursing students using Linkway: A case study. *Computers in Nursing, 13*, 71–79.

Arnold, J., & Pearson, G. (1992). *Computer applications in nursing education and practice*. New York: National League for Nursing.

Badger, K. (1996). Selecting a clinical information system that will grow with the institution. *Computers in Nursing, 14*, 23–24.

Bailey, D. R. (1988). Computer applications in nursing. *Computers in Nursing, 6*, 199–203.

Ball, M. J., Simborg, D. W., Albright, J. W., & Douglas, J. C. (Eds.). (1985). *Healthcare information management systems: A practice guide* (2nd ed.). New York: Springer-Verlag.

Ball, M. J., Snelbecker, B., & Schechter, S. (1985). Nurses' perceptions concerning computer uses before and after a computer literacy lecture. *Computers in Nursing, 3*(1), 23–32.

Bellinger, K., & Laden, J. (1985). Nurse use of general-purpose microcomputer software. *Nursing Outlook, 33*(1), 22–25.

Benford, M. S., & Slack, C. S. (1989). Development of a statewide maternal and child health information network. *Computers in Nursing, 7*, 9–14.

Billings, D. (1995). Computer-based instruction for critical care nurse educators. *Critical Care Nurse, 15*(5), 76–78.

Bloom, C. (1995). Information services: When management loses control. *healthcare Informatics, 12*(6), 101–108.

Bloom, K. C., Leitner, J. E., & Solano, J. L. (1987). Development of an expert system prototype to generate nursing care plans based on nursing diagnoses. *Computers in Nursing, 5*, 140–145.

Bongartz, C. (1988). Computer-oriented patient care. *Computers in Nursing, 6*, 204–210.

Bradburn, C., Zeleznikow, J., & Adams, A. (1993). FLORENCE: Synthesis of case-based and model-based reasoning in a nursing care planning system. *Computers in Nursing, 11*, 20–24.

Brazile, R., & Hettinger, B. (1995). A clinical information system for ambulatory care. *Computers in Nursing, 13*, 151–158.

Brown, S., Cioffi, M. A., Schinella, P., & Shaw, A. (1995). Evaluation of the impact of a bedside terminal system in a rapidly changing community hospital. *Computers in Nursing, 13*, 280–284.

Chase, S. K. (1988). Knowledge representation in expert systems. *Computers in Nursing, 6*, 58–64.

Curran, M. A., & Curran, K. E. (1995). *Informatics resources for nurses*. Raleigh: North Carolina Nursing Association Council on Nursing Informatics.

Day, R., & Payne, L. (1987). Computer-managed instruction: An alternative teaching strategy. *Journal of Nursing Education, 26*, 30–36.

Devine, E. C., & Werley, H. H. (1988). Test of the nursing minimum data set: Availability of data and reliability. *Research in Nursing & Health, 11*, 97–104.

Dick, R. S., & Andrew, W. F. (1995). Point of care: An essential technology for the CPR. *healthcare Informatics, 12*(5), 64–66, 78.

Fitzpatrick, J. J. (1988). How can we enhance nursing knowledge and practice. *Nursing & Health Care, 9*, 517–521.

Gaston, S. (1988). Knowledge, retention, and attitude effects of computer-assisted instruction. *Journal of Nursing Education, 27*, 30–34.

Gleydura, A., Michelman, J., & Wilson, C. (1995). Multimedia training in nursing education. *Computers in Nursing, 13*, 169–175.

Graveley, E., & Murphy, M. A. (1995). Nursing informatics: Making financial management come alive. *Computers in Nursing, 13*, 217–220.

Graves, J., Amos, L., Huether, S., Lange, L., & Thompson, C. (1995). Description of a graduate program in clinical nursing informatics. *Computers in Nursing, 13*, 60–70.

Halloran, L. (1995). A comparison of two methods of teaching: Computer managed instruction and keypad questions versus traditional classroom lecture. *Computers in Nursing, 13*, 285–288.

Hendrickson, G., & Kovner, C. T. (1990). Effects of computers on nursing resource use: Do computers save nurses time? *Computers in Nursing, 8*, 16–22.

IVD–CD-ROM–CD-I: Where do we go from here? (1995). *FITNE Newsletter, 8*(1), 1.

Joos, I., Whitman, N., Smith, M., & Nelson, R. (1992). *Computers in small bytes.* New York: National League for Nursing.

Khoiny, F. (1995). Factors that contribute to computer-assisted instruction effectiveness. *Computers in Nursing, 13*, 165–168.

Koch, B., & McGovern, J. (1993). EXTEND: A prototype expert system for teaching nursing diagnosis. *Computers in Nursing, 11*(1), 35–40.

Krawczak, J., & Bersky, A. (1995). The development of automated client responses for computerized clinical simulation testing. *Computers in Nursing, 13*, 295–300.

Lancaster, L. (1987). A care planning system based on nursing diagnosis. *Input/Output, 3*(3), 3.

O'Donohue, N. (1986). How to evaluate staffing software. *American Journal of Nursing, 86*, 1407–1408, 1412.

Ozbolt, J. G. (1987). Developing decision support systems for nursing. *Computers in Nursing, 5*(3), 105–111.

Poston, I. (1993). How to develop computer-assisted instruction programs. *Nursing & Health Care, 14*, 344–348.

Probst, C., & Rush, J. (1990). The careplan knowledge base. *Computers in Nursing, 8*, 206–213.

Rizzolo, M. A. (Ed.). (1994). *Interactive video: Expanding horizons in nursing.* New York: American Journal of Nursing.

Rizzolo, M. A. (1995). The American Journal of Nursing Network. *Interactive Healthcare Newsletter, 11*(7/8), 11–12.

Romano, C., Ryan, L., Harris, J., Boykin, P., & Power, M. (1985). A decade of decisions: Four perspectives of computerization in nursing practice. *Computers in Nursing, 3*, 64–76.

Ronald, J. S., & Skiba, D. J. (1987). *Guidelines for basic computer education in nursing.* New York: National League for Nursing.

Sinclair, V. G. (1988). Database management: Solving information overload. *Nursing & Health Care, 9*, 493–495.

Sparks, S. (1994). E. T. Net. *Nursing & Health Care, 15*, 134–141.

Staggers, N. (1995). Essential principles for evaluating the usability of clinical information systems. *Computers in Nursing, 13*, 207–213.

Thede, L., Taft, S., & Coeling, H. (1994). Computer-assisted instruction: A learner's viewpoint. *Journal of Nursing Education, 33*, 299–305.

Tomaiuolo, N. (1995). Accessing nursing resources on the Internet. *Computers in Nursing, 13*, 159–164.

Walker, D., & Ross, J. (1995). Therapeutic computing: Teaching therapeutic communication using a videodisc. *Computers in Nursing, 13*, 103–108.

White, J. (1995). Using interactive video to add physical assessment data to computer-based patient simulations in nursing. *Computers in Nursing, 13*, 233–235.

White, J., & Valentine, V. (1993). Computer assisted video instruction and community assessment. *Nursing & Health Care, 14*, 349–353.

Yoder, M. (1994). Preferred learning style and educational technology: Linear vs. interactive video. *Nursing & Health Care, 15*, 128–132.

Moral and Ethical Dimensions of Nursing Practice

Shaké Ketefian

The nursing profession now defines itself as a scientific field, comprised of components that make it both a discipline and a profession. The disciplinary dimension concerns itself with the development of the science of nursing, its knowledge and theory; the professional dimension is concerned with the practice of nursing, the delivery of services to meet societal needs. These two dimensions of nursing are not isolated from each other; indeed, it is a challenge of the greatest magnitude to meld one with the other, so that the disciplinary and professional components enrich and benefit each other.

This chapter focuses mainly on the professional dimension of nursing, but points of articulation with the disciplinary component are identified and discussed where appropriate. The chapter deals specifically with ethical concerns in the profession and lays a foundation for how such concerns may be addressed.

NURSING AS A PROFESSION

Nursing has been defined by various individuals over a number of generations; the commonality among the definitions relates to the focus of providing care to promote the health and well-being of individuals. The goal of nursing is the welfare of people. This goal is a moral rather than a scientific end. It implies human interactions and the seeking of what is good and what leads to health and welfare. Nursing science is expected to serve this goal (Curtin, 1979, p. 2).

Viewed in this light, therefore, ethical practice is integral to professional practice. It is not part of it, it is not related to it, but it is the essence of professional practice. The terms *ethics* and *morals* often are used interchangeably in the literature; yet, there are differences. Morals are seen as the conventions and norms of society—what ought to or should be done; ethics concern the reasoned analysis and disciplined inquiry underlying a moral code. In this spirit, Thompson and Thompson (1981) state their view that the 11 tenets of the Code for Nurses (ANA, 1985) are the moral code of the profession, whereas the Interpretative Statements are the ethical principles that explain, interpret, and analyze the statements (p. 1). Ethical dilemmas are created when a choice must be made between unsatisfactory alternatives or when important principles conflict.

MORAL REASONING

In recent years moral reasoning has come to be considered an important approach intended to assist individuals in reflecting and critically analyzing situations of moral conflict. This approach is generally relevant in analyzing both social and professional issues.

The idea of moral reasoning has been developed by social scientists and is now extensively used in nursing. Moral reasoning is grounded in the traditions of cognitive and developmental psychology; it is characterized by the sequential transformation in the way in which social arrangements are interpreted. Three levels and six stages have been identified, conceived in a hierarchical manner. Each successive stage in the developmental process of moral reasoning is more complex, comprehensive, differentiated, and effective than the preceding stage. Each stage reflects a distinctive way in which moral dilemmas and problems are evaluated.

The intellectual lineage of moral reasoning can be traced to the works of Dewey (1964) and Piaget (1965). Extending the work of these authors, Kohlberg (1971, 1978) has formulated moral reasoning following longitudinal and cross-cultural studies over a 20-year period. Kohlberg focused on the developmental and cognitive processes involved in reasoning about moral choice, rather than on the content of moral choice (Kohlberg, 1971, 1978). This reasoning is said to reveal the structure of the person's moral judgment.

Levels and Stages of Moral Reasoning

Stages of moral reasoning, according to Kohlberg (1978, pp. 50–51) are as follows:

- *Preconventional level of moral development.* Externally established rules determine right or wrong action.

Stage 1: Punishment–obedience orientation. The child focuses on avoiding punishment or negative physical consequences; deference to authority is strong.

Stage 2: Instrumental-relativist orientation. Whatever provides personal satisfaction is viewed as the right action. Elements of fairness are present, but these are interpreted in a pragmatic way.

- *Conventional level of moral development.* Expectations of family and group are maintained; loyalty and conformity to the existing social order are considered important.

Stage 3: Interpersonal concordance or "good boy–nice girl" orientation. Whatever is pleasing and brings approval from others is considered good behavior.

Stage 4: "Law and order" orientation. One has to do one's duty and actively maintain the social order because of respect for its underlying morality.

- *Postconventional level of moral development.* The individual autonomously examines and defines moral values and principles apart from the group norms or the culture.

Stage 5: The social-contract, legalistic orientation. Individual rights and standards agreed to by the whole society are critically examined and are used as the basis for determining right action. The person is aware of the relativist nature of values and opinions and emphasizes the "legal point of view" but with the idea that the law can be changed if rational considerations so indicate. The American government and Constitution are said to belong to this stage of morality.

Stage 6: Universal ethical principle orientation. Decisions of conscience dictate what is right. The person chooses ethical principles that appeal to logical comprehensiveness, universality, and consistency; they are abstract rather than concrete. The universal principles observed are those of justice, reciprocity of human rights, and respect for the dignity of individuals.

These stages are characterized in three ways: They are "structured wholes," organized systems of thought that make people consistent in their levels of moral judgment; they have "invariant sequence," by which people tend to move forward rather than backward; and they are "hierarchical integrations," in which higher-stage thinking incorporates all levels of lower-stage thinking (Rest, 1974, p. 242).

Kohlberg also has proposed that certain conditions may stimulate or account for the level of moral development. Among these are the individual's stage of intellectual/cognitive development and the concurrent social and educational climates to which the individual is exposed. Environments that provide opportunities for group participation, shared decision making, and assumption of responsibility for the consequences of action tend to stimulate the development of higher levels of moral reasoning. When education is structured so as to create cognitive conflict and disequilibrium by showing inadequacies in a person's mode of thinking, the individual is stimulated to seek higher and more adequate ways to reason about moral choice (Kohlberg, 1971, p. 183; Rest, Turiel, & Kohlberg, 1969). Although implicitly it is thought to be desirable for individuals to be at the postconventional level of morality, it appears to be the case that the majority of the American public are, and remain at, the conventional level of morality, where social roles and rules are important considerations.

Kohlberg (1978) has suggested that moral reasoning centers on 10 universal values; these are punishment, property, roles and concerns of affection, roles and concerns of authority, law, life, liberty, distribution of justice, truth, sex (p. 39). A conflict between two or more of these universal values necessitates a moral choice and its subsequent justification by the individual, requiring systematic use of the person's cognitive thought processes.

Proponents of this cognitive-developmental approach conceptualize the aims and purposes of education in a distinctive way, by placing emphasis on developing problem-solving strategies and decision-making capabilities. To this end, the educational process is designed to provide experiences that will enable the individual to learn principles and to perform "synthesizing operations" (Rest, 1974, p. 242). These ideas are consistent with those expressed by Bruner (1960), who stated that education should teach problem solving, fundamental concepts, and the essential structure of a discipline, because these are the tools of thought that enable one to make sense of one's experiences and to organize a plan of action for decision making. It needs to be noted that the focus of Bruner's work was not moral reasoning per se, but rather what education should aim to accomplish. Flexner (1915) contended that the professions involve intellectual operations and are characterized by the assumption of a large degree of intellectual responsibility. The similarities in these ideas underscore the point that the capabilities called upon in reasoning about moral choice are cognitive and intellectual in nature, developed and nurtured through educational experiences.

The connection between moral reasoning and moral behavior is not always clear nor is it direct. When moral behavior occurs, Rest, Bebeau, and Volker (1986) have theorized that four processes are presumed to have occurred in the person. The individual has: (1) interpreted the situation in terms of possible actions and who might be affected (moral sensitivity); (2) made a judgment about the right course of action (moral reasoning); (3) given priority to moral values inherent in the situation (moral commitment); and (4) shown perseverance and skills to pursue his intention to behave morally (moral implementation) (pp. 3–4).

In describing professional education, nurse educators have stated that it should be concerned with theoretical and research-based knowledge (Rogers, 1970, p. 138; Reilly & Oermann, 1992) and the development of intellectual skills and operations so that the professional nurse can assess a broad range of cues (Schlotfeldt, 1965), engage in complex problem solving (Johnson, 1968), make decisions autonomously, and assume individual responsibility for the consequences of his or her acts (Kohnke, 1978). Qualities valued for professional nurses are those that, according to Murphy (1976), enable a person to engage in postconventional level of moral reasoning and to act as a morally responsible agent, advocating patient rights.

In recent years the above conceptualization of moral reasoning by Kohlberg has been challenged on the grounds that it reflects a male-oriented perspective of morality. According to Gilligan (1982), women tend to see morality in the context of particular relationships, which she called the "ethic of care"; she further argued that a conception of morality as justice, viewed in terms of obligations and rights, fairness and impartiality, depicts a male view and obscures female reality. Gilligan's challenge or Kohlberg's view of morality can be viewed within the broader context of the feminist literature. In a field that is predominantly female, serious attention needs to be given to these alternative perspectives. However, at present there are no measurement tools to address this alternative theoretical conception, and further research is needed to validate these claims, although they remain viable theoretical conceptions.

ETHICAL THEORIES AND PRINCIPLES

Ethical theories and principles provide the decision maker with cognitive maps, a point of view, if you will, that assist in determining whether actions are morally appropriate; thus, they are concerned with the content of the moral choice. Moral reasoning deals with the process of thinking about moral choice and the adequacy of the thought process and justifications. There is increasing empirical support for the notion that the higher the reasoning process, in terms of level/stage, the more appropriate the moral choice is likely to be (Ketefian, 1981). This distinction between the two concepts is important to note, although frequently one is likely to read authors who use them interchangeably.

A number of ethical principles and theories have been discussed in the literature. The two most influential ethical theories are utilitarianism and deontology.

Ethical Theories

Utilitarianism

Utilitarianism holds that the basic principle in ethics is the principle of utility, which maintains that we ought to produce the greatest balance of value over disvalue for all those affected. If all possible outcomes are thought to be bad, then the utility principle would have us act so as to produce the least possible balance of disvalue. A decision is justified if it produces more good for the largest number than alternative methods. A feature of utilitarianism is that duty or right conduct are subordinated to what is good or that which produces good (Beauchamp & Childress, 1983, pp. 19–21). From the utilitarian perspective, the point of morality is to promote what is intrinsically good by maximizing benefits and minimizing harms. The principle of utility is in much evidence in health care practices, in institutional policies, as well as in the arena of public policy, as legislators consider and decide issues such as allocation of resources and what is likely to be of benefit to the larger society.

Deontology

The concepts of duty and the inherent rightness or wrongness of actions are central to deontological thinking. Deontologists maintain that the concept of duty or right does not necessarily depend on the idea of good. Some acts are wrong because of wrong-making characteristics regardless of consequences, such as deceiving and breaking promises. Some acts are right because of right-making characteristics, such as fidelity to promises, truth telling, and justice. In the deontological system, these right-making characteristics determine right acts and duties (Beauchamp & Childress, 1983, p. 33).

Many tenets of the profession of nursing are deontologically oriented, such as the emphasis on respect for all persons, confidentiality, and the like. Implicit commitments made between health care providers and individual patients are important indeed and must be honored. They cannot be abrogated in order to maximize goods for others. The implications of these commitments are enormous and give rise to many ethical conflicts, especially in the resource allocation and staffing areas. Consider the occasions in an understaffed unit where a nurse wishes to meet the complex needs of an individual patient, while the needs of other patients might not be met without his or her care.

Ethical Principles

The Principle of Autonomy

The term *autonomy* is quite broad and can refer to persons, will, thought, or actions. It embodies the idea of self-rule or self-governance. The principle of autonomy can be stated to mean that persons should be free to perform and decide on whatever actions they wish, as long as these do not infringe on the autonomous actions of others. Embedded in the concept appears to be the freedom to act or not to act. Nurses and other health professionals are urged to respect the autonomy of their patients. Indeed, this principle has gained wide currency and recognition in recent years. Respecting the autonomy of patients, in matters such as treatment decisions, what should be done to their persons, and the like, is the exact opposite of paternalism, which holds that someone, such as an expert, knows best what is for the good of the patient. In the not-too-distant past, information about a diagnosis such as cancer was frequently withheld from patients on grounds that "it would be too upsetting."

The Principles of Nonmaleficence and Beneficence

These may be viewed as opposite sides of the coin, although some authors treat each of these as distinct ethical principles. Nonmaleficence is viewed as the duty not to inflict harm, and beneficence is the duty to do or promote good. Where one cannot promote good, one ought to prevent harm or remove harm. There are frequent conflicts between these principles, and philosophers have developed rules for carrying out detriment–benefit, costs–risks–benefits, analyses that might be of assistance in specific decision making. For example, under certain circumstances, it may be permissible to harm, such as cause pain or disability, in order to prevent death. Many of the arguments around withdrawal of life support systems attempt to balance the burdens (harms) and benefits of treatment.

The Principle of Justice

There are many meanings and conceptions of justice. The most compelling type of justice in health care relates to issues of resource allocation, referred to as *distributive justice*. In this context, the meaning of justice as "fairness" is held to be central. How are benefits and burdens distributed in society? Who has claims or rights to certain benefits that might take precedence over others and on what grounds? Most likely, these issues would not arise if goods and resources were limitless. As this is not the case, claims must be settled, and a system of ordering priorities must be determined. Rules of justice are established to strike a balance between conflicting claims and interests.

One classification of such rules identifies the relevant property on the basis of which benefits and burdens are to be distributed (Beauchamp & Childress, 1983, p. 187). These are as follows:

- To each person *an equal share*
- To each person according to *individual need*
- To each person according to *individual effort*
- To each person according to *societal contribution*
- To each person according to *merit*

One or more of these principles may be relevant as the basis for judgment, but this depends on particular circumstances and whether there are other compelling and/or overriding considerations that need to be accounted for. For example, an employer seeking to hire an employee from among a number of applicants would be morally justified in selecting the best qualified individual, thus, using merit as the basis of selection. A nurse caring for a group of patients might devote more time and attention to one patient on a given day if she or he assesses that the patient's physiological or psychosocial needs are most compelling, thus using individual need as the basis for allocating care and ministration.

Other Relevant Principles

The theories and principles presented earlier give rise to other derivative rules or principles. These are *fidelity* (keeping promises), *veracity* (truth telling), and *confidentiality* (respecting privileged information). These derivative rules are grounded in one or more principles and are highly relevant to professional nursing practice.

The Concept of "Rights"

Many moral controversies are couched in terms of "rights." These can be understood in terms of justified claims that individuals can make on others. Legal rights are claims justified by legal principles, whereas moral rights are claims that are justified by moral principles (Beauchamp & Childress, 1983).

There is a relationship between rights and obligations, in that if a person has a justified claim, then it can be inferred that someone has a correlative obligation. Therefore, one can infer certain rights from obligations or infer certain obligations or duties from rights. For example, to say that a patient has a right to participate in his or her own treatment decisions implies that someone has an obligation to involve the patient in such decisions. Professional codes tend to be expressed in terms of the duties or obligations of professionals to their patients. They suggest, however, that patients have the right to expect the expressed behaviors once they enter into a relationship with health care providers.

The American Hospital Association has adopted "A Patient's Bill of Rights," which explicitly states the parameters of what patients have a right to expect. For example, they are said to have a right to respectful care, information on treatment, privacy, confidentiality, and the like (AHA, 1973, 275–277).

However, one often finds rights ascribed somewhat loosely or encounters debates in the literature that assume the presence of rights when they do not *necessarily* exist or lead to related obligations of the health professional. For example, if one argues that a woman has a right to decide to have an abortion and determine what shall be done to her body, it does not follow from such argument that the state or a federal agency has an obligation to pay for her abortion. There is extensive literature arguing the matter of whether there exists a right to health care irrespective of ability to pay. The nursing profession generally has taken the philosophical position that such a right does exist. Others have argued, however, that such a right does not necessarily exist and that if it did exist, it is not evident whose obligation it is to pay for health care or provide it.

PROFESSIONAL CODES AND GUIDELINES

Code for Nurses

There is general consensus that one of the identifying features of the professions is an ethical code; authors define its purpose variously, but in the main, a code serves as a means of professional self-regulation and of accountability. Jennings, Callahan, and Wolf (1987) have stated that "ethical standards are the linchpins of public trust in a profession. They transform the career of selling services into the calling of providing services" (p. 4).

The American Nurses Association (ANA) posits that "a code of ethics indicates a profession's acceptance of the responsibility and trust with which it has been invested by society" (ANA, 1985, p. iii). The professional association first adopted a "Code for Nurses" in 1950; this document is periodically revised and interpreted to reflect present-day practice. The purpose of the Code is "to inform both the nurse and society of the profession's expectations and requirements in ethical matters" (ANA, 1985, p. iii). The code provides a framework for ethical decision making and offers general principles that guide nursing actions.

The most basic principle reflected in the Code is respect for persons; other principles are autonomy (self-determination), beneficence (doing good), nonmaleficence (avoiding harm), veracity (truth telling), confidentiality (respecting privileged information), fidelity (keeping promises), and justice (treating people fairly) (ANA, 1985, p. i). Table 9–1 lists the eleven tenets of the "Code for Nurses."

TABLE 9–1. CODE FOR NURSES

1. The nurse provides services with respect for human dignity and the uniqueness of the client, unrestricted by considerations of social or economic status, personal attributes, or the nature of health problems.

2. The nurse safeguards the client's right to privacy by judiciously protecting information of a confidential nature.

3. The nurse acts to safeguard the client and the public when health care and safety are affected by the incompetent, unethical, or illegal practice of any person.

4. The nurse assumes responsibility and accountability for individual nursing judgments and actions.

5. The nurse maintains competence in nursing.

6. The nurse exercises informed judgment and uses individual competence and qualifications as criteria in seeking consultation, accepting responsibility, and delegating nursing activities to others.

7. The nurse participates in activities that contribute to the ongoing development of the profession's body of knowledge.

8. The nurse participates in the profession's efforts to implement and improve standards of nursing.

9. The nurse participates in the profession's efforts to establish and maintain conditions of employment conducive to high-quality nursing care.

10. The nurse participates in the profession's efforts to protect the public from misinformation and misrepresentation and to maintain the integrity of nursing.

11. The nurse collaborates with members of the health professions and other citizens in promoting community and national efforts to meet the health needs of the public.

Reprinted from American Nurses Association. (1985). Code for nurses with interpretive statements. Kansas City, MO: Author, with permis-

In addition to the Code, the ANA periodically develops and publishes position statements on timely and pressing ethical concerns facing the profession. One example of this pertains to guidelines governing withdrawal of food and fluids (ANA, 1988).

Other Codes and Guidelines

In addition to guidance provided by the nursing profession, it is important for nurses to be aware of relevant codes, guidelines, and statements issued by a variety of professional organizations, governmental or private agencies, commissions or task forces. These provide important information and guidance on topical issues in health care that health professionals can utilize as a resource in their work.

A few examples will suffice. A presidential commission issued a report on access to health care that has been used as an important reference on discussions by health professionals and philosophers alike on this issue (President's Commission, 1983). Similarly, a task force appointed by the Secretary of Health and Human Services presented a report on a series of issues and recommendations concerning organ transplantation that has been read, studied, and followed extensively around the country on ethical issues pertaining to organ transplantation (U.S. Department of Health and Human Services, 1986). The Hastings Center (1987) issued guidelines concerning life-sustaining measures and care of the dying that have been used extensively by professional societies in formulating their own positions on these thorny issues.

Public Duties of the Professions

Historically, a great deal of emphasis has been placed in professional education programs and ethical codes on the duties of professionals to those they serve and their ethical responsibilities for conduct and behavior in the interest of the client. An emerging body of literature has enlarged the duties of professionals to include the larger public and concern for the public "good."

Much of the expert knowledge in society is held by professionals. Because of this professionals exert significant influence in the decision making of major social institutions. Society as a whole has come to depend on professionals; therefore, one might conclude that it is important to hold the professions and professionals to public duties as well as private ones (Jennings, Callahan, & Wolf, 1987, p. 3).

The nursing profession recognizes community responsibility in its ethical code. Tenet 11 states, "The nurse collaborates with members of the health professions and other citizens in promoting community and national efforts to meet the health needs of the public" (ANA, 1985). In the interpretive statements to this tenet, the following concepts are highlighted: collaborative planning with others at many levels to promote equitable access to health care for all; active participation in decision making in institutional and political domains to ensure the just distribution of health care; and collaborative planning to ensure the availability and access of high-quality health services to all whose health needs are unmet.

The nursing profession, through its professional organizations, has been active in collaborative planning and in efforts to influence health care legislation that is just and equitable. Yet, the number of individual nurses who espouse a conception of their role as incorporating the common good is limited at present.

One might argue that by serving the interests of individual clients one serves the public. Although in a sense this is true, it is too limited a view as a conception of public duty. Nurses, by virtue of their work, have special insights into the functioning of health care institutions, into factors—personal or social—that are conducive to health or illness. They have special understanding of the impact of acute or chronic illness on families, and they have intimate understanding and knowledge of the impact a major illness has on individuals who are uninsured or underinsured. It is the public duty of nursing to stimulate public discourse on these issues, expose the underside of a system that does not seem to work for segments of society, press for reform, and engage in public advocacy on broad health policy issues.

Role of Practicing Nurses in Research

Tenet 7 addresses the responsibilities of nurses in the ongoing development of knowledge. This tenet often has been misunderstood by practicing nurses and needs special attention and interpretation, given that various types of research are actively being pursued in many health care settings.

Expectations in this regard need to be consistent with goals at each educational level, so that nurses can function appropriately at their level of competence. The undergraduate curriculum in nursing should include instruction on the research process and its contribution to nursing. The research process in nursing is discussed in Chapter 10. Nurses at the ADN and BSN levels are not expected to carry out investigations. However, they have a number of important responsibilities in terms of nursing research:

1. By virtue of their insights into patients and clinical problems, nurses can identify areas of patient care where certain interventions are carried out with insufficient scientific basis or with unfruitful results. Such insights can be the basis of clinical investigations if appropriately communicated to individuals qualified to conduct research.

2. Nurses are in a position to use research findings to improve patient care and can communicate their clinical judgments of whether such use of research is effective with regard to patient responses and outcomes. This type of systematic approach to care makes an important contribution to both clinical care and research.

3. Nurses act as advocates to their clients in instances where they are

asked to be subjects of research. Investigators, nurses or other, and institutions have formalized obligations in this regard. The nursing profession has guidelines for investigators (ANA, 1975); the Department of Health and Human Services has guidelines as well, which are mandated and followed by health care institutions. Although nurses caring for patients are not expected to take on these burdens, they have special responsibilities toward their clients that they must fulfill. Nurses need to ascertain that patients fully understand the implications of the protocol; that they are not coerced into participation; and that their right to privacy, confidentiality, and self-determination are observed and respected.

4. In cases where nurses are asked to participate in research conducted by others, such as in data gathering or administering specified protocols, they need to ascertain that (1) the research is indeed approved by the appropriate institutional committees and (2) they themselves fully understand the intent and nature of the research, its risks, and its benefits. As individually licensed professionals, they are personally accountable for all actions in which they engage, and it would be irresponsible to carry out actions prescribed by others without full knowledge and understanding. Nurses may also refuse to participate in research if they are not satisfied about its merit, safety, or for other good reasons.

ETHICAL DECISION MAKING

Nurses encounter situations on a daily basis where they must make judgments and decisions and act on them. Decision making is not a solitary endeavor and frequently involves other parties, such as patients, family members, and other health professionals. Whether the nurse participates in dialogue and collective decision making or needs to act alone, it is important to be knowledgeable in order to bring to bear the best thinking to the situation.

A number of authors have described ethical decision making at length. According to Aroskar (1980), three decision elements must be considered. These are (1) the specific facts of the situation, (2) identification of the questions that require a decision, and (3) the underlying ethical theories or principles. The reader is referred to the works of Bandman and Bandman (1985, 1995) and Thompson and Thompson (1981, 1985) for further discussion of ethical decision making. It is beyond the scope of this chapter to detail this process; however, the decision-making steps, in summary form, are presented here.

The nurse–patient decision-making process, according to Bandman and Bandman (1985), includes the following steps:

1. The nurse and patient develop a dialogue in which they interact about the patient's health concerns and problems and in which the nurse helps to frame a therapeutic setting showing concern for the patient.
2. The nurse makes data evident to the patient.
3. The nurse presents proposed alternatives and consequences of the patient's health problems in discussion with the patient and in conjunction with physicians and relevant others.
4. The dialogue between patient and nurse includes the implementation of treatment alternatives and their relative costs, risks, and benefits.
5. Finally, the nurse encourages the patient to come to the best possible resolution. (p. 79)

Presenting a somewhat different perspective, Thompson and Thompson (1985) describe a 10-step bioethical decision-making model, as follows:

1. Review the situation to determine health problems, decision needed, ethical components, and key individuals.
2. Gather additional information to clarify situation.
3. Identify the ethical issues in the situation.
4. Define personal and professional moral positions.
5. Identify moral positions of key individuals involved.
6. Identify value conflicts, if any.
7. Determine who should make the decision.
8. Identify range of actions with anticipated outcomes.
9. Decide on a course of action and carry it out.
10. Evaluate/review the results of decision/action. (p. 99)

In the first model, the focus is on assisting the patient in making a decision; in the second, the focus is on decisions that the nurse needs to make. In either case, the general approaches expressed bear close resemblance to the nursing process, described in Chapter 5.

IMPACT OF TECHNOLOGY

Technological developments in health care have given rise to new forms of ethical dilemmas. It is now possible to prolong life almost indefinitely, raising questions about quality of life and whether or not, and when, to terminate life-sustaining interventions. Organ transplantation techniques make it possible to transplant vital organs to those in need. Ethical questions in this domain pertain to allocation of organs (a scarce resource), given a great demand and limited supply; criteria for eligibility and selection of potential recipients and for rank-ordering according to priority patients who are deemed eligible; and questions pertaining to which individuals and groups should be considered appropriate donors and when life begins and ends. Another area of fast-moving technology pertains to gene research; serious questions have arisen about the potential for genetic manipulation. Our ability to deal with the ethical issues raised by scientific and technological advances has not kept pace with the rapidity with which these advances are affecting the social fabric of society. These issues are likely to become more and more compelling.

RESPONSIBLE SCIENCE

No chapter on ethical dimensions of nursing can be complete without some mention of ethics in research (also referred to by the terms *responsible conduct in science* and *scientific integrity*). In recent years a number of cases of scientific misconduct have been highly publicized in the media and have focused the attention of the scientific community, funding agencies, and legislative bodies on the ethical issues involved in conducting science and on the responsibilities of scientists. Various monitoring mechanisms have been put into place by institutions where scientists work and by governmental and other funding agencies.

The most important element in promoting responsible science has to do with sound education during the training period of young scientists. To this end, attention has been given to the development of guidelines by disciplines and departments to articulate the scope of responsible science appropriate to a discipline. This approach is intended to prevent the occurrence of scientific misconduct, to guide the work of scientists, and to provide mentorship to students while they are in training.

Many of the general ethical principles and theories discussed are relevant to this area of ethical practice and to scientific integrity. The Midwest Nursing Research Society, one of the largest regional scientific societies in nursing, has taken the leadership in developing and promulgating guidelines for scientific integrity. This document is highly recommended for those who wish to study this area of ethical practice (MNRS, 1996).

SUMMARY

This chapter introduced ethical aspects of nursing practice. It presented foundational content addressed to professional nurses to heighten awareness of ethical issues in nursing practice and nursing research; enable the reader to appreciate the centrality of ethics to professional practice; assist nurses in critically analyzing ethical issues they encounter in their practice; utilize relevant resources in ethical dilemma situations; and enhance nurses' ability to engage in ethical decision making.

It is impossible to present all material relevant to ethics in one chapter.

It is hoped, however, that the reader will use this broad exposure as the basis for pursuit of independent study.

REFERENCES

American Hospital Association. (1973). A Patient's Bill of Rights. In E. L. Bandman & B. Bandman (1985), *Nursing ethics in the life span* (pp. 275–277). Norwalk, CT: Appleton-Century-Crofts.

American Nurses Association. (1975). *Human rights guidelines for nurses in clinical and other research*. Kansas City: Author.

American Nurses Association. (1985). *Code for nurses with interpretive statements*. Kansas City: Author.

American Nurses Association, Committee on Ethics. (1988). *Guidelines on withdrawing or withholding food and fluid*. Kansas City: Author.

Aroskar, M. (1980). Anatomy of an ethical dilemma's theory and practice. *American Journal of Nursing, 80*, 658–663.

Bandman, E. L., & Bandman, B. (1985). *Nursing ethics in the life span*. Norwalk, CT: Appleton-Century-Crofts.

Bandman, E. L., & Bandman, B. (1995). *Critical thinking in nursing* (2nd ed.). Norwalk, CT: Appleton & Lange.

Beauchamp, T. L., & Childress, J. F. (1983). *Principles of biomedical ethics* (2nd ed.). New York: Oxford University Press.

Bruner, J. S. (1960). *The process of education*. Cambridge, MA: Harvard University Press.

Curtin, L. L. (1979). The nurse as advocate: A philosophical foundation for nursing. *Advances in Nursing Science, 1*(3), 1–10.

Dewey, J. (1964). What psychology can do for the teacher. In D. R. Archambault (Ed.), *John Dewey on education: Selected writings* (pp. 195–211). New York: Random House.

Flexner, A. (1915). *Is social work a profession?* (Studies in Social Work, No. 4). New York: New York School of Philanthropy.

Gilligan, C. (1982). *In a different voice*. Cambridge, MA: Harvard University Press.

Hastings Center. (1987). *Guidelines on the termination of life-sustaining treatment and the care of the dying*. Bloomington, IN: Indiana University Press.

Henderson, M. L., & McConnell, E. S. (1988). Ethical considerations. In M. A. Matteson & E. S. McConnell (Eds.), *Gerontological nursing concepts and practice* (pp. 93–121). Philadelphia: Saunders.

Johnson, D. C. (1968). Professional practice and specialization in nursing. *Image, 2*, 2–7.

Jennings, B., Callahan, D., & Wolf, S. M. (1987). The professions: Public interest and common good. *Hastings Center Report, 17*(1), Supplement, 3–10.

Ketefian, S. (1981). Critical thinking, educational preparation, and development of moral judgment among selected groups of practicing nurses. *Nursing Research, 30*, 98–103.

Kohlberg, L. (1971). From is to ought: How to commit the naturalistic fallacy and get away with it in the study of moral development. In T. Mischel (Ed.), *Cognitive development and epistemology* (pp. 151–235). New York: Academic Press.

Kohlberg, L. (1978). The cognitive-developmental approach to moral education. In P. Scharf (Ed.), *Readings in Moral Education* (pp. 36–51). Minneapolis: Winston Press.

Kohnke, M. F. (1978). *The case for consultation in nursing: Designs for professional practice*. New York: Wiley.

Midwest Nursing Research Society. (1996). *Guidelines for scientific integrity*. Scientific Integrity Committee of the Midwest Nursing Research Society. Glenview, IL: Author.

Murphy, C. P. (1976). *Levels of moral reasoning in a selected group of nursing practitioners*. Unpublished doctoral dissertation, Teachers College, Columbia University, New York.

Piaget, J. (1965). *The moral judgment of the child*. New York: The Free Press. (Original work published 1932.)

President's Commission for the Study of Ethical Problems in Medicine and Biomedical and Behavioral Research. (1983). In *Securing Access to Health Care* (Vol. 1). Washington, DC: U. S. Government Printing Office.

Reilly, D. E., & Oermann, M. H. (1992). *Clinical teaching in nursing education* (2nd ed.). New York: National League for Nursing.

Rest, J. (1974). Developmental psychology as a guide to value education: A review of "Kohlbergian" programs. *Review of Educational Research, 44*, 241–258.

Rest, J., Bebeau, M. J., & Volker, J. (1986). An overview of the psychology of morality. In J. Rest (Ed.), *Moral development: Advances in research and theory* (pp. 1–39). New York: Praeger.

Rest, J., Turiel, E., & Kohlberg, L. (1969). Levels of moral development as a determinant of preference and comprehension of moral judgments made by others. *Journal of Personality, 37*, 225–252.

Rogers, M. E. (1970). *The theoretical basis of nursing*. Philadelphia: Davis.

Schlotfeldt, R. M. (1965). A mandate for nurses and physicians. *American Journal of Nursing, 65*, 102–105.

Thompson, J. B., & Thompson, H. O. (1981). *Ethics in nursing*. New York: Macmillan.

Thompson, J. B., & Thompson, H. O. (1985). *Bioethical decision making for nurses*. Norwalk, CT: Appleton-Century-Crofts.

U. S. Department of Health and Human Services, Report of the Task Force on Organ Transplantation. (1986). *Organ transplantation: Issues and recommendations*. Washington, DC: Office of Organ Transplantation.

BIBLIOGRAPHY

Bandman, E., & Bandman, B. (1979). The nurse's role in protecting the patient's right to live or die. *Advances in Nursing Science, 1*(3), 21–35.

Beauchamp, T., & Walters, L. (Eds.). (1982). *Contemporary issues in bioethics* (2nd ed.). Belmont, CA: Wadsworth.

Brody, H. (1981). *Ethical decisions in medicine* (2nd ed.). Boston: Little, Brown.

Caplan, A., & Callahan, D. (Eds.). (1981). *Ethics for hard times*. New York: Plenum.

Davis, A. J., & Aroskar, M. A. (1983). *Ethical dilemmas and nursing practice* (2nd ed.). Norwalk, CT: Appleton-Century-Crofts.

Frankena, W. (1973). *Ethics* (2nd ed.). Englewood Cliffs, NJ: Prentice-Hall.

Ketefian, S. (1981). Moral reasoning and moral behavior among selected groups of practicing nurses. *Nursing Research, 30,* 171–176.

Ketefian, S. (1985). Professional and bureaucratic role conceptions and moral behavior among nurses. *Nursing Research, 34,* 248–253.

Ketefian, S. (1987). A case study of theory development: Moral behavior in nursing. *Advances in Nursing Science, 9*(2), 10–19.

Ketefian, S. (1989a). Moral reasoning and ethical practice. *Annual Review of Nursing Research, 7*(9), 173–195.

Ketefian, S. (1989b). Moral reasoning and ethical practice in nursing: Measurement issues. *Nursing Clinics of North America, 24*(2), 509–521.

Ketefian, S., & Lenz, E. (1995). Promoting scientific integrity in nursing research, Part II: Strategies. *Journal of Professional Nursing, 11,* 263–269.

Ketefian, S., & Ormond, I. (1988). *Moral reasoning and ethical practice in nursing: An integrative review.* New York: National League for Nursing.

Kohnke, M. F. (1982). *Advocacy: Risk and reality.* St. Louis: Mosby.

Lenz, E., & Ketefian, S. (1995). Promoting scientific integrity in nursing research, Part I: Current approaches in doctoral programs. *Journal of Professional Nursing, 11*(4), 213–219.

Macklin, R. (1987). *Moral choices: Ethical dilemmas in modern medicine.* Boston: Houghton Mifflin.

Ramsey, P. (1971). *The patient as person.* New Haven: Yale University Press.

Rawls, J. (1971). *A theory of justice.* Cambridge, MA: Harvard University Press.

Spicker, S. F., & Gadow, S. (Eds.). (1980). *Nursing images and ideals.* New York: Springer.

Steele, S. M., & Harman, V. M. (1983). *Values clarification in nursing* (2nd ed.). New York: Appleton-Century-Crofts.

Nursing Research and Its Relationship to Practice

Fredericka P. Shea

The value and importance of nursing research were first recognized by Florence Nightingale, who is credited as the founder of nursing and who was an ardent proponent of the use of statistics to show the "impact of disease and the effects of improved sanitary conditions" (Cohen, 1984, p. 133). Influenced by the Belgian astronomer-statistician Lambert-Adolphe-Jacques Quetelet and the English physician and statistician William Farr, Nightingale collected and analyzed data on the effect of her reforms (i.e., improved sanitary conditions) on the British Army in Crimea. Cohen (1984) writes:

> Calculated on an annual basis as a percentage of the patient population, the death rate at the Scutari hospital reached an incredible 415 percent in February, 1855. In March, however, Nightingales's [sic] sanitary reforms began to be implemented and mortality among the patients declined precipitously. By the end of the war, according to Nightingale, the death rate among sick British soldiers in Turkey was "not much more" than it was among healthy soldiers in England. (p. 133)

Questions posed by Nightingale could be classified under the rubric of investigations on the outcomes of nursing actions designed to promote the health of individuals, families, and communities. From Nightingale's time until the 1950s, little nursing research was conducted. A principal explanation for the dearth of nursing research may be societal norms prevailing during those years on the appropriate "place" of women. In particular, the rigors of science were considered much too taxing for women's perceived "frail" intellectual abilities. Therefore, because most nurses were women, they were not viewed as capable of becoming scientists.

Further support for this interpretation is seen in the history of nursing education, which took place in nurse training schools until the advent of baccalaureate education in 1909. The differentiation between *training* and *education* is important because it is believed to have delayed the progress of nursing research. Training refers to forming by instruction, discipline, or drill, or to teach to be fit, qualified, or proficient. Education refers to the process of acquiring knowledge and developing cognitive and other skills (Reilly & Oermann, 1992). Reflecting on the meaning of these words suggests that trained nurses were taught, disciplined, or drilled to be fit, qualified, or proficient in their narrowly defined, somewhat static role, which was subservient to male-dominated medicine. Educated nurses, however, were expected to acquire new knowledge and to develop their cognitive abilities to create and evaluate new nursing roles that would evolve in response to societal needs. Autonomy over nursing practice was envisioned as a key characteristic of new nursing roles, and nurses were seen as equals among others, including physicians, who provide health care.

The distinction between trained and educated nurses is not intended to imply that "trained" nurses were not thinkers—they were. Training schools placed insufficient value on the importance of nurses acquiring and developing intellectual abilities; acquiring the requisite knowledge and skills essential for conducting scientific investigations; and subsequently, changing nursing practice as a result of new knowledge. With the advent of social changes, for instance, the women's movement, and with the persistent efforts of visionary nurse leaders, a new value system began to evolve. As a result, nurses increasingly are becoming academically prepared to accept the responsibility for developing, evaluating, and using scientific knowledge as the basis of nursing practice.

This chapter describes the research process used in quantitative studies. Other topics covered are the meaning of research, reasons for doing nursing research, who does nursing research, and future directions for nursing research. Exploration of the research process is intended to encourage the reader to learn more about research, actively participate in nursing investigations, read the nursing research literature and evaluate its rigor and relevance for nursing practice, and incorporate new knowledge in giving nursing care, in nursing education, and in conducting further nursing research.

WHAT IS RESEARCH?

Definitions of research abound; one is set forth here. Research is the systematic process of answering questions by generating new knowledge (Figure 10–1). Analysis of the definition reveals an emphasis on research as a systematic process, a set of thoughtfully planned, interrelated, and interde-

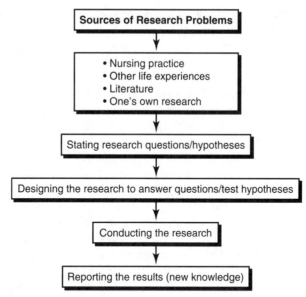

Figure 10–1. Relationship Between Research Ideas and Research Results

pendent actions as contrasted to haphazard or chance actions. The second part of the definition emphasizes research as a way of answering questions. Before questions can be answered, they need to be clearly and precisely stated. Although this may seem relatively simple and straightforward, it is one of the most creative and challenging tasks of doing good research. Clear, specific, and justified research questions drive scientific inquiry; consequently, they are of crucial importance to the entire conduct of investigations. The third part of the definition focuses on the product of doing research, the generation of new knowledge. The value of research, the very reason for doing research, is to learn something previously not known or to confirm or refute previous research findings.

On occasion, research is referred to as being synonymous with problem solving. Research involves discovering new knowledge, whereas problem solving involves using existing knowledge to respond to a perplexity, puzzlement, or bafflement. Previous research has generated much of the knowledge used in problem solving. If existing knowledge is found to be inadequate in solving a problem, then the problem may lend itself to scientific investigation.

WHY DO RESEARCH?

Scientists do research for many reasons. Richard Feynman (1988), a world-renowned physicist and Nobel Prize winner, said that doing research is "the pleasure of finding things out" (p. 7). Feynman speaks to the excitement, enlivenment, and challenge of intellectual inquiry. Nurses since Nightingale have spoken to the need for knowledge to improve nursing care in order to promote the health and well-being of people; to care in a knowing way for those who are ill and their loved ones; and to comfort, in light of known facts, those who are dying and their family and friends. In essence, one of the foremost reasons for doing nursing research is to provide care based on scientific evidence rather than on hunches, guesses, trial and error, or established, but unscrutinized, practices.

Nurses also have embraced another reason for doing research—the need and responsibility to explicate a body of knowledge that defines nursing as a unique practice discipline. The focus is on developing and testing nursing theories through research. Nursing theories and research results derived from those theories will increasingly form the basis for nursing education, practice, and subsequent research.

Another reason for doing research is to distinguish nursing as a profession from an occupation. For nursing to be appropriately designated a profession, nurses have a social obligation to develop scientific knowledge as a basis for nursing interventions and, in the absence of such knowledge, to discover it.

Other reasons for doing research include generating knowledge to solve a problem, for instance, nursing management of symptoms such as wasting, diarrhea, fatigue, depression, and social isolation, in persons living with AIDS; to develop and evaluate new products, procedures, or programs, such as a program designed to increase access to prenatal care among medically underserved pregnant women; and to provide useful information for policymakers who allocate resources. Abdellah and Levine (1994) list three areas about which policymakers need information in formulating health policies:

1. How to define policy problems in the context of health promotion, attitude change, and behavior modification, and how to gain the public's support
2. How to select the most effective policy instruments to address priority health issues and how to promote the use of these instruments
3. How to develop strategies that will ensure the effective implementation and adoption of these instruments (p. 199)

WAYS NURSES CONTRIBUTE TO RESEARCH

It is not uncommon for nurses to wonder whether they are qualified to conduct nursing investigations. Generally, the recognized research credential is that of an earned doctorate. Before colleges of nursing began granting a doctoral degree in nursing, nurses earned the doctorate in such fields as anatomy, physiology, chemistry, biology, microbiology, psychology, sociology, anthropology, and education. With the advent of and subsequent growth in the number of nursing programs granting the doctorate, the number of nurses prepared to assume leadership for conducting research has increased substantially. Although the number of nurses who have earned a doctorate is increasing, they represent a small percentage of all RNs. Thus, the principal responsibility for generating new knowledge relevant to nursing practice rests with a small fraction of all nurses. Nurses, however, can participate actively in research in many ways. The following is a partial list of how nurses in clinical practice can further the aims of nursing research:

- Observe and theorize about nursing phenomena
- Generate practice-based research questions or hypotheses derived from a theory or a conceptual framework
- Analyze, evaluate, and synthesize literature on a topic of inquiry
- Contribute to the design of a study and/or to the design of data-collection instruments
- Participate in data collection and/or in data processing
- Assist in data analysis
- Contribute to explaining or interpreting research results
- Write or contribute to the preparation of research-based papers for publication or presentation and to poster presentations
- Assist nurse researchers in gaining access to people who will be studied
- Provide nurses, as part of their practice, with the time needed to participate in research
- Seek funds to support nursing research
- Fund positions for nurse researchers or buy a portion of their time to provide leadership in assisting staff nurses in doing studies of interest to them

Students enrolled in baccalaureate and graduate (master's and doctoral) nursing programs often are expected to avail themselves of opportunities to work with faculty doing research. Because today's students are tomorrow's researchers, they are encouraged to participate in conducting research as an important way of learning how to do research. Clearly, it would be ideal if the student's and faculty's interests were similar. However, if they are not, students still can have extremely valuable experiences in learning the research process by participating in ongoing research. Invariably students who conduct research report that it "comes alive," "becomes less mysterious," and that concepts that were difficult to understand or were unclear become understandable and clear. Often, researchers, in nursing and other fields, say that participation in research helps to solidify or to clarify knowledge acquired through classroom instruction and reading. Consequently, it is not uncommon for researchers to recommend to students that they become active participants in doing research to complement the knowledge they acquire in other ways.

QUANTITATIVE RESEARCH PROCESS

Although this section focuses on the research process used in quantitative studies, it should be pointed out that nurses are increasingly conducting qualitative research and that some researchers use both. Numerous books (Denzin, 1994; Leininger, 1985; Morse, 1991; Munhall and Boyd, 1993; Parse, Coyne, and Smith, 1985; Streubert and Carpenter, 1995) describe qualitative research, and journals publish articles on qualitative approaches and research results. Among the approaches used in qualitative research are phenomenology, ethnography, grounded theory, historical studies, field studies, and case studies.

Numerous writers (LoBiondo-Wood & Haber, 1994; Polit & Hungler, 1995; Wilson, 1989; Woods & Catanzaro, 1988) describe the research process used in quantitative studies. Examining these and other sources provides the reader with a sense of how others conceptualize the research process. One conceptualization of the process used in quantitative research is that of an inverted pyramid, wherein the first step forms the foundation and each subsequent step builds on the preceding step (Figure 10–2). The steps of the process are interrelated in such a way that each one is affected by its predecessor and must be consistent with it. The reason for portraying the re-

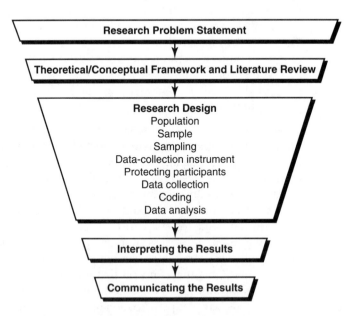

Figure 10–2. The Research Process: Sequence of Interrelated Steps. *Note:* Although the research process proceeds sequentially, each step is related to its predecessor. The results address the research problem by answering the research questions and/or confirming or refuting the hypotheses. They also give direction for future research.

search process as an inverted pyramid is to convey the notion that the research problem is the broad area of inquiry, the research process narrows the focus of inquiry, and the research results are specific findings about (and perhaps generalizable to) the research problem. A description of the five central steps of the research process follows.

Statement of the Research Problem

The statement of the research problem specifies the broad context of the proposed research. Specific objectives, derived from the overall purpose of the study, state what the research is expected to achieve (i.e., its outcomes). The researcher delineates the theory or conceptual framework guiding the research and explains its relationship to the research questions to be answered or hypotheses to be tested. Hypotheses are statements about a relationship between two or more variables; a variable is something that changes or varies and, as such, can be observed and measured.

Theoretical/Conceptual Framework and Review of the Literature

The researcher sets forth the theory or conceptual framework guiding the proposed research and its relationship to results from previous research. Relevant literature is critically analyzed, synthesized, and evaluated to determine what is known, how well it is known (i.e., how certain that knowledge is), and what is not known. The researcher attends to discerning conflicting findings, offers plausible explanations for the conflicts, and discusses how the proposed study will address them. The results of this thorough analysis help to justify why the research needs to be done—what new knowledge will be generated and why that knowledge is important.

Research Design and Data Collection and Analysis

The researcher determines the design that will be used to acquire the data (i.e., information) that then will be analyzed, synthesized, and presented as the research results or findings. The research design is the overall plan or blueprint used in conducting the investigation. It describes who will be studied, what will be done, how data will be collected, and when and where the study will be conducted. The design selected must be congruent with the study's objectives. Designs can be descriptive, correlational, experimental, or quasi-experimental.

Initially, the researcher specifies the characteristics of the population to be studied and distinguishes between the target and accessible population. The target population comprises all members of the population who meet the study's inclusion criteria. Seldom does the researcher have access to all members of the population; therefore, those who are accessible constitute the population from which the study sample is drawn.

The researcher samples or selects a small subset of members who meet the study's inclusion criteria from the accessible population. Sampling is the way in which people are chosen to be studied; those who are selected are referred to as the sample. Sampling requires that the researcher deliberately select from the array of sampling methods the one most appropriate for achieving the study's overall purpose and objectives and for answering the research questions or providing evidence that either confirms or refutes the hypotheses. Sampling methods are of two types: (1) probability and (2) nonprobability.

Probability sampling, which is based on probability theory, refers to methods by which members of the accessible population have a known and nonzero probability, or chance, of being selected into the sample. Nonprobability sampling refers to sampling methods wherein the probability of elements being drawn into the study is unknown. Probability sampling allows the research findings to be generalized to the population, whereas nonprobability sampling allows the findings to be generalized only to the sample studied. In addition, different kinds of statistics are appropriate for probability and nonprobability samples.

Develop the Data-Collection Instrument

Research involves collecting data on the variables being investigated. A form, generally referred to as the data-collection instrument or tool, is developed; the instrument lists the variables and their values. Instruments commonly used include self-administered questionnaires, interview schedules, recording forms on which observations are entered, diaries, and logs. It is crucial that the data-collection instrument contain all the variables required for the study. The data-collection instrument should be both reliable and valid. *Reliability* refers to the accuracy and consistency of measurements. *Validity* refers to the correspondence between what the instrument actually measures and what the researcher intends it to measure.

Conduct a Pilot Study

Before investing time, money, and energy in carrying out a full-fledged investigation, it is a good idea to conduct a pilot study or trial run. The purpose of a pilot study is to evaluate the correspondence between the research problem being addressed and the research design or to collect preliminary data. Often, a pilot study provides information on both anticipated and unforeseen problems, and, consequently, the proposed research design can be modified to overcome or mitigate the problems when the full-scale investigation is done. For example, if there are too few subjects at a selected site, alternative sites need to be found. A pilot study also may show that the data-collection instrument, for example, a self-administered questionnaire or interview schedule, is too long or that some questions are ambiguous or vague. With this information, the researcher can revise the instrument before doing the actual study.

In addition, a pilot study also helps the researcher to (1) identify other research questions that can be investigated with slight modifications in the research design; (2) estimate more accurately resources needed to do the study, such as the number and types of personnel, supplies, and equipment; (3) make a more realistic estimate of the amount of time needed to do the actual study; and (4) identify others who may be helpful in implementing the study. Many funding agencies expect researchers, as part of their research proposals, to demonstrate that they have done a pilot study and to show how it influenced the proposed study.

Safeguard the Rights and Welfare of Research Participants

Before conducting any investigation, including a pilot study, the researcher needs to ensure that the rights and welfare of people or animals who participate in the research are protected. Six tasks a researcher needs to perform to safeguard the rights and welfare of research participants are:

1. The researcher describes the characteristics, such as age range, gender, race/ethnicity, and health, of the population to be studied. The number of people to be studied and criteria for including or excluding them are given. If the research is to be done on members of special populations, fetuses, pregnant women, children, prisoners, or institutionalized individuals, then the researcher also must provide the rationale for studying them.

2. The researcher needs to identify the source of data, such as records, interviews, questionnaires, and specimens; whether the data will be obtained solely for research purposes; and whether existing data, for instance, records and specimens, will be used.

3. A detailed description is given on how potential participants will be recruited into the study and the procedure to be used for eliciting and obtaining their informed consent to participate in the research. Specific areas addressed include who will seek consent and what prospective participants will be told about the research; what is expected of them; the nature, seriousness, and likelihood of risks to them; precautions that will be taken to minimize the risks; and anticipated benefits of the research to them and to the generation of new knowledge that may result from their contribution to the study.

4. The researcher thoroughly describes any potential risks, physical, psychological, social, and legal, and provides an assessment of their seriousness and the likelihood of their occurring. If alternative treatments or procedures might be beneficial to the research participants, they must be described.

5. For each of the potential risks, procedures that will be taken to prevent the risks or to minimize the chances of their occurring are described. If appropriate, the researcher also describes monitoring procedures to ensure the safety of the research participants.

6. The researcher explains why the risks to the participants are reasonable in relation to the expected benefits. If it is unlikely that the

participants will benefit from participating in the study, then they should be told so. Another component of the risk–benefit assessment is to describe potential risks to participants in relation to the importance of new knowledge that may result from the study. (U.S. Department of Health and Human Services, 1992, pp. 22–25)

Collect the Data

The next part of the research design involves collecting the data. Sometimes it is necessary to use more than one instrument. For instance, the researcher might record data contained in a chart on to another form and also use a self-administered questionnaire or an interview schedule. The instruments should be completed or administered consistently across subjects. For instance, in conducting an interview, the order in which questions are asked should be the same for all subjects, as should the way in which the questions are asked. If an interview contains open-ended questions in which response categories are not prescribed in advance, then it is imperative that the interviewer write the responses verbatim. The interviewer does not alter a response to make it grammatically correct, to omit slang, or to delete socially unacceptable language. The rationale for verbatim recording is that the person's responses are the data, whereas alterations of a response by the interviewer may distort the meaning of the respondent's reply and thus introduce bias.

In collecting data, the researcher needs to respect the study participants so that their involvement corresponds directly to what they consented to; is not too demanding of their energy, time, and other resources; respects their right to privacy; and makes sense to them. For example, if the interviewer asks people about their dietary or sexual behaviors or many detailed questions about household income and expenditures, the respondents may question the purpose of the study and the type of information they consented to provide.

In collecting data, it is important that the researcher be sensitive to the needs of participants. If someone is becoming tired, anxious, or upset during an interview, the interviewer needs to assess the participant's well-being and use sound judgment in deciding what action to take, such as stopping the interview or getting assistance. The rule is to do no harm, physical, psychological, legal, social, or financial, to participants in research.

When people incur expenses, such as transportation, parking, and caregiver costs, as a result of participating in a study, the researcher should try to reimburse them. Invariably the question arises about paying people as an incentive for them to participate in research. In general, researchers do not pay subjects except to reimburse them for reasonable expenses they incur. In some cases, researchers may use incentives to encourage people to participate in a study. For example, women who use cocaine may be more likely to consent to their infants being studied if they are given diapers, educational toys, infant clothing, and so forth. Of course, incentives need to be appropriate and not of a magnitude or kind to imply or constitute coercion. For example, if a researcher is studying injection drug users who are at risk for the human immunodeficiency virus and an incentive is needed to recruit them into a study, rather than giving cash, they may be given a coupon for a meal or a gift certificate for a piece of clothing up to some reasonable dollar value.

It is also important to thank people who participate in research. A letter of appreciation, a sincere thank you upon completion of an interview, or an offer to send participants a summary of the results are ways of acknowledging appreciation.

Code the Data

Preparing data for analysis is another integral part of the research design. Researchers need to analyze data carefully before coding and entering them into the computer to ensure that they are in a useable form. For example, suppose that in response to the question, "How old are you?" a respondent writes "16 1/2" years, but the researcher had chosen to use whole numbers for age. The researcher needs to make a rule about rounding fractions to whole numbers so that all occurrences are handled in the same way. As another example, suppose people are asked to circle one number on a six-point agree–disagree scale that measures how they feel about what is being asked. In reviewing completed forms, it is found that some people circled two adjacent numbers, say two and three. Again, a decision is needed on how to handle this situation. The researcher may decide to treat the responses as "missing data" or assign each number—two and three—to a side of a coin, call the coin, flip it, and then record the number that coincides with the flipped coin. The decision rule using a coin flip results in coding a response based on chance alone rather than on the researcher's beliefs about what the person meant. If, however, a person circled one and six, the response would be coded as "missing" because the numbers represent the extremes on the agree–disagree continuum and there is no way of knowing what the person thought.

Having decided how to handle unusual or missing responses, the researcher then codes all data so they are amenable to statistical analysis. The researcher prepares a codebook listing each variable along with its values and the numbers used to signify the value of the variable. Numerical values are assigned according to rules for different types of scales: nominal, ordinal, interval, and ratio (Table 10–1).

For the *nominal* scale, the values of the variables are mutually exclusive categories. Numbers are assigned to each category. For example, the variable gender has two response categories: male and female. In coding the data, the number 1 might be used to represent male and 2 to represent female. Other numbers or symbols could be used as well. Assigning a number to represent gender is not intended to make judgments about females or males. The numbers are used only to represent the values of the variable.

TABLE 10–1. LEVELS OF MEASUREMENT: CHARACTERISTICS, STATISTICS, AND STATISTICAL TESTS

Scale	Characteristics	Statistics*	Statistical Tests
Nominal	Values are mutually exclusive categories represented by a number or symbol	Frequency Mode	Nonparametric
Ordinal	Values have an ordered relation to one another	Median Range Percentile Spearman's rho	Nonparametric
Interval	Arbitrary zero point; distance between scale points is equal	Mean Standard deviation Pearson's r	Parametric
Ratio	Absolute zero point; distance between scale points is equal	Same as interval	Parametric

Note: The statistics are examples; they are not exhaustive. Note that the scales themselves are ordered in such a way that each one is like its predecessor but has one additional characteristic.

The *ordinal* scale has the same naming (i.e., classification) characteristics of the nominal scale, except that the values of the variables have an ordered relationship of greater or lesser. In this instance, the numbers represent rank ordering of the variable's values. An example of a variable with ordered values is postsurgical diet where 1 is none, 2 is clear liquid, 3 is full liquid, 4 is soft, and 5 is regular. The order is from nothing to a regular diet. Although the numbers used to signify the values of the variable differ by one (5 − 4 = 1, 4 − 1 = 3, and so forth), the amount of difference between each value of the variable is not equal. For example, the difference between a regular diet and a soft diet is not equal to the difference between a soft and a full-liquid diet.

The *interval* scale has an arbitrary zero point, and the distance between each scale point is equal to every other. Body temperature is an example of a variable measured on an interval scale (Celsius or Fahrenheit). The Fahrenheit scale is used here to illustrate the defining characteristics of an interval scale, namely, the difference between units of measurement is equal. For example, 101.8 - 100.8 = 1 and 99.8 - 98.8 = 1; in addition, there is an arbitrary zero point of 32 degrees.

One perplexity researchers face is that some variables clearly meet the criteria of ordinal but not interval measurement. For example, using a scale to measure attitudes where 1 is strongly agree, 2 is agree, 3 is disagree, and 4 is strongly disagree, there is no arbitrary zero point and the difference between scale labels (strongly agree and agree versus agree and disagree) is not equal in a conceptual sense, although the difference between the numbers used to code the data (i.e., 1, 2, 3, 4) is equal. The issue is that some statistics have interval measurement as an underlying assumption. In general, those who adhere to a strict view will not use statistics appropriate for the interval level unless the scale has the characteristics of an interval scale, whereas those who hold a less strict view are willing to assume that the scale is roughly comparable to an interval scale, unless their data show that such an assumption is unjustified.

The *ratio* scale is like the interval scale, except that it has a genuine zero point. There are many variables of interest to nurses that meet the criteria for ratio-level data, such as pulse rate. Assume that at time 1 someone's pulse is 60 beats per minute, whereas at time 2 it is 120 beats per minute. In this case, it makes sense to say that the person's pulse rate was twice as fast at time 2 than at time 1. Multiplication and division are appropriate for a ratio scale because the scale has an absolute zero point and its intervals are equal. Other examples of variables measured at the ratio level include age, height, weight, number of calories, intake and output, medication dosages, and number of pregnancies.

Analyze the Data

Data analysis is the last part of the research design. The researcher selects the statistics appropriate for analyzing the data collected to answer the research questions or test the hypotheses. Statistics also are used to describe the sample and the reliability and validity of the data-collection instrument.

The research questions or hypotheses and the type of design, including the characteristics of the sample and variables, taken as a whole have a direct bearing on selecting the statistics appropriate for data analysis. In developing the research design, the researcher needs to analyze each part of the design with respect to its implications for data analysis because each statistic has underlying assumptions, and appropriate use of a statistic means that its assumptions are not violated. For example, if a researcher has a nonprobability sample, it often is advisable not to use statistics that have assumptions about probability. Other statistics that do not have probability as an assumption generally are preferred. Another consideration is the type of scale used to measure a variable. Some statistics assume that data are going to be measured at the interval level, such as *t* tests and analysis of variance (ANOVA). If a variable were measured on an ordinal scale, then statistics appropriate for ordinal data are needed. It is generally recommended that before beginning a study, the researcher develop tables, graphs, charts, and plots that will be used to show the results. These measures help the researcher in selecting statistics most appropriate for data analysis.

Interpretation of the Meaning of the Findings

The researcher interprets the findings with respect to the study's purpose, objectives, and research questions or hypotheses. A study often has many findings; consequently, the researcher is challenged to explain how they fit together. The expected outcome is new knowledge.

At the outset, the researcher uses a theoretical or conceptual framework in developing the focus of inquiry; the framework strongly influences the study design. At this point, the researcher uses the framework as the context in which to explain the findings. The researcher compares the results with what was asserted to be the case depending on whether the theory or conceptual framework was used to describe, predict, or explain the phenomenon investigated.

If the results support assertions derived from the framework, then the researcher, in presenting them, can claim that they correspond to what was expected and explain why they do. If the results are contrary to what was asserted, then the researcher states that the results did not support the framework. In this instance, it is essential that the researcher offer plausible explanations about why the results were contrary to what was expected. It is necessary to consider whether the results imply that the theoretical or conceptual framework did not hold up and may need to be revised in light of the results or that problems occurred with the study design, such as too few subjects or an invalid data-collection instrument. In some cases, a study may have "mixed" results; that is, some results support the theoretical or conceptual framework whereas others do not. Again, the researcher reports the findings and offers explanations.

Research results help to build new knowledge and goad researchers into refining or creating new theoretical and conceptual frameworks. Both are essential to science and assist researchers in building the knowledge base for nursing practice.

Communication of the Research Results

In the last step of the research process, the researcher communicates the results, describes the limitations of the study, and discusses the meaning of the findings for nursing theory, education, practice, or health policy. New areas of research suggested by the investigation also are discussed.

Every study has limitations simply because the conduct of science, a human enterprise, is imperfect. It is imperative that the researcher make explicit the limitations of the study. For example, the sample size can be too small, the data-collection instrument's reliability or validity was less than desired, the sampling method was deficient, or problems were encountered in translating the theoretical or conceptual framework into measuring the study's variables. The researcher indicates how the limitations may have influenced the research results. If the limitations were a consequence of problems encountered in doing the study, the researcher needs to describe how the problems were handled and recommend how they may be avoided in future studies.

An investigation invariably suggests new areas of inquiry. Some ideas previously considered as needing investigation may acquire added importance or a heightened sense of urgency, and others are assigned lower priority or dismissed. Research findings can be seen as part of an unending progression wherein they generate new research questions that result in new findings and new questions. It is in this sense that scientific knowledge is cumulative. Nursing practice is increasingly, and will continue to be, based on scientific knowledge that will help in describing, explaining, or predicting nursing phenomena. Nursing education eventually will have as its corpus scientific knowledge about nursing phenomena. Nursing textbooks, based almost exclusively on nursing research results, are expected to emerge. They also will point out areas that need to be investigated.

FUTURE DIRECTIONS FOR NURSING RESEARCH

To continue building the knowledge base for nursing practice, direction is needed and priorities need to be identified. In 1986, the National Center for Nursing Research (NCNR) was established at the federal government's National Institutes of Health (NIH). In 1993, the NCNR was renamed the National Institute for Nursing Research (NINR), placing nursing on an equal footing with other NIH Institutes (Abdellah & Levine, 1994, p. 8). The NINR (and its predecessor the NCNR) determines the national nursing research agenda for studies it funds. The purpose of the agenda is to delineate scientific initiatives for nursing research and to develop further the body of knowledge underpinning nursing practice. In 1988 the National Advisory Council for Nursing Research identified seven priorities: (1) nursing care of women at risk for having a low-birthweight infant (LBWI), to prevent premature delivery, and care of LBWI to prevent complications; (2) prevention of HIV infection and care of persons living with HIV/AIDS; (3) long-term care for the elderly; (4) symptom management (e.g., pain, fatigue, nausea and vomiting) and development of measures for assessing and managing symptoms; (5) information systems; (6) health promotion; and (7) technology dependency across the lifespan (Block, 1990). Other foci include research on minority youth behavior, biobehavioral symptom management, home health care for older adults, community-based care for chronically ill older adults to delay institutionalization, management of Alzheimer's disease symptoms, long-term care of minorities as they age, and use of innovative, current biological techniques in solving nursing problems (National Center for Nursing Research, 1992).

Using Research Results in Nursing Practice

By conducting research, one discovers new knowledge as a basis for nursing practice. Implied in this statement is the belief that nurses have a responsibility, if not an obligation, to use research results in practice. Before translating research findings into practice, however, nurses need to evaluate critically the research from which the results came; new knowledge is not necessarily "good" knowledge. There is a high degree of variability in investigations: some are outstanding, some are poor, and others lie somewhere between these extremes. As a consequence, the user of research results should not apply them in practice without first critically evaluating the research to determine whether it was done in a scientific manner. If an investigation was conducted poorly, then the results are questionable. They should not be put into practice because they probably lack scientific merit. If, however, an investigation was done well, it is more likely that its results are worthy of being applied in practice.

Often, nurse researchers, like other scientists, have their work scrutinized by peers to ensure its scientific merit. This system of checks operates in many ways. For example, submission of research proposals for funding, grant applications, usually means that the proposed investigation is reviewed critically by a panel of peers to determine its scientific merit. The outcome of the review is that the proposal is either approved or not approved. In some cases, approved proposals are assigned priority scores whereby those with "better" scores are more likely to be funded if the funding agency cannot fund all of those approved. Peer review also is done when researchers submit their research for publication in refereed journals, such as *Applied Nursing Research, Advances in Nursing Science, Image: Journal of Nursing Scholarship, Journal of Nursing Education, Journal of Nursing Measurement, Nursing Research, Qualitative Health Research, Research in Nursing and Health, Scholarly Inquiry for Nursing Practice,* and *Western Journal of Nursing Research.* These journals have a panel of peers review the researcher's manuscript; the panel recommends whether or not the manuscript should be published. Using peer–review systems is one way scientists scrutinize other's research and avoid publishing poor research. Consequently, it is recommended that nurses rely on refereed journals; however, there still is a need to evaluate research-based articles before applying the results in practice.

Research results derived from the conduct of good science also need to be evaluated to determine their applicability to practice. For example, research findings on preschoolers are not applicable to adolescents, and research results on urban dwellers are not applicable to migrant farm workers.

When results are based on sound research and they also are relevant, it is necessary to determine whether it is feasible to use them in practice. Some results can be implemented easily, whereas others may require considerable change in practice. When change is introduced into practice, the situation must be monitored to ensure that the anticipated beneficial outcomes are occurring and that other consequences secondary to the change also are positive.

Increasingly, books (for example, Phillips, 1986; Tanner & Lindeman, 1989) and articles (for example, Brett, 1987; Gennaro, 1994; Janken, Rudisill, & Benfield, 1992; Stetler, 1985; Tanner, 1987) are being written on utilizing research to improve the quality of patient care. They contain helpful insights on the intimate and dynamic connection between research and practice, which is (or ought to be) bidirectional in the sense that research findings influence practice and practice is a critical source of ideas about what phenomena need to be investigated.

Examples of Nursing Research

In this section, two studies are described illustrating some of the concepts addressed in this chapter as well as implications of each study's results for nursing practice and research.

Keeling, Knight, Taylor, and Nordt (1994) studied 109 adults, ranging in age from 30 to 85 years, who had cardiac catheterization using a femoral artery approach with a size 7 French catheter and a size 8 French sheath. Of the 109 patients, 84% were white, 10% black, and 6% "other." The researchers posed two research questions: (1) "Is there a need for pressure dressings postprocedure?" and (2) "What is the optimal length of time to restrict the patient to complete bed rest after using a femoral artery approach?" (p. 14).

In providing the rationale for the study, Keeling et al. (1994) cite literature on the variability in the standards for time patients are confined to complete bed rest or have restricted activity, ranging from 3 to 12 hours or longer. They also observe that in an effort to contain costs, cardiac catheterization is increasingly being done on an outpatient basis with postprocedure recovery times ranging from 3 to 6 hours. The rationale for complete bed rest and restricted movement in patients for whom the femoral artery approach is used is "to prevent bleeding from the catheter insertion site" (p.15). Additional justification for the research came from the researchers' clinical experience wherein they observed the need for nursing interventions, such as back rub, administration of narcotic analgesics, and use of laxatives postcatheterization to relieve patients' back and leg pain and abdominal discomfort associated with lying flat in bed for a long time.

An experimental design was used to answer the research questions. Patients were randomly assigned to either the experimental or the control group. Of the 50 patients (34 men and 16 women) in the experimental group, 9 (18%) received intravenous (IV) heparin after the procedure, and 41 (82%) did not. There were 59 patients (36 men and 23 women) in the control group; 10 (17%) received IV heparin following the procedure, and 49 (83%) did not.

Postprocedure patients in both groups received instruction on keeping their leg extended; had gauze pressure dressings over the catheterization insertion site, which were removed the morning following the procedure; sandbags over the insertion site for 6 hours after the procedure; and the head of their bed elevated 30 degrees. Furthermore, patients in the control group had complete bed rest for 12 hours after the procedure, whereas those in the experimental group had complete bed rest for 6 hours. If there were no signs of bleeding, patients in the experimental group had the sandbag removed and were allowed to resume activities, as tolerated. Except for the length of time for complete bed rest, the independent variable, the researchers held other variables constant so that they could determine the effect of length of time of complete bed rest on the incidence of bleeding, the dependent variable.

Analysis of the data showed that there was no statistically significant difference between patients in the experimental group and those in the control group on the incidence of bleeding. Further, none of the patients who got out of bed after 6 hours had bleeding. Of the 109 patients, five did bleed in the postprocedure period, and of these two were in the experimental group and three were in the control group.

The researchers comment that among the patients who bled, bleeding "occurred beyond the standard 12-hour bed rest period and/or occurred in patients receiving IV heparin postprocedure" (p. 16). Of the two patients in the experimental group who bled, Keeling et al. (1994) state "that 'it' was impossible to implicate early ambulation as the cause of bleeding. In both cases, bleeding was probably caused by very high clotting times" (p. 16). Of the three patients in the control group who bled, for two of them, bleeding was believed to have been related to removal of the dressing and patient activity on the day following the procedure. These patients also had been given IV heparin. The third patient in the control group who bled had a coughing episode that may have been related to the bleeding.

This study suggested that early ambulation decreased patient discomfort. Furthermore, decreased patient discomfort may be associated with lower nursing workload. These findings translate into reducing health care costs. Moreover, this study illustrates that research findings may have implications not only for the patients' well-being and nurses' workload but also for health care policy.

Keeling and colleagues (1994) cite implications of their study for future research. For example, a larger sample needs to be studied, and there should be "stricter control of the availability of clotting times for all subjects" (pp. 16–17). With a larger sample, one could study subsets of patients who have high-risk characteristics, such as age, history of diabetes, and obesity. They also recommend that research be done on the optimal type of insertion site dressing since removal of the dressing is associated with the incidence of bleeding. Other studies are needed on patients who have prolonged bed rest and require nursing interventions (e.g., urinary catheterization, enemas, or administration of analgesics and laxatives), which themselves are costly both in terms of nurses' time and supplies/equipment and to patients who experience further anxiety, discomfort, or pain.

In another study done by Ahijevych and Bernhard (1994), health-promoting behaviors of African American women were described and compared to other cultural groups. In the introduction to the article, the researchers comment that there is a paucity of research on the health of minorities and women and that the health of African American women, specifically, has largely been neglected. Because minority populations experience relatively high morbidity and mortality rates, research is sorely needed "to develop, implement, and evaluate culturally competent health-promotion interventions" (p. 86).

A review of related literature by the researchers revealed that Duelberg (1992) found that African American women compared to white women were less likely "to engage in 'primary prevention behaviors,' such as exercising, not smoking, and maintaining a favorable weight. However, they were more likely to engage in 'secondary prevention behaviors,' such as cervical cancer screening and breast examinations" (p. 86).

The health-promoting lifestyle behaviors of the women were measured by using the Health-Promoting Lifestyle Profile (HPLP) developed by Walker, Sechrist, and Pender (1987). The HPLP consists of 48 items on health-promoting behaviors that are answered on a 4-point Likert scale, where 1 equals "never" and 4 equals "routinely." The HPLP includes six subscales: self-actualization, health responsibility, exercise, nutrition, interpersonal support, and stress management (Walker et al.). The investigators cite several studies demonstrating the reliability (internal consistency and stability) of the HPLP (Pender, Walker, Sechrist, & Frank-Stromborg, 1990; Walker et al., 1987).

All study participants were enrolled in a larger study on nicotine dependence (Ahijevych & Wewers, 1993). Consequently, they were "biologically confirmed cigarette smokers" (p. 86). The study was explained to participants, confidentiality was promised, and informed consent to participate in the research was obtained. After completing all written instruments and giving a saliva sample, which was used to confirm smoking status, the women were given $10.

There were 187 African American women in the study, all of whom reported smoking cigarettes daily. They ranged in age from 18 to 69 years with a mean or average age of 36.1 years. Nearly two thirds (61%) were single or divorced, and just over half (52%) worked full-time. Few (12%) had an annual household income above $30,000, whereas 60% had an annual income less than $15,000. With respect to education, 28% had 11 years or less, 32% had completed high school, 31% had some education beyond high school, and 9% had graduated from college. Nearly two thirds (65%) had one or more children less than 18 years old living in their household. Of the entire sample, 48 reported currently having a medical diagnosis, and of these, 56% had hypertension and 15% had heart disease. Somewhat fewer (10%) reported having multiple medical diagnoses (p. 87).

Selected results presented here on the HPLP revealed that the women scored highest on the interpersonal support (mean [*M*] = 2.90, standard deviation [*SD*] = .59) and self-actualization (*M* = 2.89, *SD* = .53) subscales. They scored lowest on exercise (M = 1.95, SD = .65). Scores on the other sub-scales were as follows: stress management (M = 2.45, SD = .55), nutrition (M = 2.37, SD = .56), and health responsibility (M = 2.34, SD = .58).

When the women's scores on the six subscales of the HPLP were com-pared to those of other groups, it was found that the women had the low-est mean score on three subscales: self-actualization, exercise, and nutrition. The second lowest mean score was on the subscale measuring interper-sonal support. Compared with the other groups, the African American women's ranking was highest on health responsibility.

The researchers discuss their findings, of which a selection is pre-sented. Findings useful for practice include the need for nurses to assess health-promotion behaviors in African American women. Nurses can jointly develop with women similar to those in this study, a *realistic* plan for im-proving lifestyle practices, such as developing an exercise regimen, en-rolling in a smoking cessation program, and developing ways to increase interpersonal support and manage stress. In developing plans, nurses must assess the women's resources—money, time, and energy—so that they can succeed in achieving their goals.

Research implications include replicating the study with a larger sample and including African American women who do not smoke. Fur-thermore, instruments need to be developed and tested on minority popu-lations so that they are culturally relevant and sensitive. One of the reasons why this research article was presented in the chapter is because it involves research with women who have not been studied adequately, including both minorities and nonminorities. The NIH requires that grant applications for research projects include women and minorities. If the proposed re-search excludes them, the researcher must provide a clear and compelling justification for the decision.

SUMMARY

This chapter emphasized the relationship between research and nursing practice and ways in which nurses can participate in doing research. Re-search is the systematic process of answering questions by generating new knowledge. The steps of the research process are interrelated in such a way that each one is affected by its predecessor and must be consistent with it. The five central steps of the research process used in quantitative studies are: (1) statement of the research problem; (2) selection of the theoretical/conceptual framework and review of relevant literature; (3) specification of the research design; (4) interpretation of the meaning of the findings; and (5) communication of the research results.

Nursing research provides the knowledge needed for nursing practice and enables nursing to continue in its development as a profession and dis-cipline. Through research, nursing is able to explicate a body of knowledge that eventually will define nursing as a unique practice discipline. Another important outcome of research is to ensure that nursing care is based on sound scientific knowledge. By conducting research, new knowledge is generated for use in nursing practice. Nurses have a responsibility to use research results derived from sound scientific studies.

REFERENCES

Abdellah, F. G., & Levine, E. (1994). *Preparing nursing research for the 21st century: Evolution, methodologies, challenges.* New York: Springer.

Ahijevych, K., & Bernhard, L. (1994). Health-promoting behaviors of African American women. *Nursing Research, 43,* 86–89.

Ahijevych, K., & Wewers, M. E., (1993). Factors associated with nicotine dependence among African American women. *Research in Nursing & Health, 16,* 283–292.

Block, D. (1990). Strategies for setting and implementing the National Center for Nursing Research priorities. *Applied Nursing Research, 3,* 2–6.

Brett, J. L. L. (1987). Use of nursing practice research findings. *Nursing Research, 36,* 344–349.

Cohen, B. I. (1984). Florence Nightingale. *Scientific American, 250,* 128–137.

Denzin, N. K. (1994). *Handbook of qualitative research.* Thousand Oaks, CA: Sage.

Duelberg, S. (1992). Preventive health behavior among black and white women in urban and rural areas. *Social Science and Medicine, 34,* 191–198.

Feynman, R. (1988). *What do you care what other people think? Further adventures of a curious character.* New York: Norton.

Gennaro, S. (1994). Research utilization: An overview. *Journal of Obstetric, Gynecologic, and Neonatal Nursing, 23,* 313–319.

Janken, J. K., Rudisill, P., & Benfield, L. (1992). Product evaluation as a research utilization strategy. *Applied Nursing Research, 5,* 188–194.

Keeling, A. W., Knight, E., Taylor, V., & Nordt, L. A. (1994). Postcardiac catheterization time-in-bed study: Enhancing patient comfort through nursing research. *Applied Nursing Research, 7,* 14–17.

Leininger, M. (Ed.). (1985). *Qualitative research methods in nursing.* Orlando, FL: Grune & Stratton.

LoBiondo-Wood, G., & Harber, J. (1994). *Nursing research: Methods, critical appraisal, and utilization* (3rd ed.). St. Louis: Mosby.

Morse, J. M. (1991). *Qualitative nursing research: A contemporary dialogue.* Newbury Park, CA: Sage.

Munhall, P. L., & Boyd, C. A. (1993). *Nursing research: A qualitative perspective* (2nd ed.). New York: National League for Nursing.

National Center for Nursing Research. (1992). *Update: National Center for Nursing Research.* Bethesda, MD: Author.

Parse, R. R., Coyne, A. B., & Smith, M. J. (1985). *Nursing research: Qualitative methods.* Bowie, MD: Brady Communications.

Pender, N. J., Walker, S. N., Sechrist, K. R., & Frank-Stromborg, M. (1990). Predicting health-promoting lifestyles in the workplace. *Nursing Research, 39,* 326–332.

Phillips, L. R. F. (1986). *A clinician's guide to the critique and utilization of nursing research.* Norwalk, CT: Appleton-Century-Crofts.

Polit, D. F., & Hungler, B. P. (1995). *Nursing research: Principles and methods* (5th ed.). Philadelphia: Lippincott.

Reilly, D. E., & Oermann, M. H. (1992). *Clinical teaching in nursing education* (2nd ed.). New York: National League for Nursing.

Stetler, C. B. (1985). Research utilization: Defining the concept. *Image, 17,* 40–44.

Streubert, H. J., & Carpenter, D. R. (1995). *Qualitative research in nursing: Advancing the humanistic imperative.* Philadelphia: Lippincott.

Tanner, C. A. (1987). Evaluating research for use in practice: Guidelines for the clinician. *Heart and Lung, 16,* 424–430.

Tanner, C. A., & Lindeman, C. A. (Eds.). (1989). *Using nursing research.* New York: National League for Nursing.

U.S. Department of Health and Human Services. (1992). *Application for public health service grant—Grant application form PHS 398* (OMB No. 0925–0001). Rockville, MD: Author.

Walker, S. N., Sechrist, K. R., & Pender, N. J. (1987). The health-promoting lifestyle profile: Development and psychometric characteristics. *Nursing Research, 36,* 76–81.

Woods, N. F., & Catanzaro, M. (1988). *Nursing research: Theory and practice.* St. Louis: Mosby.

Wilson, H. S. (1989). *Research in nursing* (2nd ed.). Redwood City, CA: Addison-Wesley.

BIBLIOGRAPHY

Abraham, I. L., Nadzam, D. M., & Fitzpatrick, J. J. (1989). *Statistics and quantitative methods in nursing.* Philadelphia: Saunders.

Artinian, B. A. (1988). Qualitative modes of inquiry. *Western Journal of Nursing Research, 10,* 138–149.

Babbie, E. (1990). *Survey research methods* (2nd end). Belmont, CA: Wadsworth.

Brockopp, D. Y., & Hastings-Tolsma, M. T. (1995). *Fundamentals of nursing research* (2nd ed.). Boston: Jones and Bartlett.

Chinn, P. L., & Jacobs, M. (1991). *Theory and nursing: A systematic approach* (3rd ed.). St. Louis: Mosby.

Christy, T. Y. (1975). The methodology of historical research. *Nursing Research, 24,* 189–192.

Cook, T. D., & Campbell, D. T. (1979). *Quasi-experimental design and analysis issues for field settings.* Chicago: Rand McNally.

Davis, L. L., & Grant, J. S. (1993). Guidelines for using psychometric consultants in nursing studies. *Research in Nursing and Health, 16,* 151–155.

Fawcett, J., & Downs, F. (1992). *The relationship between theory and research* (2nd ed.). Philadelphia: Davis.

Fowler, F. J. (1993). *Survey research methods* (2nd ed.). Beverly Hills, CA: Sage.

Frank-Stromberg, M. (Ed.). (1988). *Instruments for clinical nursing research.* Norwalk, CT: Appleton & Lange.

Fuller, E. O., Hasselmeyer, E. G., Hunter, J. C., Abdellah, F. G., & Hinshaw, A. S. (1991). Summary statements of the NIH nursing research grant applications. *Nursing Research, 40,* 346–351.

Ganong, I. H. (1987). Integrative reviews of nursing research. *Research in Nursing and Health, 10,* 1–11.

Hayes, P. (1993). Replicative studies. *Clinical Nursing Research, 2,* 243–244.

Hutchinson, S. (1990). The case study approach. In L. Moody (Ed.), *Paths to knowledge* (pp. 33–59). New York: National League for Nursing.

Jackle, M. (1989). Presenting research to nurses in clinical practice. *Applied Nursing Research, 2,* 189–191.

Kerlinger, F. N. (1986). *Foundations of behavioral research* (3rd ed.). New York: Holt, Rinehart, & Winston.

Kirchoff, K. T., & Dille, C. A. (1994). Issues in intervention research: Maintaining integrity. *Applied Nursing Research, 7,* 32–37.

Koziol-McLain, J., & Maeve, M. (1993). Nursing theory in perspective. *Nursing Outlook, 41,* 79–81.

Lambert, C. E., & Lambert, V. A. (1988). Clinical nursing research: Its meaning to the practicing nurse. *Applied Nursing Research, 1,* 54–57.

Lincoln, Y. S., & Guba, E. G. (1985). *Naturalistic inquiry.* Newbury Park, CA: Sage.

Lynn, M. R. (1986). Determination and quantification of content validity. *Nursing Research, 35,* 382–385.

Mateo, M. A., & Kirchoff, K. T. (1991). *Conducting and using nursing research in the clinical setting.* Baltimore: Williams & Wilkins.

Maurin, J. T. (1990). Research utilization in the socio-political arena. *Applied Nursing Research, 3,* 48–51.

Moody, L., Vera, H., Blanks, C., & Visscher, M. (1989). Developing questions of substance for nursing science. *Western Journal of Nursing Research, 11,* 393–404.

Morse, J. M. (1991a). Approaches to qualitative-quantitative methodological triangulation. *Nursing Research, 40,* 120–122.

Morse, J. M. (1991b). Evaluating qualitative research. *Qualitative Health Research, 1,* 283–286.

Munhall, P. L. (1988). Ethical considerations in qualitative research. *Western Journal of Nursing Research, 10,* 150–162.

Munro, B. H., & Page, E. N. (1993). *Statistical methods for health-care research* (2nd ed.). Philadelphia: Lippincott.

Pettengill, M. M., Gellies, D. A., & Clark, C. C. (1994). Factors encouraging and discouraging the use of nursing research findings. *Image: Journal of Nursing Scholarship, 26,* 143–147.

Pugh, L. C., & DeKeyser, F. G. (1995). Use of physiologic variables in nursing research. *Image: Journal of Nursing Scholarship, 27,* 273–276.

Reineck, C. (1991). Nursing research instruments: Pathways to resources. *Applied Nursing Research, 4,* 34–45.

Rempusheski, V. F. (1991). Elements, perceptions, and issues of informed consent. *Applied Nursing Research, 4,* 201–204.

Rossi, P. H., & Freeman, H. E. (1993). *Evaluation: A systematic approach* (5th ed.). Beverly Hills, CA: Sage.

Ryan, N. M. (1989). Developing and presenting a research poster. *Applied Nursing Research, 2,* 52–55.

Ryan-Wenger, N. M. (1992). Guidelines for critique of a research report. *Heart & Lung, 21,* 394–401.

Selby, M., Tornquist, E., & Finerty, E. (1989). How to present your research. *Nursing Outlook, 37,* 172–175.

Spector, P. E. (1981). *Research designs.* Beverly Hills, CA: Sage.

Tanner, C. A. (1987). Evaluating research for use in practice: Guidelines for the clinician. *Heart & Lung, 16,* 424–430.

Thurber, F. W., Deatrick, J. A., & Grey, M. (1992). Children's participation in research: Their right to consent. *Journal of Pediatric Nursing, 7,* 165–170.

Topham, D. L., & DeSilva, P. (1988). Evaluating congruency between steps in the research process: A critique guide for use in clinical nursing practice. *Clinical Nurse Specialist, 2,* 97–102.

Tornquist, E. M., & Funk, S. G. (1990). How to write a research grant proposal. *Image: Journal of Nursing Scholarship, 22,* 44–51.

Waltz, C. F., Nelson, B., & Chambers, S. B. (1985). Assigning publication credits. *Nursing Outlook, 33,* 233–238.

Waltz, C. F., Strickland, O., & Lenz, E. (1991). *Measurement in nursing research* (2nd ed.). Philadelphia: Davis.

Washington, C. C., & Moss, M. (1988). Pragmatic aspects of establishing interrater reliability in research. *Nursing Research, 37,* 190–191.

Wilson, H., S., & Hutchinson, S. A. (1996). *Consumer's guide to nursing research: Exercises, activities, tools and resources.* Albany, NY: Delmar.

Leadership in Nursing

Kate Moore

Nursing leadership focuses on improving health care delivery wherever nurses work. Nurses can learn about leadership concepts and how to use them in their daily work. Even when nurses prefer "just" to do patient care and leave the leadership to someone else, knowledge of current concepts in leadership is important for every nurse to understand how work is successfully accomplished.

This chapter presents a discussion of contemporary issues on leadership that are useful to nursing as it stands on the edge of change in health care delivery. Traditional and current leadership theories, the concept of followership, a comparison of leadership and management, the concepts of power and influence, the context of leadership (which includes current financing systems, restructuring, and nursing care delivery models), and the shift to community are discussed.

TRADITIONAL LEADERSHIP THEORY

Traditional leadership theory has focused on characteristics of leaders, the environment, and the interaction of the two. It has examined leadership behaviors, style, and relationships with followers. Traditional leadership theory has been replaced by contemporary perspectives of leadership for two reasons. First, traditional theory has been unable to explain or predict leadership effectiveness in a variety of settings (Conger & Kanungo, 1994). Traditional leadership theory development and evaluation took place under conditions in which businesses were stable, with long career trajectories for employees, and a growing economy that benefited many. Changes in the work setting could be planned and controlled. Second, American business practices are far more complex than they have ever been. The information age, multiculturalism, new meanings to job flexibility, and technological wizardry require new and different leadership skills.

State versus Trait

One classic leadership theory, known as the "state versus trait" argument, provides a useful introduction for understanding some of the early leadership concepts. This theory is based on whether one believes that leadership is a *trait* inherent in individuals from birth or whether leadership is a product of the *state* or circumstance in which individuals find themselves. The *trait* argument says that true leaders possess certain internal qualities and will act as leaders regardless of circumstances. The *state* argument proposes that individuals act as leaders based primarily on chance events; only the nature of these events makes it possible for a certain person to step forward and act as a leader. Those who act as leaders under one set of circumstances may not be able to do so under a different set of circumstances. The "state versus trait" argument is perhaps best used as a springboard to examine how each factor contributes to leadership. For example, one might ask the following questions: Which traits are found in individuals identified as leaders? Under which conditions are such traits enhanced or minimized? Which traits, if any, can be adopted to increase a person's effectiveness if she or he is called on to act as a leader? Which states or circumstances can nurses create, support, or modify to improve opportunities for nursing leadership? How can nurses effectively combine their leadership traits and the state of health care to advance goals for better patient care and professional ideals?

Theories X and Y

A theory proposed in the early 1960s and developed since that time is one suggested by McGregor (1960). He called the prevailing attitude of management toward workers Theory X. Theory X suggested that employees did not enjoy work and preferred to avoid responsibility and accountability. Supervisors, in turn, had to monitor closely the processes and quality of the work. McGregor disagreed with these assumptions and suggested that people did enjoy work and would be willing to assume responsibility if given the opportunity and support to do so. He called this theory Theory Y. McGregor recommended that managers reduce supervision and increase support for employees and employee-driven standards and goals.

More recently a balance of Theories X and Y was suggested and referred to as Theory Z (Ouchi, 1981). This theory combined the humanistic perspective of McGregor (1960) and his support of employee involvement and accountability with the expectation that some supervision and monitoring are useful. Such monitoring was important to communicate expectations and let employees know how they were performing. This integrated perspective held more appeal for both management and staff. It appealed to managers because they are responsible for monitoring the productivity and well being of employees as they work toward organizational goals. It appealed to staff who need to know if their performance and productivity meet standards and want to have input into decisions that affect their work life. This "new" way of looking at management/staff relationships initiated distinctive changes in how leadership was viewed. Even though these theories actually represent management rather than leadership theories, they provide a bridge between the long-dominant position that employees are passive, resistant, uninterested in performance, and unwilling to be accountable for their work and the view that employees are committed, want to be actively involved in decisions, and are the most valuable of all resources.

CURRENT PERSPECTIVES

Current perspectives emphasize transformational and charismatic leadership. Transformational leadership is represented in the work of Bennis and Nanus (1985). Conger and Kanungo (1994) discuss charismatic leadership, an important component of transformational leadership.

Transformational Leadership

From interviews of 90 leaders in public and private industry, Bennis and Nanus (1985) identified four major strategies used by successful leaders: (1) attention through vision, (2) meaning through communication, (3) trust through positioning, and (4) deployment of self. These strategies became the basis of transformational leadership.

The first strategy, attention through vision, is used by leaders to express a clear picture of the world they want to create. They are certain about the future and what will happen. These leaders are not naive; in fact, they consider past history, competing forces, details of their vision, and the visions of others as they create their own. Leaders are well aware of the uncertain conditions in which they promote their vision but can maintain the vision through the turbulence of change and growth. Nursing leaders demonstrate vision when they evaluate the changes occurring in health care and role of the nurse. They sustain their vision as they develop systems of care and staff to meet the health care needs of people in varied settings.

The second strategy, meaning through communication, is used as leaders inform others about their vision and show how it can be accomplished. Communication is a dynamic, transactional process (Northouse & Northouse, 1992). Leaders are skilled communicators who readily and consistently describe their vision and its consequences. They do not make pronouncements about the work to be done and step back with the expectation that someone else will do it. They describe their vision and demonstrate it through their intense involvement in the work. Nursing leaders are tireless in their actions to communicate and live their vision. They meet with staff to explain and listen; they use themes such as patient-focused care to symbolize their goals. Their excitement in describing the vision encourages staff to persist in their own development.

The third strategy leaders use is trust through positioning. This means that leaders take a stand about what they believe in and want to accomplish. The leader analyzes carefully forces in the environment that have an impact on their vision, including the needs and perceptions of followers. Leaders consider the needs of their followers while maintaining a commitment to their vision.

The fourth and final strategy of leadership is called deployment of self. Successful leaders engage in constant learning. They recognize that the risks they take—and ask others to take—may not always have successful outcomes. However, leaders do not see failure as defeat but as an opportunity to learn and grow. Leaders are noted for their support of colleagues and subordinates who take risks, regardless of the outcome. Leaders are open to change and innovation and are willing to take risks publicly for what they believe in.

Bennis and Nanus (1985) in their study of leaders recognized the value of empowerment that leaders used with their followers. They referred to this "magic" that some leaders were able to create in their organizations as transformative leadership. The concept is now known as transformational leadership. Leaders take advantage of opportunities at all levels of an organization and draw others to them through their commitment to a vision. Applying the strategies of leadership and providing an opportunity to involve others in decision making enable followers to gain confidence in themselves and work toward achieving organizational and personal goals. Biordi (1993) believes that involvement of nurses in decisions affecting patients and staff is more important than ever.

Charismatic Leadership

Organizations, including health care organizations, experience multiple and rapid changes that often occur all at the same time. Employees must deal with changing job requirements, new technology, reduced and redistributed resources, and the constant pressure to do more with less. Leadership is needed at every level in the organization to maintain progress, meet changing needs, and sustain morale when the changes seem overwhelming. Charismatic leadership theory (Conger & Kanungo, 1994) suggests that leaders can unite individuals in times of turmoil to work toward a common goal. Charismatic leaders are characterized by their determination to change the current state of affairs accompanied by an awareness of forces in the environment and their followers' needs.

There are three stages of development in charismatic leadership. In the first stage, leaders are recognized as those who fully understand the forces creating present conditions and who are ready to initiate changes. In the second stage, the charismatic leader engages followers in sharing a vision of the ideal situation and translates this vision in a way that energizes people. In the last stage, leaders are perceived as "giving their all" to meet the newly set goals, with dedicated followers committed to them. Followers maintain a significant role in charismatic leadership theory, as they energize the momentum of the leader.

Leadership effectiveness, then, is found in individuals who can adapt to rapid changes, have a vision for the future, generate the commitment of a critical mass of followers, inspire and empower others despite turbulent conditions, and communicate clearly with others.

Followership

Leaders need followers who may have more or less experience with the task at hand and varied commitment to goal achievement. Leaders may adjust their approaches to the group, depending on the group's needs, but always remain focused on assisting the group to achieve shared goals.

The role of followers makes a significant difference in the ways in which leaders achieve goals. Although it may be argued that leaders are not leaders without followers, the ease with which a group incorporates a leader's vision and commits itself to the leader's work affects outcomes (Ellis & Hartley, 1995). Followers may exhibit varying degrees of commitment. Professional commitment partly lies in recognizing and supporting the leader's vision and working toward organizational goals. At the same time, leaders guide, protect, and respond to followers. Followers should be regularly informed by leaders of progress and setbacks and encouraged to develop their own creative solutions to problems. Thus, as the involvement of followers increases, so does their "ownership" of the vision. In this way the vision becomes a part of each person's work in the organization.

Leaders may choose certain followers to assume specific supportive positions on the "team" in the same way a president chooses a cabinet. This team is composed of trusted advisors who have expertise in areas that the leader may not, have an exceptional network through which they can gain and distribute information, complement the leader's strength, are loyal both publicly and privately, and are willing to sacrifice personal needs and interests for their leader's cause. This inner-circle phenomenon in politics and business is evident when executives carefully choose the individuals whom they believe will best support their goals. This is reflected in nursing when the vice president of nursing selects the team of directors and department heads for their expertise in managing specialty areas as well as for their willingness to further the vice president's goals. The leader acknowledges the loyalty and dedication of followers by offering rewards such as job promotions, mentorship, and introduction to influential people who can advance the individual's career.

Leadership and Management

A discussion of leadership is incomplete without the inevitable comparison to management (Table 11–1). Leadership and management have both overlapping and distinctive characteristics (Bleich, 1995). Leadership characteristics are usually more abstract and somewhat more difficult to define. For example, leaders inspire, motivate, and challenge groups. Just how that is accomplished is still subject to debate. Managers are those individuals appointed to a *position* to accomplish particular organizational goals. The tasks of managers are usually well defined by the organization, and managers are evaluated based on how well they achieve those goals. Managerial tasks include:

1. Hiring
2. Staffing
3. Scheduling
4. Supervising
5. Delegating
6. Planning and administering a budget
7. Orienting, training, and evaluating staff
8. Interacting with other organizational managers to coordinate efforts
9. Maintaining and improving work and work life quality
10. Ensuring consistent and accurate flow of information between staff and administration
11. Representing the unit's interests and competencies to the rest of the organization.

Leaders may not hold formal organizational positions or have job descriptions that relate specifically to leadership activity. Leaders may engage in some self-initiated managerial tasks such as organizing, delegating, coordinating, and supervising activity that contribute to their vision. Leaders who neglect or are not proficient at such tasks will be wise to have colleagues who assume those responsibilities. The chaos that can occur when no attention is paid to important managerial tasks may not cause a leader to lose her or his position, but it can be disruptive and generate dissatisfaction and conflict among followers. The emphasis of leadership in comparison to management is that leaders seem to be more easily recognized, they possess traits that attract and motivate others, and they transcend the boundaries of the formal organization.

Managers are appointed to a formal position and have a title granted by the organization that employs them. Their responsibilities are defined by the organization and their major responsibility is to meet organizational goals. Managers' goals and responsibilities change when they change positions; their authority is granted by their position. When managers leave an organization, they relinquish these goals.

Leaders, on the other hand, have goals that transcend any formal position. Although managers have a responsibility to produce for the organiza-

TABLE 11–1. COMPARISON OF CHARACTERISTICS OF LEADERS AND MANAGERS

Leaders	Managers
Inspire, motivate, and challenge followers	Direct others to carry out activities that fulfill organizational goals
May or may not hold formal position in organization	Are appointed to a position (with title) within organization
Set goals for future that transcend any formal position; have a vision for the organization	Set goals and assume responsibilities based on position in organization; relinquish goals when leave organization
Are granted authority for decisions from followers	Are granted authority for decisions based on organizational structure
May engage in self-initiated tasks that contribute to their vision	Have managerial tasks that are well defined by organization
May or may not be an effective manager	May or may not be a leader
View crisis as opportunity to create new and innovative solutions to problems	Respond to crisis in terms of established organizational norms and values
Take risks	Maintain order

tion, leaders have a vision and mission that they believe will improve conditions in the organization and for which they amass a wide range of resources. Political leaders, for example, will appeal to diverse geographical, cultural, religious, and socioeconomic groups for support for certain ideals. Such leaders deliver their messages in ways that each group can accept and that inspire them to contribute to the effort. Thus, an effective political leader will weave together a collective interest into a strong tapestry of support.

Many of the leaders' and managers' duties are routine, although one can often sense the leadership qualities of a manager through the manager's approach to new, unexpected events or crises. Managers often try to define a crisis in terms of established organizational norms and values. They attempt to subdue the crisis and return to previous, "normal" conditions. Leaders, instead, view a crisis as an opportunity to create new and unique solutions to problems and engage followers in progressing toward goals. Leaders take risks in developing strategies to cope with the crisis and establish innovative means of handling problems. Leaders increase the commitment of followers by the way in which they handle crises in the organization.

The development of leadership and management skills in nursing progresses in the same ways as clinical expertise. Leadership and management concepts are introduced in undergraduate programs to prepare students for future roles in complex health care systems. Master's and doctoral education in nursing administration are available across the country for nurses who seek careers in leadership and management and who want to prepare for research using organizational, administrative, and leadership theories. Some graduate programs combine master's degrees in nursing administration with business administration.

POWER AND INFLUENCE

Power and influence are important tools that nurses use to advance desired outcomes within an organization (Gillies, 1994).

Power

Power is the ability to achieve desired goals through the use of resources. An individual with power is one who can affect the distribution of resources such as time, materials, staff, and information. An individual with resources attracts others who desire access to some of the same resources. Individuals may decide to exchange resources so that both can achieve their own desired goals. For example, a nurse who wants a day off to attend a conference may agree to work an undesirable weekend shift; thus, the staff nurse exchanges her resource—time during a difficult staffing period—for a resource held by the nurse manager, which is the power to grant time off.

Types of Resources in Power

There are different types of resources used for developing and exerting power in an organization. Personal resources include skill in interpersonal relationships, creativity in solving problems, a sense of humor, and expertise in certain aspects of patient care. Personal resources are valuable in that they can be readily shared with the team, unit, and organization to improve working conditions and demonstrate an investment in the employer's goals. Sharing personal resources on behalf of the organization attracts the attention of others who may be willing to share both their own personal resources and the organizational resources to which they have access.

Organizational resources are those provided by a business entity, such as a hospital, health maintenance organization, community agency, clinic, or professional organization. Some organizational resources are budgetary control, personnel, positions, materials, and access to information. Creative, cost-effective use of resources enables an organization to be more productive and waste less. An organization aware of new staffing methods can offer options to nurses who want a high degree of flexibility in their schedules and may be able to attract personnel when other organizations cannot. A strong staff development department, another organizational resource, can provide on-the-job training and precepting for new nurse managers. An active research committee can bring the latest in clinical developments to the staff for use in solving difficult patient care problems. Such resources are valuable and can be used in multiple ways to achieve a variety of organizational goals.

Community resources are those associated with the geographical area in which nurses practice and with professional networks. Geographical community resources include local educational programs, support groups, and connections to media who favor nursing. A professional network includes nursing and other professional organizations that serve as a resource for nurses both professionally and personally. This network is a type of community (Vestal, 1995), providing support for nurses and offering resources to accomplish goals. Nurses who belong to professional associations extend relationships far beyond the geographical confines of their locale. Through meetings and conferences, nurses develop relationships with others and have numerous opportunities to update information and skills. Nurses may agree to speak at each others' meetings, work together on projects, introduce each other to colleagues with whom they share special interests, and exchange information about job openings. Through multidisciplinary professional networks nurses can avail themselves of a wide range of perspectives and sources of information about current issues in health care. Such an expanded network also improves the opportunity to promote nursing to those unfamiliar with the field's accomplishments.

Increasing Power

There are two perspectives on increasing power. One is that in order to increase power, nurses share resources with others to empower them. In this way, the nurse extends an original power base and gains additional power. Those individuals who have been accorded this shared power are more likely to reciprocate and to respond to the first individual's subsequent requests for assistance. As one's power base grows, nurses can accomplish more of their goals and more efficiently than without a broad base of support.

The second perspective is that keeping power and tight control over resources is the primary way to increase one's power. Nurses with this perspective seek to gain direct control over more and more resources while exchanging only what is absolutely necessary to maintain desired relationships with others (Gillies, 1994). Maintaining tight control over resources and denying others legitimate opportunities for power may come at considerable expense at a time of crisis. Individuals with whom one has traded resources (shared resources) only sparingly are not likely to remain loyal under difficult circumstances.

Influence

Influence is a more subtle form of power. It is suggestion rather than a direct manipulation of resources or active pursuit of a controversial goal. Influence is present either through words or behaviors that characterize one's positions and view (Hersey & Duldt, 1989). Using influence may be more acceptable to people not comfortable with the use of power to advance desired goals. Individuals with influence may have power, but they prefer to suggest to others possible decisions or how resources may be used in a situation. Nurses use influence by sharing opinions with key individuals, raising questions about issues, identifying possibilities for improvements, and inspiring confidence in others' ventures. Nurses who express preferences rather than demand them are viewed as having influence. Nurses also should consider whom they want to be influenced by.

Nurses decide how, when, and under which circumstances to use personal, organizational, and community resources as a means of power. They may gather and keep resources and power to themselves or share their power with others. In an organization, regardless of size and complexity, nurses may influence others by expressing and demonstrating their beliefs and identifying possible strategies for change.

CONTEXT OF LEADERSHIP

Context refers to conditions or circumstances in which an event takes place. The context may alter the way in which events are interpreted or handled. The context in which nursing and nursing leadership exists includes the financing of health care, delivery systems, and nursing models of care delivery.

Financing of Health Care

The delivery system in the United States has been defined by payment systems. The way in which care is insured and paid for governs access to care and choice in providers. Payment systems are designed increasingly to provide efficient care that will benefit the majority of individuals. At the same time, the financial burden of care has been shifted to individuals. Much of the impetus for this change in health care has come from the seemingly uncontrollable costs of care. Health care expenditures have increased at a faster pace than the overall economy. Hospital care continues to represent the largest category of health care spending, 38.4% of total health expenditures (Levit, Lazenby, Cowan, & Letsch, 1994). A large number of people also remain uninsured or underinsured and lack access to the health care system or face limited services.

Consumers pay for more than one-half of all health care expenditures through private health insurance and out-of-pocket payments for health care services. Public programs, such as Medicare and Medicaid, contributed 42% of the funding for health care (Levit et al., 1994).

Private Health Insurance

Individuals may purchase health insurance coverage that allows them to seek and choose their primary provider with minimal restrictions. Private health insurance offered through employment is less costly than if paid for without an employer's subsidy. Unemployed individuals, therefore, are less likely to have private health insurance, which reduces their access to some providers. Patients with private health insurance can make appointments with providers whose fees are paid by a combination of the insurance coverage and direct fee from the patient.

Health Maintenance Organizations

Individuals who enroll in a health maintenance organization (HMO) may choose from several types of coverage depending on the type of plan an employer selects, the amount of the premium the employee is willing to pay, and the copayments and covered services selected. Patients enroll for a specific time for services of the HMO. Physicians, advanced practice nurses, and other professionals and paraprofessionals are employed by the HMO. Patients may visit their primary caregiver as needed, but referrals to other specialists are determined by the primary caregiver. Referrals are made to specialists who have formal agreements with the HMO to provide services for a predetermined fee. A similar arrangement exists for diagnostic testing and treatment services. Patients are covered only for services by professionals with whom the HMO has a contract and only when referred by their primary provider. Several HMOs may have arrangements with specialist groups and health care organizations that provide diagnostic testing and treatment. The primary provider, that is, the physician or advanced practice nurse, acts as a gatekeeper for patients in assessing and authorizing the need for further services.

Today HMOs cover approximately 15% of the population and are distributed unevenly across the United States (Morrison & Luft, 1994). Morrison and Luft suggest that even though HMOs have not grown to the level predicted, they have been significant agents of change in the health care system.

Preferred Provider Organizations

A preferred provider organization is a group of physicians and health care systems who have a formal arrangement to offer services on a fee-for-service basis. This group of providers offers services at a discounted rate to insurance companies in exchange for the assurance that a minimum number of patients will use their services and their fees will be paid promptly (Hicks, Stallmeyer, & Coleman, 1992).

Managed Care

Managed care is a generic term that represents a large-scale approach to health care. Used by insurers and providers, managed care defines the care patients receive according to predetermined guidelines based on their complaints, symptoms, or tentative diagnoses. Guidelines, developed by the insurer or provider, suggest the type and extent of services needed to treat the patient based on expected responses. The guidelines aim for a specific level of quality that can be achieved while containing costs. In managed care, the needs of the average or typical patient with a particular diagnosis are estimated in advance and form the basis for reimbursable services. Each service has to be justified by the provider to keep costs within the bounds set by the organization.

Capitation

Capitation refers to the method of allotting a certain amount of money per person, "per capita," to the health care provider to meet all of that person's health care needs. The provider is responsible for how the funds are used (Finkler & Kovner, 1993). Any additional amount spent on patient care above the predetermined amount allotted for all enrollees is not reimbursed by the insurance company and, instead, is paid for by the provider. Capitation is considered a long-term financing mechanism. For example, a provider may have 800,000 people enrolled for 10 years under such a system. The provider assesses the enrollees to determine their current level of wellness, prevalence of high-risk behaviors and conditions, and types of preventative care needed by them. Under capitation, wellness programs, such as exercise and stress management, save the insurer in the long term by keeping enrollees healthy and avoiding costlier illnesses and treatments.

Delivery Systems

Reengineering, restructuring, retooling, and redesign are terms used today to describe significant changes in health care organizations. These changes include reducing the number of managers and licensed personnel, increasing the number and responsibilities of unlicensed personnel, training employees to do multiple tasks (cross-training), and altering the processes of care delivery (Dienemann & Gessner, 1992). With fewer managers in health care organizations, those remaining assume increasing responsibilities and have more staff reporting to them. Although the manager can control and coordinate a wider range of services, she or he is not able to oversee activities closely, must rely on the ability of staff to work independently, and is less available to staff who need assistance (Pabst, 1993).

One example of restructuring is to place a satellite pharmacy close to a unit, such as an intensive care unit, that uses many medications on a daily basis. Rather than sending medication orders to a central pharmacy, waiting as they are processed and the medications are returned to the unit, the intensive care nurse works closely with the pharmacist stationed in the unit to obtain medications as needed.

Training employees to do multiple tasks is known as *cross-training*. A nurse's aide or patient care assistant may be taught not only to take vital signs but also to do electrocardiograms, insert catheters, and assist in minor procedures. A cross-trained staff member benefits the health care team by increasing its flexibility. It also frees the registered nurse for activities that require an advanced level of education and clinical expertise. There are risks, however, that accompany the use of cross-trained personnel. For instance, patient care may be seen as a series of tasks rather than a holistic approach to meeting client needs; principles of safety may not be incorporated in care provided by personnel with limited education for their role; and careful supervision is required by the RN to ensure that proper procedures are followed by staff for whom the nurse is responsible.

Nursing Care Models

There are a variety of models for the organization and delivery of nursing care. The following lists the most common ones:

- Case Management
- Team Nursing
- Modular Nursing
- Primary Nursing
- Case Nursing
- Functional Nursing

One of these models, *case management,* focuses on the allocation of health services. Strictly speaking, case management is not purely a nursing model in that other disciplines collaborate to provide care. Case management represents a major advance in care delivery as it emphasizes this multidisciplinary approach to patient care (Moore, 1992). Case management is the process of deciding in advance, based on evidence from the literature and provider experience, the precise types and timing of services that will be needed according to a particular patient diagnosis and status. Case management care plans, also known as clinical paths, recovery paths, maps, and a variety of other terms, are organized so that assessments, expected outcomes, interventions, and evaluations are plotted against a time line. A multidisciplinary team develops the case management care plan so that a complete picture of the patient's expected experience is clear to all providers. The patient's progress is monitored carefully and frequently with untoward responses handled by the case management team to ensure that standards of quality are met. The keys to successful case management are realistic expectations, close coordination of services, prompt intervention in response to patient progress, teamwork among disciplines, and short- and long-term evaluation of outcomes.

There are numerous models of case management (Lyon, 1993). The individual who acts as case manager may or may not be a nurse. This fact is often a surprise to nurses who assume that they are rightful heirs to the coordination and management of patient care. Some institutions have social workers or nonprofessionals act as case managers, with nurses represented as a member of the team. When nurses are case managers, they are likely to act in one of three roles: (1) they may be staff who work at the bedside giving hands-on care on a daily basis; (2) they may be unit-based nurses who do not provide hands-on care but oversee the management of many different patients; or (3) they may be advanced practice nurses prepared at the master's level who manage a caseload of patients with specific diagnoses pre- and posthospitalization.

Team nursing generally refers to a group of staff who work together and share responsibility for the care of a specific group of patients (Hyams-Franklin, Rowe-Gillespie, Harper, & Johnson, 1993). The team can consist of RNs, assistive personnel, and others such as social workers. Patients are assigned to the team, and team members are scheduled on a given day to care for patients on their team.

Modular nursing is similar to team nursing in that the unit is subdivided into geographical areas, and a team of caregivers care for patients only in that area (Abts, Hofer, & Leafgreen, 1994). This is especially useful on units that have long hallways or are spread over a large area. The use of modules reduces the physical distance that staff have to cover to care for their patients. Patients belong to a module depending on the room to which they are assigned. The disadvantage for both patients and staff is that assignments are arbitrary because they are based on patient location rather than consistency in care or patient needs.

In *primary nursing*, the RN assumes responsibility for all the care provided to patients for whom the nurse is "primarily" responsible. This model was popular in the days when hospitals used their resources to hire professional caregivers rather than other types of personnel (Manthey, 1980).

Case nursing is used primarily outside the hospital, such as in home care, in which the nurse provides most, if not all, of the patient's care (Komplin, 1995). In this method, the nurse has a caseload of patients for whom he or she is responsible and communicates needs to physicians and supervisory personnel.

In *functional nursing*, each nurse on a unit is responsible for certain tasks to be performed for all patients on the unit (Ellis & Hartley, 1995). Tasks such as administering medications, performing wound care, processing orders, and giving baths are divided among the staff. Such care, however, is fragmented, and it may not be clear who is responsible for individual patients. Patients have several nurses each shift and lack a specific person to whom they can direct their concerns.

In reality, most health care settings use a combination of these methods; it is rare to have any of these in place in pure form. For example, some patients who are at risk for readmission or lengthy stays may be case-managed to prevent treatment delays that increase hospital expense. Case management uses team concepts that may cross unit and institutional boundaries and include a broad range of personnel. Patients on the same unit may be treated by a combination of primary nursing and functional models. Staff, managers, and nursing service leaders need to take into consideration the resources available, unit design, types of patients treated, preparation of staff, and access to other services in determining the model most appropriate for a specific setting.

SHIFT TO COMMUNITY

Future models of care delivery will not resemble the models of the past (Lamb, 1995). Information systems and community-based care will change forever the ways in which nurses deliver care to clients. Smaller, more geographically dispersed families mean that individuals do not have as much assistance at home as they recover from illnesses and cope with chronic illnesses as in past years. The support nurses and others provide needs to keep patients as independent as possible. The impetus to hospitalize patients only as long as absolutely necessary gives nurses a wealth of opportunities to become more involved in community-based care (Batra, 1992). Well-integrated community services assist hospitals to overcome the shortfalls of abrupt discharges and uneven follow-up care.

Nursing practice began in homes and settings external to hospitals. Nurses were physically and geographically mobile to attend to patients, making their way through crowded streets and tenements and riding on horseback to isolated rural settlements. As hospitals grew, nurses moved their practice into the institutional setting, leaving matters of organization, budgets, and management to others. Nursing services external to hospitals began to be seen as an afterthought; indeed, community nursing services in New York City went bankrupt because nurses neglected to document care so they could be reimbursed and be involved in the financial side of providing services (Hamilton, 1988). The current emphasis on community-based care requires nurses who understand how to evaluate the health needs of newly discharged patients and of diverse groups of individuals within the community; how to link services in a way that accommodates cultural norms; and how to access community resources. Nurses will care for patients in many settings, such as physician offices, industry, schools, shopping malls, day care, nursing centers, fitness centers, fairgrounds, and churches. Patient records will be readily available through sophisticated information systems that will enable practitioners to deliver care at remote sites. Access to advanced clinical information will be available in the same way through information systems that will connect practitioners to a database of updated knowledge that can be used to assist the patient, family, and nurse to make health care decisions. Nurses will work in multidisciplinary systems in an interdependent role in managing patients' care. Nurses who are able to demonstrate expertise in managing systems, using information systems, and practicing outcome-oriented and theory-based care will emerge as leaders in the 21st century.

SUMMARY

Perspectives on leadership have changed distinctly since leadership was first regarded as a unique phenomenon. Early debates about the nature of leadership were "either/or" debates. That is, leadership was assumed to be either a product of natural ability only (trait) or the circumstances that gave rise to opportunities for leadership (state). Leadership is viewed now as transformational and charismatic in nature. To sustain commitment through complex and rapid change, leaders in health care need to be visionaries who can communicate with inspiration, are immersed in their work, and encourage trust through visible commitment to common goals. Leaders differ from managers in that they are not necessarily constrained by formal position, and leaders' goals transcend the organization. Leaders are sensitive to their followers' needs; in order to sustain momentum toward a vision, the leader cultivates the active, thoughtful support of followers while fulfilling their needs.

Influence and power are useful concepts for nurses to learn. Nurses can develop skills to affect the outcome of issues that are important to them. As nurses become influential, they develop skills in how to use power resources. Personal, organizational, and community resources are readily available to nurses for use in attaining professional goals. The responsible use of resources (power) assists nurses in carrying out the everyday tasks of decision making, negotiation, problem solving, and delegating.

The context of nursing practice is affected by the financing of health care, delivery systems, and nursing models used in the provision of direct care. The financing of health care has a major effect on nurses' roles and goals for patient care. Care delivery has to take into account the types of personnel available, settings in which the care is delivered, accessibility of resources, and consumer need.

Nurses in the 21st century will practice in open, community-based health care systems rather than the closed system of hospitals. Nursing's proven capacity for meeting patient needs in multiple settings will enable nurses to practice in these newer community-based systems. Nursing has only to gain from the myriad opportunities for leadership in health care.

REFERENCES

Abts, D., Hofer, M., & Leafgreen, P. K. (1994). Redefining care delivery: A modular system. *Nursing Management, 25*(2), 40–43, 46.

Batra, C. (1992). Empowering for professional, political, and health policy involvement. *Nursing Outlook, 40*, 170–176.

Bennis, W., & Nanus, B. (1985). *Leaders: The strategies for taking charge.* New York: Harper Perennial.

Biordi, D. L. (1993). Ethical leadership. In A. Marriner-Tomey (Ed.), *Transformational leadership in nursing* (pp. 51–68). St. Louis: Mosby.

Bleich, M. R. (1995). Managing and leading. In P. Yoder-Wise (Ed.), *Leading and managing in nursing* (pp. 2–21). St. Louis: Mosby.

Conger, J. A., & Kanungo, R. N. (1994). Charismatic leadership in organizations: Perceived behavioral attributes and their measurement. *Journal of Organizational Behavior, 15*, 439–452.

Dienemann, J., & Gessner, J. (1992). Restructuring nursing care delivery systems. *Nursing Economics, 10*, 253–258, 310.

Ellis, J. R., & Hartley, C. L. (1995). *Managing and coordinating nursing care* (2nd ed.). Philadelphia: Lippincott.

Finkler, S. A., & Kovner, C. T. (1993). *Financial management for nurse managers and executives.* Philadelphia: Saunders.

Gillies, D. A. (1994). *Nursing management: A systems approach* (3rd ed.). Philadelphia: Saunders.

Hamilton, D. (1988). Faith and finance. *IMAGE: Journal of Nursing Scholarship, 20,* 124–127.

Hersey, P., & Duldt, B. W. (1989). *Situational leadership in nursing.* Norwalk, CT: Appleton & Lange.

Hicks, L., Stallmeyer, J. M., & Coleman, J. R. (1992). Nursing challenges in managed care. *Nursing Economics, 10,* 265–275.

Hyams-Franklin, E. M., Rowe-Gilliespie, P., Harper, A., & Johnson, V. (1993). Primary team nursing: The 90's model. *Nursing Management, 24*(6), 50–52.

Komplin, J. (1995). Care delivery systems. In P. Yoder-Wise (Ed.), *Leading and managing in nursing* (pp. 410–435). St. Louis: Mosby.

Lamb, G. (1995). Early lessons from a capitated community-based model. *Nursing Administration Quarterly, 19*(3), 18–26.

Levit, K. R., Lazenby, H. C., Cowan, C. A., & Letsch, S. W. (1994). National health expenditures. In C. Harrington, & C. L. Estes (Eds.), *Health policy and nursing* (pp. 14–27). Boston: Jones and Barlett.

Lyon, J. C. (1993). Models of nursing care delivery and case management: Clarification of terms. *Nursing Economics, 11,* 163–169.

Manthey, M. (1980). *The practice of primary care.* Boston, MA: Blackwell Scientific.

McGregor, D. (1960). *The human side of enterprise.* New York: McGraw-Hill.

Moore, K. (1992). Case management provides flexibility, opportunity for nurse managers. *Midwest Alliance in Nursing Journal, 3*(3), 13–18.

Morrison, E. M., & Luft, H. S. (1994). Health maintenance organization environments in the 1980s and beyond. In C. Harrington, & C. L. Estes (Eds.), *Health policy and nursing* (pp. 113–124). Boston: Jones and Barlett.

Northouse, P. G., & Northouse, L. L. (1992). *Health communication: Strategies for health professionals.* Norwalk, CT: Appleton & Lange.

Ouchi, W. (1981). *Theory Z: How American business can meet the Japanese challenge.* Reading, MA: Addison-Wesley.

Pabst, M. K. (1993). Span of control on nursing inpatient units. *Nursing Economics, 11,* 87–90.

Vestal, K. W. (1995). *Nursing management: Concepts and issues* (2nd ed.). Philadelphia: Lippincott.

BIBLIOGRAPHY

Bernhard, L. A., & Walsh, M. (1995). *Leadership: The key to the professionalization of nursing* (3rd ed.). St. Louis: Mosby.

Flarey, D. L. (1995). *Redesigning nursing care delivery. Transforming our future.* Philadelphia: Lippincott.

Fralic, M. F. (1993). The new era nurse executive: Centerpiece characteristics. *Journal of Nursing Administration, 23*(1), 7–8.

Gardner, K. (1991). A summary of findings of a five-year comparison study of primary and team nursing. *Nursing Research, 40,* 113–117.

Gipson, J. L., Ivancevich, J. M., & Donnelly, J. H. (1994). *Organizations* (8th ed.). Burr Ridge, IL: Irwin.

Hampton, D. C. (1993). Implementing a managed care framework through care maps. *Journal of Nursing Administration, 25*(5), 21–27.

Marquis, B. L., & Huston, C. J. (1996). *Leadership roles and management functions in nursing: Theory and application* (2nd ed.). Philadelphia: Lippincott.

Michaels, C. (1992). Carondolet St. Mary's nursing enterprise. *Nursing Clinics of North America, 27*(1), 77–85.

Simms, L. M., Price, A. A., & Ervin, N. E. (1994). *Nursing administration* (2nd ed.). Albany, NY: Delmar.

Spitzer-Lehman, R. (1994). *Nursing management desk reference: Concepts, skills, and strategies.* Philadelphia: Saunders.

Yoder-Wise, P. (1995). *Leading and managing in nursing.* St. Louis: Mosby.

Future Perspectives

Marilyn H. Oermann

Predicting the future for professional nursing is risky, particularly given the many changes that are occurring in the health care system and in society at large. Forecasts of the future are fragile at best, reflecting the biases and personal views of the forecaster. Yet forecasts are important if nursing is to carve an essential role for itself in the health care system in years to come. Nursing must continue to take an active role in shaping changes in the health care system in ways that will advance its development as a recognized profession.

Preparation for practice today also needs to prepare the nurse for tomorrow. The future has both change and constancy. Change represents risk taking and challenge; constancy is familiarity and comfort (Bolles, 1983, p. 7). Both components need to be incorporated into a future perspective of nursing. Nursing's continued development as a profession depends on understanding trends in the health care system and society and their potential impact on nursing and its practice.

This chapter examines selected trends that affect the health care system and nursing, such as changing demographics and settings for care, cost of health care, technology, health promotion, and the shift toward community care. The impact of these changes on nursing practice and the role and responsibilities of the professional nurse are considered.

CHANGING DEMOGRAPHICS

Many authors have written about the graying of America and its implications for the health care system and nursing practice. The current health care system is acute care oriented, yet elderly people face chronic health problems that require nursing rather than acute medical care and technology. In 1900, 3.12 million people were older than 65 (4% of the U.S. population; Mann, 1987, p. 10). In 1984 people over 65 years of age made up 12% of the population (Dimond, 1990, p. 336). During the next 25 years, the number of people 65 years and older will increase, and the number of people 85 years and older will increase even more significantly. By 2030, people over 65 years of age are expected to make up 21% of the total population (Dimond, 1990, p. 336).

As the proportion of older people increases, their need for health care also increases, as does their use of hospital and other health care resources. This phenomenon will create an unprecedented demand for facilities and services to meet the need of an aging population. As individuals, elderly people are healthier than people of that age at earlier points in history. Thus, although overall health care resources will be taxed because of the increasing number of aged persons and their problems, these individuals are expected to enjoy a better health status than in the past.

Elderly people have more chronic diseases and use more health care services than people in other age groups. Elderly patients already occupy a large portion of hospital beds; with an anticipated increase in the elderly population, more and more older people will occupy beds in hospital settings and require care in the home and community. As a result, nurses will need to be knowledgeable about and possess skills for care of the elderly in various settings. Currently, patients admitted to hospitals are more ill, require more intensive nursing care than in the past, and are certain to require such care in the future. This increasing acuity of patient needs will create a demand for nurses who are educated not only in the care of elderly people in general but also in providing intensive care to them.

The future is clear; nurses need skills in caring for the aging and a theoretical framework for planning and delivering such care. de Tornyay (1992) suggests that nursing will be central to care of the elderly in the future. Providing technical care without understanding the aging process and nursing interventions specifically geared to elderly people will not meet the needs of this age group, particularly when they face a critical illness. Issues associated with high technology and its use at the end of life must be resolved, as must other ethical decisions in terms of quality of life and treatments to prolong life. The cost of prolonging life through technology, aside from consideration of other implications, will be a factor in evaluating this type of intervention for elderly people who face a critical illness. Discovering more humane approaches to dying in hospitals is becoming increasingly more important.

Problems of elderly people, however, tend not to be acute but rather chronic in nature. In the beginning of the 20th century, acute infectious diseases were prevalent and created most of the illnesses faced by the population. Tuberculosis, for instance, was the number-one disease. Today, the problems are of a chronic nature, such as arthritis, atherosclerosis, and diabetes. Chronic illnesses require more care and care over a longer period. The aging process itself, resulting in decreased hearing and sight, slowed reflexes, memory loss, and other typical changes, creates the need for nursing care. These changes are not illnesses affecting elderly people but are responses to aging that require nursing management. Nurses need to be skilled in promoting self-care and independence among elderly people, considering the physiological and other changes these people face.

Hospital and medical care in general are not only expensive, but also are not geared to meet the needs of elderly people with an array of chronic problems and other changes associated with aging. Elderly people will continue to require services outside of hospital settings; these services are best provided by nurses in outpatient and long-term care settings, the home, and through other community agencies. Care in these settings can more effectively deal with the chronic nature of an older person's health problems.

The role of nursing in the future in providing long-term care will continue to expand. As the number of aged persons increases, the demand for nurses in nursing homes and other long-term care settings also will increase. With the projected continued growth in the nursing home population, clinical experiences for students in nursing homes and long-term care are important in preparing them for a future role in caring for the elderly. Tagliareni, Sherman, Waters, and Mengel (1991) described a collaborative effort between associate degree nursing programs and nursing homes to provide clinical experiences for students and to improve patient care.

In addition to the demand for nurses skilled in care of the aged in hospitals and long-term care settings, there will be an increased need for nurses in outpatient and other ambulatory settings, such as adult day care centers, day treatment facilities, and community mental health centers. The need for nursing care of elderly people in the home also will continue to grow. Home care includes providing skilled nursing care to clients, with the goal of avoiding hospitalization and improving health status, and expanded home care programs. Because of the increased elderly population being cared for in the home and through other community settings, nurses prepared to care for this population will be in great demand.

Elderly and other people with chronic illnesses need *nursing* care; care provided by nurses in the home and other outpatient and community settings serves as one strategy for avoiding hospitalization and improving health status. Home care also is more cost-effective than inpatient care. Brooten and coworkers (1988) developed and tested a model designed to discharge patients early from the hospital with the help of nurse specialists who provide transitional follow-up care in the home. Studies have documented the cost effectiveness of this model. For instance, in research with low-birthweight infants, the mean savings in hospital and physician charges was $18,560 for each infant discharged early and followed in the home by a perinatal nurse specialist prepared at the master's level. No differences were found in infant mortality, morbidity, or growth between infants in the early discharge group and those in the control group (Brooten et al., 1989, pp. 315–316). The New York Visiting Nurse Service demonstrated that acquired immunodeficiency syndrome (AIDS) patients could be cared for in the home for $800 per day compared with $3,000 per day in the hospital (Maraldo, 1989, p. 303). Other research also documents the cost effectiveness of nurses providing home care rather than inpatient acute care.

The provision of adequate care to infants and children will continue to be a priority in addition to the increased number of aged people and their need for nursing care and other health services. The infant mortality rate is particularly high for minorities and other groups such as teenage mothers. Infants in the United States continue to die because of low birthweights; many of these deaths could be prevented with prenatal care. Providing effective prenatal care is essential not only to improve the outcomes of the pregnancy and health of the infant but also in terms of cost-effectiveness. Prenatal care is less expensive than an early delivery and premature birth.

Nurses assume an important role in providing care to mothers and children. Their responsibilities include, among others, health education, health promotion, providing access to the services needed, counseling, and direct care. This role will continue in the future. Nursing's Agenda for Health Care Reform (NLN, 1991), nursing's proposal for reform in the health care system, provides for improved access to prevention services for mothers and children, including prenatal and perinatal care, infant and well-child care, school-based prevention services, and health screening for children. Prevention not only improves the health of the population but also is less costly than illness care. It is far less expensive for a child to be immunized than to be treated for the illness. Nursing's role in health promotion and prevention of illness is well established and will become more important in the future in terms of maternal and child care as well as care of other age groups. This care of mothers and children will be community based, delivered through various community agencies, in homes, neighborhood clinics, schools, and other community settings (Oermann, 1994a, b).

HEALTH CARE COSTS

One of the greatest problems in health care today is its high cost. Annual health care costs in the United States are the highest in the world (Schieber, Poullier, & Greenwald, 1994, p. 36). Since the mid-1980s, health care expenditures in the United States have continued to increase. Levit, Lazenby, Cowan, and Letsch (1994) reported that national health expenditures grew at a substantially faster pace than did the overall economy, consuming a rising percentage of the gross national product. Medicare costs continue to increase; some health care experts suggest that the system will collapse. Rising health care costs have made care unaffordable for many Americans; many remain either without medical insurance coverage or with inadequate coverage. Adequate prenatal care remains inaccessible for many women; even some private insurers do not cover prenatal care.

For health care reform to be effective, Schieber et al. (1994) suggest that three problems must be resolved. First, health care services must be available and provided to the poor and disadvantaged. Second, a mechanism should be developed to pool health risks and reform private health insurance, for example, eliminating preexisting conditions and nonrenewable clauses. Last, mechanisms must be found to control the costs of health care (p. 36).

Health care has moved from individual hospitals and solo physician practice to large corporate entities and varied types of health care organizations. One important force in the health care delivery system is the growing number of managed care organizations such as health maintenance organizations (HMOs) and preferred provider organizations (PPOs). The number of enrollees in HMOs and PPOs, both of which are described in Chapter 11, has increased significantly (Estes, Harrington, & Davis, 1994). Nurses will move more and more into practice in these managed care organizations. Physician practice patterns also have changed rapidly, moving toward large partnerships and group practices.

Nursing's Response to Costs

Nursing has the opportunity to respond to rising health care costs. In the hospital, long-term care settings, and the home, nursing care offers both tremendous cost savings and meets clients' needs. In hospitals, particularly given the decreased length of stay for patients, nursing care can prevent the occurrence or exacerbation of health care problems. For example, nursing interventions can prevent decubitus and other skin problems. Nurses assist patients and families in acquiring knowledge and skills for engaging in self-care both in and out of the hospital; other nursing interventions that focus on health promotion and prevention of additional problems in the long term reduce costs of illness care. These nursing interventions in the hospital setting can mean cost savings. In ambulatory and long-term care settings and the home, studies have documented the cost savings of nursing care. Not only can nursing save costs, but also in many instances nursing management is more appropriate for the client than is acute medical care, such as with chronic illness care, health promotion, and health education.

Nurses today and in the future must be reimbursed for their services. Third-party reimbursement for nursing services benefits clients in their pursuit of both quality and cost-effective care. The ANA and other nursing groups and individuals have supported direct reimbursement for nursing services for years (Streff & Netzer, 1990). Payment for nursing services should include hospital and other acute care settings as well as the many other settings in which nurses deliver care. Maraldo (1989) proposed that services be reimbursed either in a fee-for-service arrangement or managed care arrangements with nurses as primary providers of care (p. 303). Direct payment to nurses is more cost-effective and would make more services available to clients. Nurses need to market their services as primary providers who can lower costs and provide the needed health care.

The number of physicians is anticipated to increase from a physician-to-population ratio of 144 per 100,000 in 1986 to 176 per 100,000 in 2000. This represents an increase of 22%. By 2000 there will be an excess of 90,000 physicians needed to maintain a constant physician-to-population ratio (Grumbach & Lee, 1994). Some experts indicate that a surplus of physicians currently exists in selected geographic areas and specialties. As competition for health care dollars increases, physicians will compete with nurses, particularly nurse practitioners and nurse midwives, for the same health care dollars and, in some areas of the country, for patients. An oversupply of physicians may change the roles of nurses and other health professionals. Physicians may need to alter their traditional practices to secure enough patients; care by physicians may include providing more services to clients such as teaching and counseling, creating greater access to care, and making their services more convenient.

Prospective Payment System

In hospitals today, patients are more acutely ill and stay for shorter periods than in the past. Care has shifted gradually from hospitals to community agencies and care within the home. A major change occurred in 1983 when a prospective rather than retrospective reimbursement system for Medicare patients was instituted. This prospective payment system, which is based on diagnosis-related groups (DRGs) for all hospitals receiving Medicare, was enacted to decrease hospital expenditures. Before its enactment, efforts had been made to decrease costs for care of hospitalized patients. However, in a retrospective reimbursement system, hospitals are paid after services are provided at a cost determined by the hospital. When few restrictions on costs exist, there is limited incentive to reduce them.

A prospective payment system based on DRGs attempts to define types of cases similar in their amount of use of hospital services using length of stay as a measure of hospital services (Plomann & Shaffer, 1983). The DRGs focus on resources consumed during a hospital stay (Roos, Wennberg, & McPherson, 1988) and are determined according to patient diagnoses, age, treatments, including surgery, discharge status, and gender (Reilly & Oermann, 1992). Reimbursement is based on DRGs and occurs in terms of rates set in advance for these various categories of medical diagnoses.

The intent of DRG policy was to create a competitive environment among hospitals, link payment to diagnosis, and reduce hospital costs, as well as maintain quality (Bull, 1988, p. 415). In this system, there is an incentive to move clients quickly out of hospitals and other health care agencies. If patients are discharged before the designated length of stay, the hospital keeps the difference in cost; if the client extends the length of stay, the hospital does not receive full reimbursement for the extension. Prospective reimbursement limits hospitalization to clients with documented needs and restricts the use of nonessential diagnostic tests and other medical services.

Findings from a study by Bull (1988) suggest that DRGs have influenced discharge planning, professional nursing practice, and overall patient care. Following implementation of DRGs in the study hospitals, discharge planning became more routine, communication increased among health care workers, and there was increased collaboration reported among nurses, social workers, physicians, and family members (Bull, 1988, p. 417). Other changes in patient care included greater family involvement in discharge planning, emphasis on self-care, and promotion of independence among patients. In contrast, nurses also reported greater stress on clients and their families in relation to performing care at home.

The prospective payment system provides an opportunity for nursing to determine the nursing intensity required for each DRG classification. This determination serves as a basis to account for the cost of nursing services. Shortened hospital stays create the need for research on early discharge, the discharge planning process and care of the patient in the home; this type of research is needed to document the effectiveness of nursing care in preparing the client for discharge and providing transitional and follow-up care in the home. Nurses need to resolve conflicts between the demands to discharge clients within an average length of stay and the nurses' own judgments about the care the client still needs and most appropriate setting for receiving that care.

Clients today often require more acute care at home; the need for this type of nursing care will continue. An array of community and home care services need to be both available and accessible to clients after hospitalization. Nurses in the community have identified a shift in the nature of client problems, with more first home visits needed immediately after discharge and more complex care being required. In addition, more intensive care nurses are being hired to provide this care (Phillips, Fisher, MacMillan-Scattergood, & Baglioni, 1989, p. 325). Findings of a study by Phillips and associates (1989) suggest that following the introduction of DRGs, home health care agencies began serving a different population. Clients required more visits and a greater number of services. The need for services that require more time and are more complex also increased. Nurses now provide more services per visit, including those that require more time and skill (Phillips et al., 1989).

The movement of health care out of hospitals into the community and home signifies a different nurse–patient relationship, one established and carried out in the client's own environment rather than the captive hospital setting. In the home, the client has a greater say in care and decision making. In addition, acutely ill clients cared for in the home require, along with physical care, an array of technical services once available only in the hospital. Teaching clients and family is a major nursing intervention. Planning client care requires extensive coordination of services, often on a 24-hour basis. Planning among agencies is increasingly important, particularly as the nurse assists clients and families in gaining access to care needed and providing for continuity of care.

TECHNOLOGY

Nursing functions in a health care system that is ever changing and continually expanding its knowledge base. The health care system is at the center of much new technology in terms of instrumentation of care and computerization. Technology is an important part of health care and nursing practice in and out of hospital settings. "One of the most noteworthy developments in medical technology is the growth in outpatient applications" (Hull & American Hospital Association, 1994, p. 164), with many procedures and treatments now available on an outpatient basis.

Technology, even though it has improved care for many, presents its own problems. High technology means high cost. In industry, technology often reduces costs for labor; in the health care system, however, technology contributes to an increase in costs. The cost of technology also is high ethically, in terms of "rightness" of an intervention and eligibility of a person to receive it. Use of technology has become a resource issue; questions such as who should receive costly and limited technologies and who should make these decisions need to be answered. Technology prolongs life, sometimes without improvement in quality; issues associated with cost and quality of life need to be addressed.

The integration of technology throughout the health care system will continue. Nurses working in high-tech environments also must develop "high-touch" skills (Reilly & Oermann, 1992). The need to provide humanistic care, particularly as the nurse faces increasingly more complex technological care, will remain important. Responding to the patient's individualized needs and providing supportive care to the family and others are essential in a high-tech environment. High-touch skills are most vulnerable in any environment where the client's stay is short (Reilly & Oermann, 1992). Nurses need to participate in decisions on the use of new technology for clients, considering not only patient needs but also the potential impact on nursing resources and practice.

Improved and expanded technology in health care will continue to require more technological skills among nurses. Nurses will use these skills not only in critical care units but also throughout hospitals and in other agencies and the home. New technology calls for new knowledge and skills; nurses will face the need to update their own knowledge base and skills (Oermann, 1994a). Although some technology saves nursing time, other interventions require more skilled practice and greater time spent in carrying out care.

Hospitals and other types of health care agencies will continue to develop information systems for managing data and carrying out their functions. The use of computers and their impact on health care and nursing practice were discussed in Chapter 8. The role of the computer in nursing will continue to increase, requiring yet another type of nursing knowledge and skill.

HEALTH PROMOTION

More emphasis in the future will be on health promotion and the use of economic incentives to prevent illness and remain healthy. Many health problems are preventable through education and maintenance of healthy lifestyles. Consumer involvement in health care will continue. The public has become increasingly better informed about the effect of a healthy lifestyle on the prevention of illness and self-care measures. Consumers will seek information about health promotion and disease prevention even more. Many people are serious about assuming responsibility for maintaining their own health.

Nursing has a significant role in health promotion and prevention of illness. Nurses provide health education and are involved in many health promotion activities; this involvement will become even greater as more and more consumers assume an active role in maintaining their health. Health education and promotion are far less expensive than illness care. Nurses have the knowledge and skill to provide this education and health promotion to clients and families (NLN, 1992). Many of the competencies for future health professionals identified by the Pew Health Professions Commission (1991) reflect skills in health promotion and disease prevention.

In schools, nurses will assume a leading role in developing and implementing school health programs. Health education is particularly important at an early age when health values are formed. Sigsby and Campbell (1992) highlight the role of the nurse in schools as providing access to basic health services and health education for children.

Nurses increasingly will be required to provide health education and promotion at the workplace. Nursing services can keep employees healthy and on the job. Health screening, teaching, health promotion programs, stress management, and follow-up care, among other interventions, are particularly appropriate for nurses to carry out in the employee's own setting. Opportunities for occupational health nursing will increase; as the field develops, advanced education will be needed for carrying out this role. Nursing research will need to document the impact of nursing services on health outcomes and promoting health in varied settings.

SHIFT TO COMMUNITY

A significant change in the health care system is the shift toward the community as a primary setting for the delivery of care. Greater numbers of patients are cared for in their homes and through varied community agencies. Patients cared for in the home often have complex health problems, and the nurse may be faced with managing acutely ill patients discharged early from hospitals. O'Neill and Pennington (1996) describe this shift in patient care from the hospital to the home and the resulting demand for home care nursing. Neighborhood health centers, nurse-managed clinics, homes, outpatient facilities, day care, schools, and shelters are important settings for the delivery of care.

The nurse plays an essential role in caring for the community's health and participating in primary care in community systems (NLN, 1991; Oermann, 1994a, b). Primary health care, which includes essential health services such as adequate nutrition, maternal and child health care, immunization, and health education, is by its nature community based (Mooney, 1995). To provide primary care and to practice in community systems, nurses need an understanding of the community, of the factors influencing their clients' health and that of the community, of resources in the community and how to access them, and of the culture and values of the particular community (Oermann, 1994b). The Pew Health Professions Commission (1991) emphasizes the important role of the health professional in caring for the community's health and the need for skills in working with others in the delivery of health care. The nurse in the future will work in multidisciplinary arrangements and will need to collaborate with other health providers to manage care and deliver health services. Other competencies of future health professionals are as follows:

1. Care for community's health.
2. Expand access to care and improve public's health.
3. Provide contemporary clinical care.
4. Emphasize primary care.
5. Participate in coordinated care.
6. Ensure cost-effective and quality care.
7. Emphasize prevention.
8. Involve patients and families in decision making.
9. Promote healthy lifestyles.
10. Use technology appropriately.
11. Improve health care system.
12. Manage information.
13. Understand role of physical environment on health.
14. Provide counseling on ethical issues.

15. Be responsive to increased public, governmental, and third-party participation in health care.
16. Participate in culturally diverse society.
17. Continue to learn.*

* Adapted from Pew Health Professions Commission. (1991). *Healthy America: Practitioners for 2005.* Durham, NC: Author.

Reilly and Oermann (1992) suggest that the movement of health care toward the community signifies a different client–nurse relationship from the type encountered in the hospital. Knowledge of and respect for various cultural groups and their values, beliefs, and patterns of behavior are essential for nurses in the community. Humanistic nursing care requires sensitivity to these cultural patterns and values (Reilly & Oermann, 1992, p. 472).

SUMMARY

The future of nursing already is evident today. Current trends need to be examined for their impact on the present and future practice of nursing. Changes in nursing are occurring as a result of rapid transformations in the health care system and in society at large. The increase in the number of elderly people requiring care will continue to create more demands on health care resources. Nurses are caring for more acutely ill elderly clients in hospitals, community settings, and the home. The elderly face chronic illness best managed by nurses outside the acute care setting; nursing will continue to play an important role in the care of elderly people. Technology now extends the life of many who would have died in the past; use of technology is associated with high costs both financially and ethically.

Cost containment will remain an issue in the future. The high costs of health care already have resulted in significant changes in care delivery and services. Cost considerations in all dimensions of health care and nursing practice will continue. Hospitalization is reserved only for those who are acutely ill, and patients are finding themselves discharged to community settings earlier than in the past. Early discharge has placed a burden on community agencies and changed the focus of care for many nurses who practice in these settings.

High technology continues to be infused in hospitals and increasingly is being used in the home, thus necessitating that nurses have advanced knowledge and technological skills as well as the ability to provide humanistic care in this environment. Questions about the value of technology, its cost, and its impact on the client and family need to be addressed.

Nurses will practice in a multitude of settings; many health care problems, such as those associated with chronic illness, are best managed by nurses. Nursing's role in health promotion and education will continue. Prevention needs to be a nursing priority to improve the health of the population and from a cost perspective. The cost of illness far exceeds the cost of prevention. The need for nurses, and especially nurses prepared for this changing practice, will continue.

In a rapidly changing world, innovative skills are needed; problem solving cannot rely on past solutions but rather must rely on new ideas. Change in the knowledge and skills needed by nurses for future practice and in the settings in which they will deliver care and constancy in the goal to serve the health needs of society are important to the future of professional nursing.

REFERENCES

Bolles, R. N. (1983). Life/work planning: Change and constancy in the world of work. *The Futurist, 17*(6), 7–11.

Brooten, D., Brown, L. P., Munro, B. H., York, R., Cohen, S. M., Roncoli, M., & Hollingsworth, A. (1988). Early discharge and specialist transitional care. *Image: Journal of Nursing Scholarship, 20*, 64–68.

Brooten, D., Munro, B. H., Roncili, M., Arnold, L., Brown, L. P., York, R., Hollingsworth, A., Cohen, S. M., & Rubin, M. (1989). Developing a program grant for use in model testing. *Nursing & Health Care, 10*, 315–318.

Bull, M. J. (1988). Influence of diagnosis-related groups on discharge planning, professional practice, and patient care. *Journal of Professional Nursing, 4*, 415–421.

de Tornyay, R. (1992). Reconsidering nursing education: The report of the Pew Health Professions Commission. *Journal of Nursing Education, 31*, 296–301.

Dimond, M. (1990). Health care and the aging population. In C. A. Lindeman & M. McAthie (Eds.), *Nursing trends and issues* (pp. 336–338). Springhouse, PA: Springhouse.

Estes, C. L., Harrington, C., & Davis, S. (1994). The medical-industrial complex. In C. Harrington & C. L. Estes (Eds.), *Health policy and nursing* (pp. 54–69). Boston: Jones and Bartlett.

Grumbach, K., & Lee, P. R. (1994). How many physicians can we afford? In C. Harrington & C. L. Estes (Eds.), *Health policy and nursing* (pp. 284–293). Boston: Jones and Bartlett.

Hull, K., & American Hospital Association. (1994). Hospital trends. In C. Harrington & C. L. Estes (Eds.), *Health policy and nursing* (pp. 150–168). Boston: Jones and Bartlett.

Levit, K. R., Lazenby, H. C., Cowan, C. A., & Letsch, S. W. (1994). National health expenditures. In C. Harrington & C. L. Estes (Eds.), *Health policy and nursing* (pp. 14–27), Boston: Jones and Bartlett.

Mann, G. J. (1987). Beyond the hospital: Building for a healthier future. *The Futurist, 21*(1), 9–10, 12–13.

Maraldo, P. J. (1989). Home care should be the heart of a nursing-sponsored national health plan. *Nursing & Health Care, 10*, 301–304.

Mooney, M. M. (1995). Primary care is no place for physicians. *Nursing & Health Care, 16*, 84–86.

National League for Nursing. (1991). *Nursing's agenda for health care reform.* New York: Author.

National League for Nursing. (1992, October). *An agenda for nursing education reform in support of nursing's agenda for health care reform.* New York: Author.

Oermann, M. H. (1994a). Professional nursing education in the future: Changes and challenges. *Journal of Obstetric, Gynecologic, and Neonatal Nursing, 23,* 153–159.

Oermann, M. H. (1994b). Reforming nursing education for future practice. *Journal of Nursing Education, 33,* 215–219.

O'Neill, E. S., & Pennington, E. A. (1996). Preparing acute care nurses for community-based care. *Nursing & Health Care, 17,* 62–65.

Pew Health Professions Commission. (1991). *Healthy America: Practitioners for 2005.* Durham, NC: Author.

Phillips, E. K., Fisher, M. E., MacMillan-Scattergood, D., & Baglioni, A. J. (1989). DRG ripple and the shifting burden of care to home health. *Nursing & Health Care, 10,* 325–327.

Plomann, M. P., & Shaffer, F. A. (1983). DRGs as one of nine approaches to case mix in transition. *Nursing & Health Care, 4,* 438–443.

Reilly, D. E., & Oermann, M. H. (1992). *Clinical teaching in nursing education* (2nd ed.). New York: National League for Nursing.

Roos, N. P., Wennberg, J. E., & McPherson, K. (1988). Using diagnosis-related groups for studying variations in hospital admissions. *Health Care Financing Review, 9*(4), 53–62.

Schieber, G. J., Poullier, J. P., & Greenwald, L. M. (1994). U. S. health expenditure performance: An international comparison and data update. In C. Harrington & C. L. Estes (Eds.), *Health policy and nursing* (pp. 28–39). Boston: Jones and Bartlett.

Sigsby, L. M., & Campbell, D. W. (1992). Public schools as a clinical setting for RN students. *Nurse Educator, 17*(5), 19–21.

Streff, M. B., & Netzer, R. (1990). Third-party reimbursement. In J. C. McCloskey & H. K. Grace (Eds.), *Current issues in nursing* (3rd ed. pp. 363–368). St. Louis: Mosby.

Tagliareni, E., Sherman, S., Waters, V., & Mengel, A. (1991). Participatory clinical education. *Nursing & Health Care, 12,* 248–250, 261–263.

BIBLIOGRAPHY

Aiken, L. H. (1995). Transformation of the nursing workforce. *Nursing Outlook, 43,* 201–209.

Alford, D. M., & Futrell, M. (1992). Wellness and health promotion of the elderly. *Nursing Outlook, 40,* 221–226.

Alspach, J. G. (1990). Critical care nursing in the 21st century. *Critical Care Nurse, 10*(9), 8–16.

American Association of Colleges of Nursing. (1993, March). *Addressing nursing education's agenda for the 21st century* (Position statement). Washington, DC: Author.

American Organization of Nurse Executives. (1993). Eight premises for a reformed health care system. *Nursing Management, 21*(11), 42–44.

Baker, C. M. (1994). School health: Policy issues in the 1990s. *Nursing & Health Care, 15,* 178–184.

Barger, S. E., & Crumpton, R. B. (1991). Public health nursing partnership: Agencies and academe. *Nurse Educator, 16*(4), 16–19.

Bless, C., Murphy, D., & Vinson, N. (1995). Nurses' role in primary health care. *Nursing & Health Care, 16,* 70–76.

Brenneman, S. K. (1995). A critical review of health care for an aging population. *Issues on Aging, 18*(2), 10–13.

Cousins, M., & McDowell, I. (1995). Use of medical care after a community-based health promotion program: A quasi-experimental study. *American Journal of Health Promotion, 10*(1), 47–54.

DeCorte, P., Gunther, J., Harrison-Woodside, T., Jewell, D., & Kaloti, F. (1995). Health insurance: Impact on hospitalization rates for asthma. *Nursing Connections, 8*(3), 33–42.

de Tornyay, R. (1993). Nursing education: Staying on track. *Nursing & Health Care, 14,* 302–306.

Dracup, K., & Bryan-Brown, C. W. (1993). Critical care and healthcare reform. *American Journal of Critical Care, 2,* 351–353.

Fagin, C. M., & Lynaugh, J. E. (1992). Reaping the rewards of radical change: A new agenda for nursing education. *Nursing Outlook, 40,* 213–220.

Farley, S. (1993). The community as partner in primary health care. *Nursing & Health Care, 14,* 244–249.

Fink, S. V., & Picot, S. F. (1991). Nursing home placement decisions and postplacement experiences of African-American and European-American caregivers. *Journal of Gerontological Nursing, 21*(12), 35–42.

Girouard, S. A., & Smoot, M. D. (1994). Health care reform and nursing resource policy: The North Carolina experience. *Nursing & Health Care, 15,* 412–416.

Graff, W. L., Bensussen-Walls, W., Cody, E., & Williamson, J. (1995). Population management in an HMO: New roles for nursing. *Public Health Nursing, 12,* 213–221.

Harrington, C. (1991). Why we need a teaching home care program. *Nursing Outlook, 39*(1), 10–29.

Helmer, D. C., Dunn, L. M., Eaton, K., Macedonio, C., & Lubritz, L. (1995). Implementing corporate wellness programs: A business approach to program planning. *AAOHN Journal, 43,* 558–563.

Hills, M. D., & Lindsey, E. (1994). Health promotion: A viable curriculum framework for nursing education. *Nursing Outlook, 42,* 158–162.

Kraft, J. L., & Durnham-Taylor, J. (1995). Quality oversight: How much is too much? *Nursing Economics, 13,* 272–275.

McEwen, M. (1994). Promoting interdisciplinary collaboration. *Nursing & Health Care, 15,* 304–307.

Mundinger, M. O. (1994). Health care reform: Will nursing respond? *Nursing & Health Care, 15,* 28–33.

Mohr, W. K. (1996). Ethics, nursing and health care in the age of reform. *Nursing & Health Care, 17,* 16–21.

Oermann, M. H. (1991). Effectiveness of a critical care nursing course: Preparing students for practice in critical care. *Health & Lung, 20,* 278–283.

Oermann, M. H., Dunn, D., Munro, L., & Monahan, K. (1992). Critical care education at the baccalaureate level. *Nurse Educator, 17*(2), 20–23.

Oermann, M. H., & Provenzano, L. M. (1992). Students' knowledge and perceptions of critical care nursing. *Critical Care Nurse, 12*(1), 72–77.

Packard, N. J. (1993). The price of choice: Managed care in America. *Nursing Administration Quarterly, 17*(3), 8–15.

Porter-O'Grady, T. (1994). Building partnerships in health care: Creating whole systems change. *Nursing & Health Care, 15*, 34–38.

Prescott, P. A. (1993). Nursing: An important component of hospital survival under a reformed health care system. *Nursing Economics, 11*, 192–199.

Primas, P. J., Mileham, T., Toronto, C., & McCoy, B. J. (1994). Breaking the cycle of disadvantage: A nursing system of health care. *Nursing & Health Care, 15*, 10–17.

Schuster, C. (1995). Have we forgotten the older adults? An argument in support of more health promotion programs for and research directed toward people 65 years and olders. *Journal of Health Education, 26*, 338–344.

Sigsby, L. M., & Campbell, D. W. (1995). Nursing interventions classification: A content analysis of nursing activities in public schools. *Journal of Community Health Nursing, 12*, 229–237.

Tallon, R. (1996). Technology assessment: Analytical product research. *Nursing Management, 27*(1), 24–25, 29.

Whittaker, S., & Minich, L. (1995, October). Pew efforts seek to change how health professions are regulated. *American Nurse, 27*(7), 1, 14.

Witmer, A., Seifer, S. D., Finocchio, L., Leslie, J., & O'Neill, E. H. (1995). Community health workers: Integral members of the health care work force. *American Journal of Public Health, 85*, 1055–1058.

Functional Health Pattern Assessment Form: Adults

NURSING HISTORY

I. *Health perception–health management pattern*

a. How has general health been?

b. Any colds in the past year? If appropriate, absences from work/school?

c. Most important things done to keep healthy? Think these things make a difference to health? (Include family folk remedies, if appropriate.) Breast self-examination? Use cigarettes? Drugs? Ever had a drinking problem? When was your last drink?

d. Accidents (home, work, driving)?

e. In past, been easy to find ways to follow suggestions of doctors or nurses?

f. If appropriate: What do you think caused this illness? Action taken when symptoms perceived? Results of actions?

g. If appropriate: What is important to you while you are here? How can we be most helpful?

2. *Nutritional–metabolic pattern*

a. Typical daily food intake? (Describe.) Supplements?

b. Typical daily fluid intake? (Describe.)

c. Weight loss/gain? (Amount) Height loss/gain? (Amount)

d. Appetite?

e. Food or eating: Discomfort? Swallowing? Diet restric..ons? If appropriate: Breastfeeding? Problems with breastfeeding?

f. Heal well or poorly?

g. Skin problems: Lesions, dryness?

h. Dental problems?

3. Elimination pattern

a. Bowel elimination pattern. (Describe.) Frequency? Character? Discomfort? Problem in control? Laxatives?

b. Urinary elimination pattern. (Describe.) Frequency? Problem in control?

c. Excess perspiration? Odor problem?

4. Activity–exercise pattern

a. Sufficient energy for desired/required activities?

b. Exercise pattern? Type? Regularity

c. Spare time (leisure) activities? Child: Play activities?

d. Perceived ability for: (code for level according to key below)

Feeding _____   Grooming _____

Bathing _____   General mobility _____

Toileting _____   Cooking _____

Bed mobility _____   Home maintenance _____

Dressing _____   Shopping _____

Functional Levels Code

Level 0:   Full self-care

Level I: Requires use of equipment or device

Level II: Requires assistance or supervision of another person

Level III: Requires assistance or supervision of another person and equipment or device

Level IV: Is dependent and does not participate

5. Sleep–rest pattern

a. Generally rested and ready for daily activities after sleep?

b. Sleep-onset problems? Aids? Dreams (nightmares)? Early awakening?

c. Rest/relaxation periods?

6. Cognitive–perceptual pattern

a. Hearing difficulty? Aid?

b. Vision? Wear glasses? Last checked?

c. Any change in memory lately?

d. Easy/difficult to make decisions?

e. Easiest way for you to learn things? Any difficulty learning?

f. Any discomfort? Pain? How do you manage it?

7. Self-perception–self-concept pattern

a. How would you describe yourself? Most of the time, feel good (not so good) about yourself?

b. Changes in your body or the things you can do? Are these problematic for you?

c. Changes in way you feel about yourself or your body (since illness started)?

d. Find things frequently make you angry? Annoyed? Fearful? Anxious? Depressed? What helps?

e. Ever feel you lose hope? Not able to control things in life? What helps?

8. Role–relationship pattern

a. Live alone? Family? Family structure (diagram)?

b. Any family problems you have difficulty handling? (Nuclear/Extended)

c. How does family usually handle problems?

d. Family depend on you for things? How managing?

e. If appropriate: How family/others feel about your illness/hospitalization?

f. If appropriate: Problems with children? Difficulty handling?

g. Belong to social groups? Close friends? Feel lonely (frequency)?

h. Things generally go well for you at work? (School?) If appropriate: Income sufficient for needs?

i. Feel part of (or isolated in) neighborhood where living?

9. Sexuality–reproductive pattern

a. If appropriate to age/situation: Sexual relationships satisfying? Changes? Problems?

b. If appropriate: Use of contraceptives? Problems?

c. Female: When menstruation started? Last menstrual period? Menstrual problems? Para? Gravida?

10. Coping–stress-tolerance pattern

a. Any big changes in your life in the last year or two? Crisis?

b. Who's most helpful in talking things over? Available to you now?

     c. Tense a lot of the time? What helps? Use any medicine, drugs, alcohol?

     d. When (if) have big problems (any problems) occur in your life, how do you handle them?

     e. Most of the time, is this (are these) way(s) successful?

11. Value–belief pattern

     a. Generally get things you want out of life? Important plans for the future?

     b. Religion important in your life? If appropriate: Does this help when difficulties arise?

     c. If appropriate: Will being here interfere with any religious practices?

12. Other

     a. Any other things that we have not talked about that you would like to mention?

     b. Questions?

SCREENING EXAMINATION FORMAT

(May add other pattern indicators to expand the examination)

General appearance, grooming, hygiene _____

Oral mucous membranes (color, moistness, lesions) _____

Teeth: Dentures _____ Cavities _____ Missing _____

Hears whisper? _____

Reads newsprint? _____ Glasses? _____

Pulse (rate) _____ (rhythm) _____ (strength) _____

Respiration _____ (depth) _____ (rhythm) _____ Breath sounds _____

Blood pressure _____

Hand grip _____ Can pick up pencil? _____

Range of motion (joints) _____ Muscle firmness _____

Skin: Bony prominences _____ Lesions _____ Color changes _____

Gait _____ Posture _____ Absent body part _____

Demonstrated ability for: (code for level)

Feeding _____ Grooming _____

Bathing _____ General mobility _____

Toileting _____ Cooking _____

Bed mobility _____ Home maintenance _____

Dressing _____ Shopping _____

Intravenous, drainage, suction, etc. (specify)

Actual weight _____   Reported weight _____

Height _____   Temperature _____

During history and examination:

Orientation _____   Grasp ideas and questions (abstract, concrete?) _____

Language spoken_____   Voice and speech pattern _____

Vocabulary level _____

Eye contact _____   Attention span (distraction)_____

Nervous or relaxed (rate from 1 to 5) _____

Assertive or passive (rate from 1 to 5) _____

Interaction with family member, guardian, other

(if present) _____

From Gordon, M. (1995). Manual of nursing diagnosis: 1995–1996 (7th ed.). St. Louis: Mosby, with permission.

Nursing Health History Form

NURSING/PATIENT/FAMILY PROFILE

Obtained from:			Reviewed by:	Unit:	Date:	
Conducted by:	Unit:	Date:	Reviewed by:			
Age:	Sex:					

ADMISSION VITAL SIGNS					
Temperature	Pulse	Respirations	Blood Pressure	Height	Weight

Previous hospitalization? When? Where? Why?

Admitting Medical Diagnosis:	Admission Date:	Related Diagnosis:

Surgical Procedure:	Date:	Admitting Physician:

"Why are you here?"	Allergies:

Current Prescription and Non-prescription medications (type, dose, frequency and time taken at home, reason)

Language spoken:	Translator:

Significant other:	Phone # (Home):	(Work):	Do they know you are here? ☐ Yes ☐ No ☐ Notified

Where do you anticipate going after discharge?

SELF-CONCEPT MODE

1. How would you like to be addressed?_____

2. How do you feel about being in the hospital?_____
   Why?_____

	No	Yes	If yes, describe:	Update*
3. Has there been a marked change in your mood in the previous 3–4 months?	☐	☐		
4. Are you depressed?	☐	☐		
5. Are you having problems with anxiety?	☐	☐		

6. What, if any cultural or spiritual/religious practices are important
   to you or your family while you are here?_____

PHYSIOLOGICAL MODE

Oxygenation	No	Yes	If yes, describe:	Update*
1. Any problems with your breathing?	☐	☐		
2. Do you smoke?	☐	☐		
3. Do you use alcohol/drugs?	☐	☐		

*See progress notes

PHYSIOLOGICAL MODE continued

Oxygenation (*continued*)	No	Yes	If yes, describe:	Update*

1. Any problems with:

your heart? ☐ ☐ _____

your blood pressure? ☐ ☐ _____

your circulation? ☐ ☐ _____

2. Any bleeding problems? ☐ ☐ _____

Nutrition/fluids and electrolytes

1. Any recent weight loss or gain? ☐ ☐ _____
2. How has your appetite been? _____

3. When did you last eat or drink? _____
4. Special diet/intolerances? ☐ ☐ _____

5. Dental appliances or problems? ☐ ☐ _____

Elimination

1. Any problems with urinating? ☐ ☐ _____

2. Any problems with your bowels? ☐ ☐ _____

3. What is your normal bowel pattern? _____

4. Date of last bowel movement? _____
5. Any ostomy appliances? ☐ ☐ _____

Activities of Daily Living (ADL) and Rest

1. Are you able to manage ADL independently? ☐ ☐ _____
2. Assistive devices for above? ☐ ☐ _____

3. **Risk for falls assessed?* ☐ ☐ _____
   If yes, followup with Standards for
   Fall Prevention
4. Any problems sleeping lately? ☐ ☐ _____
5. Do you take/do anything to help you sleep? ☐ ☐ _____

Protection

1. Any problems with your skin? ☐ ☐ _____

2. **High risk for skin breakdown?* ☐ ☐ _____
3. If yes, inspect: (check if intact)

☐ Heels ☐ Head ☐ Hips ☐ Coccyx ☐ Elbows ☐ Nails ☐ Back ☐ Ears ☐ Other
Describe affected areas: _____

If yes to 2 or 3, utilize Standards for Potential or Actual Impaired Skin Integrity

1. Senses and Neurologic function

Any changes or difficulties with the following:
☐ Vision ☐ Hearing ☐ Memory ☐ Smell ☐ Taste ☐ Sensation ☐ Speech
Describe: _____

Assistive devices: _____

**Must be assessed by nurse, do not ask patient   **See progress notes*

2. **Mental Status:* ☐ Alert ☐ Oriented ☐ Disoriented ☐ Confused ☐ Semi Conscious ☐ Comatose
Describe: _____

	No	Yes		Update*

3. Do you have pain? ☐ No ☐ Yes
Where? _____ Describe: _____ When did it start? _____
Rating (0-10) _____ What helps it? _____ How long does it last? _____
What makes it worse? _____

4. Have you noticed any changes from the
way you usually, think, feel, behave? ☐ No ☐ Yes _____

Endocrine function

1. Do you have: If yes, describe:
Diabetes? ☐ No ☐ Yes _____
Thyroid problems? ☐ No ☐ Yes _____
Other hormonal problems? ☐ No ☐ Yes _____
Sexual functioning problems? ☐ No ☐ Yes _____

Other

2. Communicable diseases? ☐ No ☐ Yes _____

ROLE FUNCTION

1. Secondary role (occupation, marital status, etc.): _____
Significant relationships: (list) _____

2. Tertiary role (hobbies, interests, life style): _____

3. Do you foresee any financial concerns ☐ No ☐ Yes
in relation to your illness? _____

INTERDEPENDENCE MODE

1. What are your living arrangements?
☐ Alone ☐ Shared If shared, with whom: _____
☐ House ☐ Apartment ☐ Other (describe): _____

2. Of your significant others, who would you like to be included in decisions about your care and/or teaching?

3. Do you anticipate any difficulty caring for yourself after leaving the hospital? ☐ No ☐ Yes If yes, how?

4. Are there any nurses or agencies visiting you in the home? ☐ No ☐ Yes

5. Are you currently involved with other health care related services? ☐ No ☐ Yes
(e.g., clinics, chiropractor) _____

Are there any other issues related to your health or hospital stay that you ☐ No ☐ Yes
would like to discuss? _____

General Impressions/Second Level Assessment

_____
_____
_____

What are your main goals while here? (See Care Plan) _____

*See progress notes

NURSING/PATIENT/FAMILY PROFILE

PATIENT SUMMARY

Physiological Mode

Review Date

Vital Signs:
☐ Do not resuscitate
☐ Accucheck

Weight

Allergies:

Nutrition

Diet: _____ NPO after midnight _____

Feeding: ☐ Complete ☐ Assist
☐ Self ☐ Assistive devices:

Intake: _____ Output: _____

Activity and Rest

Bath: ☐ Complete ☐ Assist
☐ Self ☐ Specify: _____

Grooming: ☐ Complete ☐ Assist
☐ Self ☐ Specify: _____

Ambulation: ☐ Complete bedrest ☐ Bathroom privileges ☐ Up ad lib
☐ Full weight bearing ☐ Partial weight bearing
☐ Non weight bearing
☐ Assistive device(s):

☐ Transfer assist   Number of persons required _____
☐ Ambulift

Patient name: _____
Identification Number: _____
Attending _____
Physician: _____

Oxygenation

Oxygen Therapy:

Tube/Trach Care:

Elimination

Routine Bladder

Bowel

Consults

Medical diagnosis: _____
Surgical procedure: _____
Admitting date: _____ **Anticipated discharge date:** _____

Protection

Safety:

Dressing:

Fluids & Electrolytes

I.V. Therapy

Site change date:

Other

Room number: _____
Primary nurse: _____
Associate nurse(s): _____

Nursing health history form patterned on Roy's adaptation model. Reprinted with permission from Mount Sinai Hospital, Nursing Department, Toronto, Canada.

Assessment of Self-Care
Requisites Form

Name:_____ ID #_____

Caregiver 1. _____ Relationship_____
Caregiver 2. _____ Relationship_____

D = Deficit	P = Potential	✓ = No Deficit	NA = Not Assessed	R = Resolved
A. UNIVERSAL SELF CARE	Assessment Guide Used			
	DATE			
1. Maintenance of Sufficient Intake of Air				
2. Maintenance of Sufficient Intake of Fluid				
3. Maintenance of Sufficient Intake of Food				
4. Provision of Care Associated with Elimination				
5. Maintenance of Sleep/Activity Balance				
6. Maintenance of Social/Solitude Balance				
7. Prevention of Hazards				
8. Promotion of Normalcy				
B. DEVELOPMENTAL SELF-CARE REQUISITES				
1. Provides Conditions that Promote/Support Development				
2. Prevents Conditions that Affect Development				
C. HEALTH DEVIATION SELF-CARE REQUISITES				
1. Seeks and Secures Medical/Community Resources				
2. Attends to Effects of Pathological State				
3. Carries Out Prescribed Measures				
4. Regulates Deleterious Effects of Prescribed Measures				
5. Modifies Self Concept in Acceptance of a Particular Health State				
6. Learns to Live with the Effects of the Condition				
CHN INITIALS				

DETAILED ASSESSMENT OF SELF-CARE AGENCY

NAME:_____ ID#_____

CODE: ✓ = Adequate   **N = Not Adequate**   **D = Declining**   **NA = Not Assessed**

COMPONENT	DATE/CODE/INITIAL	COMMENT
1. Ability to maintain attention and be vigilant in self-care		
2. Controlled use of available physical energy for self-care		
3. Ability to control body movement and position of parts		
4. Ability to reason within a self-care frame of reference		
5. Motivation to care for self		
6. Ability to make and to act on decisions about care of self		
7. Ability to acquire technical knowledge about self-care from authoritative sources and to use it		
8. A repertoire of skills for self-care (cognitive, perpetual, manipulative, communicative and interpersonal)		
9. Ability to order self-care actions to achieve goals of self-care		
10. Ability to consistently perform self-care actions integrating them with relevant aspects of personal, family and community living		

FOUNDATIONAL CAPABILITIES AND DISPOSITIONS

	DATE/CODE/INITIAL	COMMENTS
Sensation		
Attention		
Perception		
Memory		
Learning		
Self Awareness		
Self Value		
Self Acceptance		
Self Image		
Future Directed Value System		
Ability to Work With Body and its Parts		

Nursing assessment form patterned on Orem's self-care model for community health. Reprinted from Vancouver Health Department, Vancouver, British Columbia, Canada, with permission.

Patient Database Forms

PATIENT DATA BASE
Department of Nursing

Date _____ Time _____ Room No. _____

Age _____ Sex ☐ M ☐ F

Doctor Notified _____

Notified At _____ By _____

Primary Language _____

Contact Person _____ Phone # _____

Contact Person _____ Phone # _____

Information Obtained from _____ Relationship _____

ADMIT FROM: ☐ E.R. ☐ Home ☐ Admitting VIA: ☐ Ambulatory ☐ Stretcher
☐ Dr. Office ☐ Extended Care Facility ☐ Wheelchair ☐ Other _____

VITAL SIGNS: T _____ P _____ R _____ BP _____ HEIGHT _____ WEIGHT _____

ORIENTED TO: POLICIES EXPLAINED   VALUABLES DISPOSITION
☐ Call Light   ☐ Telephone / TV   ☐ Visiting Hours   ☐ Electric Appliances   ☐ Home
☐ Bed Operation   ☐ Unit Routines   ☐ No Smoking   ☐ Tele - Safe   ☐ Safe
☐ Meal Times   ☐ Other _____   ☐ ID Bands   ☐ Bedside Rail Release Form ☐ Other _____
                  _____   ☐ Eyeglass / Denture Release Form
                                                                                          ☐ None

ALLERGIES (Medication, Food, Tape, Dye, etc. What reaction?) _____
_____
_____

Reason for admission and duration of illness (patient's own words) _____
_____
_____

Previous illnesses, hospitalizations, surgeries? _____
_____
_____

Previous Blood Transfusion? ☐ Y ☐ N   Reaction? ☐ Y ☐ N   Explain: _____

CURRENT HEALTH PROBLEMS:

1. Diabetes	☐ Y ☐ N	5. Thyroid	☐ Y ☐ N	9. Blood Disorder	☐ Y ☐ N	13. Arthritis ☐ Y ☐ N
2. Respiratory	☐ Y ☐ N	6. Cardiac Problems	☐ Y ☐ N	10. Stroke	☐ Y ☐ N	14. Renal ☐ Y ☐ N
3. Glaucoma	☐ Y ☐ N	7. Hypertension	☐ Y ☐ N	11. Seizure Disorder	☐ Y ☐ N	15. S T D ☐ Y ☐ N
4. Sickle Cell	☐ Y ☐ N	8. G I	☐ Y ☐ N	12. Cancer	☐ Y ☐ N	16. Mental Illness ☐ Y ☐ N
						17. Other ☐ Y ☐ N

Comments _____

CURRENT MEDICATIONS

(Prescribed and Over the Counter)	DOSE	FREQUENCY	REASON FOR TAKING	TIME OF LAST DOSE
1.				
2.				
3.				
4.				
5.				
6.				
7.				
8.				
9.				

Do you have your medication with you? ☐ Y ☐ N   Disposition _____

SKIN INTEGRITY

☐ Burns   ☐ Abrasions   ☐ Intact

☐ Bruises   ☐ Rash   Turgor _____

☐ Scars   ☐ Fragile   _____

☐ Laceration   ☐ Pressure Sores

Describe / Additional Assessment: _____

_____

_____

_____

ELIMINATION

Abdomen (Describe): _____ Bowel Sounds:_____

Time Food / Fluid Last Ingested:_____

Additional Assessment:_____

Urinary: ☐ No Problems ☐ Urgency ☐ Burning / Dysuria ☐ Nocturia ☐ Incontinent ☐ Hematuria

☐ Other _____

Bowel: Usual Frequency _____ ☐ Constipation ☐ Diarrhea ☐ Hemorrhoids Last BM _____

☐ Elimination Aid _____

Stool Appearance: ☐ Normal ☐ Tarry ☐ Bloody ☐ Other _____

Additional Assessment: _____

_____

REPRODUCTION

Female: ☐ Normal Menses ☐ Abnormal Bleeding ☐ Practices Breast Self Exam ☐ L M P _____

☐ Mammogram (Yr.) _____ ☐ Gravida _____ ☐ Para _____ ☐ Last Pap Smear _____

☐ Would you like more information regarding self breast exam   ☐ Yes   ☐ No

☐ Other _____

Male: ☐ Denies Problems ☐ Penile Discharge ☐ Prostate Problem ☐ Practices Testicular Self Exam

☐ Would you like more information regarding testicular self exam   ☐ Yes   ☐ No

☐ Other _____

Additional Assessment: _____

_____

NUTRITION

Intake / Appetite: ☐ Adequate ☐ Anorexia / Bulemia ☐ Difficulty Chewing ☐ Hyperglycemic

☐ Decreased ☐ Nausea / Vomiting ☐ Dysphagic ☐ On Insulin (Dosage) _____

☐ Increased ☐ Dentures Upper / Lower _____

☐ Other _____

Food Intolerances: _____

Food Preference (Meal Size / Frequency): _____

Previous or Special Diet: _____

Recent Weight Change (gain / loss, amount, time period): _____

Additional Assessment: _____

_____

_____

_____

_____

_____

COGNITION / SENSATION / COMMUNICATION

Level of Consciousness:
- ☐ Comatose - Not Reactive to Pain
- ☐ Semicomatose - Reacts to Pain But Cannot be Aroused
- ☐ Lethargic - Can be Aroused and Responsive to Verbal Commands
- ☐ Awake and Oriented To: ☐ Time ☐ Person ☐ Place

Muscle Weakness: ☐ Yes ☐ No
Describe: _____

Speech: ☐ Clear ☐ Slurred ☐ Unable to Speak

Additional Assessment: _____

Hearing: ☐ Normal ☐ Hearing Aid ☐ Hard of Hearing ☐ Total Loss of Hearing
Vision: ☐ Normal ☐ Glasses ☐ Contacts ☐ Total Loss of Vision

Have you noticed any changes in memory: _____

Additional Assessment: _____

VENTILATION

Respirations:
- ☐ Regular
- ☐ Shallow
- ☐ Labored
- ☐ Retractions
- ☐ Orthopnea
- ☐ Dyspnea
- ☐ Wheezing
- ☐ S O B

Breath Sounds (Location, Insp, Exp):

	Location	Insp	Exp
Crackles			
Wheezes			

☐ Clear

Cough:
- ☐ None
- ☐ Non-Productive
- ☐ Productive
- ☐ Character of Sputum _____

Additional Assessment: _____

CIRCULATION

Skin Type:
- ☐ Warm
- ☐ Cool
- ☐ Dry
- ☐ Moist
- ☐ Other _____

Skin Color:
- ☐ Normal ☐ Pale
- ☐ Cyanotic ☐ Other _____
- ☐ Jaundiced

Pulses: Irregular Regular
- ☐ Radial ☐ ☐
- ☐ Apical ☐ ☐

Edema:
- ☐ Absent
- ☐ Present

Comments: _____

Strength: R L (Use Key)
- ☐ Radial ☐ ☐ _____
- ☐ Pedal ☐ ☐ _____

KEY	
3 +	Strong
2 +	Normal
1 +	Weak
0	Absent

Additional Assessment: _____

MOBILITY

Gait: Steady ☐ Unsteady ☐
☐ Denies Problems   ☐ Contractures   ☐ Paralysis
☐ Pain   ☐ Fractures

Assign appropriate level according to patient's perceived ability to perform activities:

	Dependent	Independent	With Assistance		Dependent	Independent	With Assistance
Feeding	☐	☐	☐	Toileting	☐	☐	☐
Grooming	☐	☐	☐	Dressing	☐	☐	☐
General Mobility	☐	☐	☐	Bathing	☐	☐	☐
Bed Mobility	☐	☐	☐	Transferring	☐	☐	☐

Assistive devices used: _____
History of Falls: _____
History of Dizziness? _____
What do you do for exercise / how often? _____
Recent change in exercise tolerance? _____
Additional assessment: _____

PSYCHOSOCIAL

Behavior:

☐ Cooperative   ☐ Anxious   ☐ Crying
☐ Uncooperative   ☐ Restless   ☐ Depressed
☐ Confused   ☐ Combative   ☐ Other _____

Occupation: _____
What do you do in your leisure time? _____
Have you experienced any recent stressful events? _____
Alcohol / Drug Use? _____
Support System? _____
Role in Family: _____
Who do you live with? _____
Additional Assessment: _____
Tobacco Use?   ☐ Yes   ☐ No   If yes, type / duration: _____

COMFORT / REST / SLEEP

Resting Habits: ☐ Daily Naps   ☐ Sleep Aids   ☐ Gets up at night   ☐ Unable to Sleep

Additional Assessment: _____

Pain:
None
Location: _____
Quality / Intensity: _____
Pattern / Duration: _____
Method of Pain Management: _____

Precipitating Factors: _____

VALUE / BELIEF

Will being in the hospital interfere with any religious practices? _____
Do you have a living will? ☐ Yes ☐ No   Copy obtained ☐ Yes ☐ No   Do you want any info. ☐ Yes ☐ No
                                            and placed on chart?   regarding advanced directives / living will?
Organ donor card signed? ☐ Yes ☐ No

Is there anything we haven't talked about that you would like to mention? _____

DISCHARGE PLANNING

Easiest way for you to learn: ☐ Written   ☐ Verbal   ☐ Audio / Visual

Projected discharge teaching / educational needs:

_____
_____
_____
_____

Admitting Nurse: _____ Date: _____ Time: _____

Patient database patterned on Orem's self-care model. Reprinted with permission from Newark Beth Israel Medical Center, Department of Nursing, Newark, NJ.

PATIENT CARE FLOW SHEET

DATE:	7 am - 3 pm	3 pm - 11 pm	11 pm - 7 am
AIR BLOOD PRESSURE			
PULSE: RATE/QUALITY			
RESPIRATIONS: RATE/RHYTHM			
LUNG SOUNDS			
APICAL RATE/RHYTHM			
HEART SOUNDS			
SKIN: APPEARANCE/TURGOR			
SKIN: COLOR/TEMPERATURE			
FOOD & WATER WEIGHT			
EDEMA			
INTRAVENOUS THERAPY SITE			
SITE APPEARANCE			
IV DRESSING CHANGE			
TYPE SOLUTION			
RATE			
LIB - BEGIN SHIFT			
LIB - END SHIFT			
IV INTAKE			24°
PO FLUID INTAKE			24°
DIET			
% TAKEN			
SELF/ASSISTANCE			
ACTIVITY REST & SLEEP ACTIVITY			
TOLERATION			
RANGE OF MOTION			
SLEEP/REST PATTERN			

		7 am - 3 pm	3 pm - 11 pm	11 pm - 7 am
ELIMINATION	VOIDING			
	URINE APPEARANCE			
	OUTPUT			24°
	ABDOMEN/BOWEL SOUNDS			
	STOOL			
				24°
SOLITUDE & SOCIAL INTERACTION	COMMUNICATION			
	LEVEL OF CONSCIOUSNESS			
	ORIENTATION			
	VISITORS			
PROTECTION FROM HAZARDS	SAFETY: SIDE RAILS			
	CALL LIGHT WITHIN REACH			
	WOUNDS: LOCATION			
	TYPE			
	APPEARANCE			
	TREATMENT			
	DRESSING CHANGE			
	PAIN: TYPE/LOCATION			
	INTERVENTION			
	RESPONSE			
	EQUIPMENT			
NORMALCY	HYGIENE			
	ORAL CARE/BACK CARE			
	BEHAVIOR			
KNOWLEDGE & SKILLS	TEACHING			
	PROCEDURES			
	SIGNATURES			

Patient care flow sheet. Reprinted with permission from Newark Beth Israel Medical Center, Department of Nursing, Newark, NJ.

ADMISSION ASSESSMENT ADDENDUM

CONCLUSIONS

I. Maintenance of a sufficient intake of air

Patient's Self Care Requisite is unmet ____
Patient's Self Care Requisite is met
without assistance ____

Requires the assistance of: ____ Caregiver
____ Nurse/Staff
____ Both

II. Maintenance of adequate intake of food and water

Patient's Self Care Requisite is unmet ____
Patient's Self Care Requisite is met
without assistance ____

Requires the assistance of: ____ Caregiver
____ Nurse/Staff
____ Both

III. Provision of care associated with elimination processes

Patient's Self Care Requisite is unmet ____
Patient's Self Care Requisite is met
without assistance ____

Requires the assistance of: ____ Caregiver
____ Nurse/Staff
____ Both

IV. Maintenance of a balance between rest and activity

Patient's Self Care Requisite is unmet ____
Patient's Self Care Requisite is met
without assistance ____

Requires the assistance of: ____ Caregiver
____ Nurse/Staff
____ Both

V. Maintenance of a balance between solitude and social interaction

Patient's Self Care Requisite is unmet ____
Patient's Self Care Requisite is met
without assistance ____

Requires the assistance of: ____ Caregiver
____ Nurse/Staff
____ Both

VI. Prevention of hazards

Patient's Self Care Requisite is unmet ____
Patient's Self Care Requisite is met
without assistance ____

Requires the assistance of: ____ Caregiver
____ Nurse/Staff
____ Both

VII. Promotion of normalcy

Patient's Self Care Requisite is unmet ____
Patient's Self Care Requisite is met
without assistance ____

Requires the assistance of: ____ Caregiver
____ Nurse/Staff
____ Both

VIII. Developmental self care requisites

a. Bringing about and maintaining conditions that support life processes and promote the processes of development towards higher levels of the organization of human structures and towards maturation.

Patient's Self Care Requisite is unmet ____
Patient's Self Care Requisite is met
without assistance ____

Requires the assistance of: ____ Caregiver
____ Nurse/Staff
____ Both

b. Provision of care associated with effects of conditions that can adversely affect human development.

1. Provision of care to prevent the occurrence of deleterious effects of such conditions

Patient's Self Care Requisite is unmet ____
Patient's Self Care Requisite is met
without assistance ____

Requires the assistance of: ____ Caregiver
____ Nurse/Staff
____ Both

CONCLUSIONS (cont'd)

2. Provision of care to mitigate or overcome existent deleterious effects of such conditions

Patient's Self Care Requisite is unmet ____
Patient's Self Care Requisite is met
    without assistance ____

Requires the assistance of: ____ Caregiver
                            ____ Nurse/Staff
                            ____ Both

IX. Health deviation self care requisites

a. Seeking and securing appropriate medical assistance in the event of exposure to specific biological agents or environmental conditions or when there is evidence of genetic, physiologic or psychologic conditions known to produce or be associated with human pathology.

Patient's Self Care Requisite is unmet ____
Patient's Self Care Requisite is met
    without assistance ____

Requires the assistance of: ____ Caregiver
                            ____ Nurse/Staff
                            ____ Both

b. Being aware and attending to the effects and results of pathologic conditions and states, including effects on development.

Patient's Self Care Requisite is unmet ____
Patient's Self Care Requisite is met
    without assistance ____

Requires the assistance of: ____ Caregiver
                            ____ Nurse/Staff
                            ____ Both

c. Effectively carrying out medically prescribed diagnostic, therapeutic and rehabilitative measures directed to preventing specific types of pathology, to the pathology itself, regulation of integrated human functioning, correction of deformities or abnormalities, or to compensation for disabilities.

Patient's Self Care Requisite is unmet ____
Patient's Self Care Requisite is met
    without assistance ____

Requires the assistance of: ____ Caregiver
                            ____ Nurse/Staff
                            ____ Both

d. Being aware of and attending to or regulating the discomforting or deleterious effects of medical care measures performed or prescribed by the physician including effects of development.

Patient's Self Care Requisite is unmet ____
Patient's Self Care Requisite is met
    without assistance ____

Requires the assistance of: ____ Caregiver
                            ____ Nurse/Staff
                            ____ Both

e. Modifying self-concept (and self image) in accepting oneself as being in a particular state of health and in need of specific forms of health care.

Patient's Self Care Requisite is unmet ____
Patient's Self Care Requisite is met
    without assistance ____

Requires the assistance of: ____ Caregiver
                            ____ Nurse/Staff
                            ____ Both

f. Learning to live with the effects of pathologic conditions and states and the effects of medical diagnostic and treatment measures in a life-style that promotes continued personal development.

Patient's Self Care Requisite is unmet ____
Patient's Self Care Requisite is met
    without assistance ____

Requires the assistance of: ____ Caregiver
                            ____ Nurse/Staff
                            ____ Both

Reference   1. Orem, Dorothea: Nursing Concepts of Practice, 5th edition, 1995 Mosby, pp 196-202.

LIST THE REQUISITES THAT HAVE NOT BEEN MET IN ORDER OF PRIORITY:

_____
_____
_____
_____
_____
_____

FROM THIS LIST IDENTIFY THOSE THAT ARE THE FOCUS OF CONCERN DURING THIS HOSPITALIZATION AND ADDRESS THEM IN THE PATIENT'S PLAN OF CARE.

THOSE ITEMS WHICH REMAIN MUST BE ADDRESSED AS PART OF THE DISCHARGE PLAN FOR THE PATIENT.

Index